CONTENTS

FOREWORD

As the coauthor of *Intuitive Eating*, which was first published in 1995 and is now in its fourth edition, I have spent many years of my career helping people rediscover trust in their inner wisdom to navigate their eating lives and to discover an appreciation for their here-and-now bodies. So many people have credited *Intuitive Eating* with healing their relationship with food and their bodies.

But if we pause for a moment, we might question why it's even necessary for them to do this intensive work. Weren't they born with all of this innate wisdom? Of course they were! Babies instinctively know when they're hungry and full. They don't need an instruction book to guide them to and away from the breast or bottle. Shouldn't this intrinsic ability continue throughout life?

Unfortunately, a disconnect from this wisdom often emerges when an infant grows into an "independent" toddler who is on the path toward developing their individual identity. The well-meaning parent begins to question whether their child will make the "right" choices to keep them healthy and growing. The parent then begins to direct and often control what and how much their child is eating.

Eventually, that newborn Intuitive Eater can evolve into a teen and then an adult who has lost trust in their inner wisdom and searches for an outside source to guide them in their eating choices—one that often leads them down a misdirected path of self-judgment and despair.

There is so much at stake when a parent tries to do the "right thing" and ends up failing. This failure can appear as a food fight between child and parent, a child who ends up sneaking the foods that have been forbidden, and/or a child who eventually develops shame about their body or even an eating disorder, because they don't meet diet culture's unrealistic ideals. If only these parents could have found that instruction book that didn't come with birth, to help them achieve their best intentions and to prevent their child's diversion from inner trust. The only problem is this instruction book is nowhere to be found.

Intuitive Eating is directed toward adults, and the *Intuitive Eating Workbook for Teens* toward teens. But adults and teens have far more autonomy, for the most part, and agency in their decisions about eating than children do. I receive innumerable requests for more information about how to raise kids as Intuitive Eaters and have known for a long time that there needed to be a book that is explicit in guidance, with a solid framework of motivation for parents to take the leap of faith and jump into this uncharted territory.

Parents want simple "how-to" answers to properly guide their children's eating life and to avoid these painful problems. But "how-to" answers aren't enough to break through what are often generations-old beliefs about child-rearing. First, the parent needs preparation for this journey, which includes a deep dive into their own eating history and beliefs and a resolution to make changes in their own relationship to food and body, if needed. Also necessary is acceptance that children are born with all the wisdom they need about how to eat, a commitment to tune in to their child's signals, and respect that the child's inner wisdom will continue to guide them throughout their growing years and their entire lives.

So why this book? Rather than an instruction book, it's a comforting, reassuring safe place for parents to land that helps them release the reins and learn what it takes to help their child maintain an intuitive, self-regulating pace of eating. At the beginning of their journey, parents will find a thorough teaching and understanding of the psychology behind the negative effects of external control, as well as an appreciation for the power of role modeling. This will provide the framework and motivation to venture into a new and exciting way of guiding their children toward the joy, satisfaction, and trust that accompanies Intuitive Eating.

Before I continue describing the book that you're about to read, I'd like to circle back to the newborn infant. All animals and humans are born with a survival instinct, and the primary source of survival is food. Now, most parents are eager to listen to their newborn infant's signal that announces that they're ready to eat. Sometimes there may be confusion about the difference between a hunger signal, a sleepy signal, or simply one that says, "Notice me—I want to be held," but very quickly, parents learn what each cry means. They also become acutely aware of when the infant has had enough to eat. If a parent tries to push the baby back on the breast or bottle after the little one turns it aside, the baby will rule, and feeding will stop.

The baby's emotional journey also begins at birth. Babies are born with an ability to express their emotions. Anyone who has been around a baby knows that they express these emotions through smiles, giggles, and frequent crying. With these emotions, they're conveying their wants, needs, and joy in living. The world can be a frightening place, and this tiny infant looks to caregivers for consistent and predictable care. The attuned parent will very soon learn to honor their child's physical and emotional needs. With this, most importantly, the child is able to trust that their needs in life will be met. They'll also quickly learn that their hunger and fullness signals can be trusted.

What infants aren't born with, however, are language and beliefs about food and appearance. They emerge, instead, as a result of their environment. Infants take in language and cadence by mimicking their parents. They babble; words emerge, and finally sentences. And as time goes on, the family's beliefs become ingrained in the child.

If only it were as simple to stay present and attuned to the child's innate wisdom about eating as the infant becomes a toddler and beyond. Something often goes awry when solid food is introduced. For so many families, a disconnect begins to emerge, as the parent replaces these inborn messages with external messages about eating that come from a multitude of sources. Whether it's the pediatrician who becomes concerned that the child is gaining weight too quickly or not quickly enough, or a well-meaning grandparent who feels they know best about how to feed the child, or the persistent influx of noise from all forms of media, parents can become confused about the "right thing" to do when feeding their child.

This is why it's so crucial for families to challenge and dismantle the beliefs that they have introjected from society—especially if diet culture has intruded into their belief system about food and body. If not, these beliefs will be passed down to their children.

This book will literally save lives. As the authors document, dieting and a focus on shrinking one's body increases the risk for eating disorders. And eating disorders can be deadly.

By following the brilliant wisdom that this book contains, parents can break through the dogma they're fed that tells them it's their responsibility to help their children maintain or attain optimal health by keeping them in a smaller body. Accurate information offers them the first tools they'll need.

The authors then provide a model, which they call the "3 Keys," for embracing this new path toward protecting children's innate wisdom about eating. In a compassionate and encouraging way, this model brings parents to an unconditional love and support for their child's body, teaches them how to develop a flexible and reliable feeding routine, and helps them develop and use their own intuitive voice. Along with the 3 Keys, this book gives parents the guidance they need to provide their children with gentle nutrition and intuitive movement. Parents will also receive the reassurance that although this journey may feel difficult and even impossible at times, they'll be able to return to this book throughout their children's development to get everything they need to provide a protective environment for them, so that they can live their lives with the freedom that comes with trusting that innate wisdom about eating that arrived with them at birth.

Thank goodness that this book has finally arrived! No, it may not be that instruction book that tells parents exactly what to do. Instead, it's a course in learning to trust their own wisdom so that they can guide their children toward an emotionally and physically satisfying relationship with food and their bodies.

Elyse Resch, MS, RDN, CEDRD-S, FAND
Nutrition Therapist
Coauthor of *Intuitive Eating* and *The Intuitive Eating Workbook*
Author of *The Intuitive Eating Workbook for Teens* and *The Intuitive Eating Journal: Your Guided Journey for Nourishing a Healthy Relationship with Food*

INTRODUCTION

When you become a parent, no one hands you a guidebook that tells you how best to fulfill this new role. But everyone has opinions on how best to feed this new little life. Everyone is so afraid of messing it up. Because, frankly, feeding our kids is hard. Finding your own path through all that chaos is like trying to have a pleasant conversation at a rock concert.

Our culture has boiled food and feeding ourselves down to science. Fuel. Calories in/calories out. There is so much more to the story.

The truth is that there is more to food than just nutrition and calories. It isn't about fueling our bodies alone; it can be about connection, culture, emotions, love, family, history, joy, grief, and everything else. How humans need to eat and interact with food is much more complex than what could fit into a how-to manual. We aren't given the guidebook because no one could write it.

Not even us.

This isn't an instruction manual. This is a *manifesto*. An ode to healing the relationship with food. A path to growing up with an inherent trust in your body.

This book offers guidance to parents using the science of what we know about food and bodies and embracing our existence in those bodies. This is an introduction to embodiment and a discussion of resilience. Here, we can re-parent ourselves so we can learn how to do less harm to our future generations.

WHAT TO EXPECT

In order to facilitate this work, we've drawn inspiration and have learned from many who have done the work before us. We are dietitians and parents, and we are acutely aware of the impact that food can have on our lives. So here we will talk about food, feeding, and body image. We will also talk about the oppressive systems that led us here, that keep us here. We will examine the painful memories we strive to protect our little ones from. As well as the ways in which we may be more privileged or marginalized by the bodies and lives we inhabit.

WHO THIS BOOK IS FOR

Children and families struggle with food and eating in many different ways. This book aims to reach those parents who want to prevent disordered eating—such as restricting or binge eating—from setting in as a result of the diet mentality we are surrounded by in our culture. It was also written to help put an end to what we describe as generational dieting—if you, your parents, your grandparents, have all been passed down generations of beliefs that are tied to dieting and a focus on thinness as the goal, that will show up within your parenting around food, whether you intend it or not. This book is a tool for parents to understand what they can do to maintain or return their child's Intuitive Eating ability, to help them appreciate and respect their unique body in a world that wants us to self-loathe.

We understand that not all families who struggle with food need the same solutions. First, not every family has consistent access to enough food to eat, which means that fostering a healthy relationship with food will not feel as important as getting enough food to hungry mouths at the table. There are circumstances for many families that are beyond the individual's responsibility which are systemic barriers to food security. Intuitive Eating is not a viable solution for the millions of people experiencing food insecurity, which significantly increases one's risk for disordered eating and eating disorders. Additionally, although avoidant and extreme picky eating is certainly a significant issue families face, that isn't the focus of our work. Families who struggle more with avoidant or very anxious eaters, where parents are worried their child doesn't eat enough, and every meal has become a battle, will benefit from a more individualized and therapeutic, structured approach that helps return their child to a calmer and more competent place with eating. This book isn't intended to be advice for families who struggle specifically with avoidant/restrictive food intake disorder (ARFID) or severe picky eating, although we do offer guidance around the quite common "picky phase" of eating in the toddler and early childhood years. The 3 Keys model isn't a replacement for eating disorder treatment or medical advice from a doctor or dietitian.

NOT EVERYONE HAS SOVEREIGNTY OVER THEIR OWN BODY

As we began writing this book, it became clear that we cannot discuss how to help our children, or anyone for that matter, attain a positive relationship with food and body without acknowledging the social justice issues happening today. These issues, if left unaddressed, will continue to keep people trapped in patterns of body oppression, trauma, and violence. If we—you, us, the nutrition field, the eating disorder field, parents, caregivers, medical practitioners, public health professionals—are aiming to help people live well, with peace and confidence, and to be able to trust their bodies and food, we must go beyond just the issues that face the most privileged.

The injustice and inequity in the world related to food and bodies run deeper than any of us can measure. Many people don't have—and will never have—a sense of safety in their body. One in six children in the United States do not know where their next meal is coming from. The systems that we are led to believe are in place to create equality, justice, and fairness with food and bodies are broken, corrupt, and exclusive. Human trafficking, the trading of human bodies for forced labor or sexual exploitation and slavery, is currently robbing nearly 25 million women, men, and children of their freedom today, *in this moment*. No region of the United States is lacking in food deserts and suffering the effects of food apartheids—areas where healthful and affordable food isn't accessible to the people who live there.

Unjustly, those who experience food insecurity also face a significantly higher risk of developing disordered eating and chronic disease. This risk also increases if you're an immigrant—separated from family, familiarity, and support—are disabled, a person of color, transgender or nonbinary, or queer. The reasons why having one or more of these nondominant identities are considered risk factors aren't biological, but cultural. Racism, specifically anti-Blackness and the domination of white-supremacist sociocultural conditioning, in the United States and other first-world Western cultures, is deeply embedded in the ways many of us are robbed of our embodiment, burying our Intuitive Eating ability, and led to believe our bodies are never good enough until they are thin enough. White supremacy, homophobia, xenophobia, transphobia, ableism, and fatphobia are all direct contributing factors to why people don't have the resources they need to get enough food, have a safe place to live, or get the treatment they need for mental and physical health. Living in a marginalized body in our culture can cause PTSD, eating disorders, debilitating anxiety, maladaptive coping behaviors, or even suicide. Not having the time or resources to take care of your body, feeling the desire to have a different body, or the need to disconnect from your body all result from the ways our culture and systems tell us that all bodies aren't good bodies or worthy of respect, resources, or love.

As two white people who have experienced tremendous privilege and social power in our lives, we want to state the limitations we possess in writing about and speaking to the ways social structures and discrimination interfere with one's ability to be an Intuitive Eater. Even with the marginalization we have faced, there are many forms of discrimination we will never have to encounter. Our lack of personal experience limits the way we may understand how groups of people with one or more marginalized identities define, experience, and strive for Intuitive Eating.

One of our main goals was to write a book that was accessible to parents who have questions around feeding, disordered eating prevention, and body confidence concerns for their kids. We wanted to create a book that you can pick up, easily interpret, and then apply what you've learned to your own family based on their individual needs, neuro-wiring, biology, and competence. We suspect some readers will find that a lot has been left unanswered, specifically around individual feeding difficulties. In addition to Evelyn Tribole and Elyse Resch, the original pioneers of Intuitive Eating, the work of Ellyn Satter on division of responsibility, Niva Piran and Tracy Tylka's research on embodiment, Katja Rowell and Johanna Cormack's contributions to responsive feeding and picky eating, the attachment and childhood development work of Daniel Siegel, Tina Payne Bryson, and Janet Lansbury among countless others, and the groundwork laid by fat activists and size acceptance pioneers are just some of the many people who offer further reading and resources for you beyond *How to Raise an Intuitive Eater*. The difficulties and concerns parents face when it comes to feeding are diverse, and there isn't one solution for all.

EMBODIMENT

Let's talk about embodiment—you'll be hearing this word a lot throughout this book. When we refer to a healthy relationship with food and body, we are alluding to embodiment. Embodiment is a huge concept, and we have learned the most from Niva Piran. Intuitive Eating is one small drop in the embodiment pond. It's a vital piece, and yet there is so much more. Embodiment also accounts for the intersecting identities and lived experiences a person may have. We all inhabit multiple identities that cannot be untangled or isolated from one another. These include skin color, religion, body size, ability, gender identity, country of origin, health, socioeconomic background, and more.

INTUITIVE EATING

Newborn babies enter the world knowing how to take their first breath and when to cry for food, and innately trusting that their caregiver will give them what they need to survive. That intuitive wisdom is key to their survival. They know when it's time to eat and when they've had enough. *Quite literally, Intuitive Eating is something we are born doing. Our brains and bodies are hardwired to know when and how much to eat.* However, this is a concept that is often lost in translation. So now here we are, writing a whole book about it. We decided that it's important to begin this book with an understanding of what exactly we are referring to.

Intuitive Eating is a dynamic interplay of instinct, thought, and emotion.

It's a common misunderstanding to boil Intuitive Eating down to one of these two common incomplete descriptions:

Eat when you're hungry and stop when you're full.
Eat whatever you want, whenever you want.

Those two sentences leave out the important piece that makes Intuitive Eating such an empowering and healthful way to approach eating.

Let's take a closer look into this:
- Instinct: Our natural instinct to seek out food when we're hungry and to stop eating when we're full is what most people think about when

they first learn of Intuitive Eating. Our brain, including neurochemicals and appetite hormones, controls these instincts of how much, when, and what we feel like eating—otherwise known as our desires. We do not consciously control our instincts and appetite. Many people believe their appetites, or food cravings, are wrong or bad—thoughts that have come from a long history of messaging with puritanical roots. They aren't wrong; it's diet culture that has attached shame to them. When we attempt to override these instincts and, say, count our calories instead of satisfying our hunger, we throw off our body's communication system and send confusing messages to our brain. Our instincts are very wise, and they play an important role in Intuitive Eating.

- Thought: Our thoughts also play a big part in our eating decisions, particularly thoughts about our bodies and food. Some of the most influential thoughts that impact appetite, drive to eat, and eating choices are dieting thoughts. **Restraint theory and habituation theory are psychological influencers of Intuitive Eating, and are two of the biggest ways our thoughts dictate our behavior.** For example, when we think *I shouldn't be eating this* or *My diet starts Monday*, most people will have a very predictable behavioral response of "overeating." On the other hand, if our thought is *I can have that later when I'm hungry, no need to eat it now if I'm not*, there is no drive to eat just because something is available. **We biologically and subconsciously need to avoid famine for survival—and dieting is interpreted as famine by our brains.** When our thoughts aren't influenced by deprivation or restriction, we can focus on the present. Examples of thoughts about eating for the present that don't involve deprivation include: *How hungry am I? What sounds good? I'm allowed to eat whatever I want.* These thoughts do not create a drive to overeat, because there simply is no need to if you can have what you need or want when you get hungry again. The need to overeat comes from the threat of deprivation—thinking that you shouldn't eat something, you won't have it again for a long time, you aren't allowed to eat something, or you feel guilty for eating something. These diet-mentality thoughts have a strong impact on Intuitive Eating and are something you'll learn much more about as you read this book.

- Emotion: "Emotional eating" is often thrown around as a bad term when we talk about eating. But there is no way around it, emotions are a part of the human eating experience. There's nothing wrong with this despite emotional eating being commonly referred to as a no-no by diet culture. **Emotion, as one of the three parts of Intuitive Eating, includes how our feelings in the moment impact our appetite, cravings, and need to cope or soothe. The more in touch with our emotions we are, the more we can recognize how and why our emotions influence our desire to eat.** When we have unmet emotional needs, food often becomes a quick and effective way to cope or soothe ourselves. It is eye-opening and critical to learn how our judgment surrounding emotional eating leads us to disconnect *further* from our body's wisdom of how much to eat. Kids, just like adults, experience the need to cope and soothe and may have a drive to eat because it can feel distracting or soothing in response to their emotions. Have you ever noticed you might eat differently when you're sad versus stressed? Excited versus worried? Kids who are very anxious may resist eating, eat to soothe, or not feel hungry. Our emotions can influence eating—creating avoidance of eating or a desire to eat.

The combination of these three sources of information—our instincts, thoughts, and emotions—creates our unique Intuitive Eating experience. Intuitive Eating sources internal information from the body and mind, as opposed to external information. External rules and information are things outside of you. For example: labeling foods as good or bad, "healthy" or "unhealthy," or restricting certain "off-limits foods" or even pressure to eat from a parent. Intuitive Eating is about looking inward, trusting your body, and having permission to eat. Interestingly, humans have evolved by eating intuitively over tens of thousands of years. It has only been in the past few hundred years or so that we turned away from Intuitive Eating to dieting, and only in the last few decades that we've been using specific information, like calories, fitness trackers, and food labels, to dictate what we should eat.

This dynamic interplay of instinct, thought, and emotion is something we'll return to throughout the book.

WHY THIS BOOK NEEDED TO EXIST

We have so much compassion for the parents we see in our offices who come to us looking for guidance and have so many different concerns: *My child is sneaking food. My kid just wants to eat sweets all day. My child is afraid to eat. My child is losing/gaining weight and we're worried. I try to make them eat vegetables but they refuse. I'm afraid about their future.*

Parents and caregivers, we hear you. You want the best for your child, and you're trying to do this "right," but you're struggling to know what the next step is. Perhaps deep down you know that being strict and controlling your kids' food may not be right for them, but there is so much pressure for parents to feed their kids perfectly and raise healthy, high-achieving humans. It's almost impossible to not feel incredibly confused by it all.

We believe we've been focusing on the wrong things forever. **The biggest problem we face with feeding our kids is that early on they are losing touch with their natural, healthy relationship with food and body.** It's rare to find a book or even information from a doctor that emphasizes the positive impact having a healthy relationship with food and body has on a child throughout their life. On the other hand, you don't have to look far to find facts about how "bad" processed foods are, how important it is to limit sugar or carbs, or the risks of "childhood obesity." These messages are all around us and it would take superhuman powers to experience living, let alone parenting, without being influenced by them. Here lies the confusion. **The very strategies and solutions that have been given to parents to ensure good health and nutrition for their kids are backfiring.** What seem like harmless rules about eating develop into significant rebound behaviors many of the parents who come to us see in their homes. Parents have become so entrenched in diet mentality themselves, it's unintentionally passed down to their kids. Our societal and media messaging about bodies—size, shape, gender, skin color, beauty standards, fitness standards, and so on—are incredibly powerful and do play a role in shaping self-confidence and self-respect in young people.

We see the confusion that kids and parents have about how to eat on a regular basis. The good news is, there is a way to help kids—and the whole family—that will help them become a confident eater with a healthy relationship with food and their body.

WE HAVE TO TALK ABOUT MENTAL HEALTH

We can't write a book about health and food without talking about mental health. No matter what your child eats, or how physically healthy their body is, if they are suffering emotionally and psychologically, they will not be well. We remind parents of this often. There are so often mental health issues to address when parents notice a concern about food. **It's time we as parents, and as a society, put our children's relationship with food and body on the front burner, and appearance and weight on the back burner. This is how we refocus on mental health.**

What if all these messages and all this pressure is impacting our kids' mental health? Are we willing to sacrifice their mental health for the sake of a number on the scale or the potential to meet ever-shifting and impossible beauty standards? Of course not. And you may not have realized that you had been tricked into thinking that way until right now.

Commonly, messaging around mental and physical health is like this:

- It's important to maintain a "healthy" weight and eating habits.
- Mental health will fall in line as a result of having a healthy weight and eating healthfully (or it's just not something that is a concern at all until there is an obvious problem).

Instead, we invite you to think of things this way:

- We need to protect and promote mental health and body appreciation no matter what body size someone has.
- Intuitive Eating is proven to be protective and healthier than any mode of dieting or rigid eating.

Many things impact our health, both physical and mental. Some things we might not even realize are impacting us tremendously—including negative experiences in and near our bodies. Things like feeling unlovable, restricting food in order to change your body size, falling into "yo-yo" dieting, clinical or subclinical eating disorders, harmful overconcern about healthy eating (orthorexia), feeling shame about your body or eating habits, and feeling like you have to look a certain way in order to be successful or appreciated are common.

SELF-COMPASSION

Parenting is hard. Having to face your mistakes as a parent and try to do things differently makes parenting even harder. We are all in this struggle together. We are imperfect. We have learned that one of the most important things we can do is practice self-compassion.

So, what is self-compassion?

Instead of mercilessly judging and criticizing yourself for various inadequacies or shortcomings, self-compassion means you're kind and understanding when confronted with personal failings—after all, who ever said you were supposed to be perfect?

—KRISTIN NEFF, PHD (self-compassion.org)

You will see us bring this up again and again—it's easy to forget and beat yourself up. We can't erase the past and start over, as much as we'd love to, but what we can do is learn how to make changes and feel compassion for ourselves and for our kids.

EATING IS ABOUT FOOD *AND* BODY—NOT JUST FOOD

As we move through the book, you'll hear us mention *food and body* quite frequently. For a book that's about eating, why do we talk so much about a child's relationship with their body? Isn't this about having a good relationship with food? Well, the two really can't be separated. Our body, how we feel in it and about it, dictates thoughts and actions. How, when, what, and how much to eat are decisions we make in connection to our body. If a child has a positive relationship with their body, they will have an instinct to take care of it and feed it. If a child has a negative relationship with their body, they are more likely to ignore their body's needs, deny their cravings or desires, or even inflict pain upon themselves. With awareness of these associations, you can begin to get a sense of how closely connected physical and mental health are, particularly when it comes to a person's relationship with food.

WHAT DOES IT LOOK LIKE TO HAVE A HEALTHY RELATIONSHIP WITH FOOD?

That's a big question. It's the one that we are going to try to help you answer for yourself and for your child. Although the following most certainly isn't a complete list, some of the ways a healthy relationship with food can be described are:

- You don't worry about "good" or "bad" eating, or feel a pressure to eat any certain way.
- To the extent you're able, you're willing to eat an amount of food your

body needs for energy and satisfaction, and in the case of younger eaters, for growth and development.

- When you're hungry you can sense it most of the time and allow yourself to eat without feeling bad or guilty.
- You can prioritize getting enough food over having to get certain "healthy" foods.
- You have permission to be flexible and spontaneous with food decisions.
- You're able to stop eating when you feel you've had enough because you know you'll have more food later when you need it. *(Here we have to acknowledge that for those living with food insecurity—not knowing when, if, or how substantial the next meal will be—this might not be true. Having a healthy relationship with food is still possible, but we have to note that it's a privilege to have that confidence in where your next meal is coming from.)*
- What you eat and what your body looks like aren't getting between you and your life.

Read the points listed above again, only this time, picture a young toddler or an infant. Would you say these things describe how a very young child eats? Probably yes! Young children naturally have a positive relationship with food and their bodies unless there has been an interruption in their environment or by their caregiver, such as being denied food when hungry.

How about an unhealthy relationship with food? How do those thoughts and beliefs show up for us? For most people, there are many different rules floating around inside our heads. These are just a small sample of some of the ways an unhealthy relationship with food can show up as problematic beliefs or rules:

- Parents believe they should control their child's food intake because kids can't control it themselves.
- Thinking a certain weight, size, or shape is an important factor in your health.
- You don't think you deserve to eat what you want or need unless you have achieved weight or exercise goals.
- Assuming that everyone should be striving to be healthier and "in shape."

- Feeling guilty for eating.
- Believing that managing your weight or your child's weight is simple; it's about calories in versus calories out.

How do you feel after reading the two lists? Chances are you would hope that more items on the first list describe your child's relationship to food. You may be noticing that some or all of those things have already been lost by your child and you'd love to help them get them back.

That is what we need to talk about. Our kids deserve to feel lovable, worthy, and accepted no matter what their bodies look like. They do not need to spend their energy worrying about calories or food rules. They deserve to be free to explore their passions, without the distraction of weight control and body image distress. We know you do love your child unconditionally. We also know that the messages can get mixed.

That is why we are here with our *manifesto*.

PART I

THE PROBLEM WE ARE FACING

1

THE PROBLEM YOU'RE
NOT ABLE TO SEE

The pressure to be the best parent possible is staggering. Feeling like every choice you make can impact your child for the rest of their life is overwhelming. Every time our child doesn't take our advice, doesn't listen, gets hurt, is rude, or any other relatively human behavior—we take it hard. It feels like proof that we have no idea what we are doing. With all of that pressure, what if we could find some peace and freedom?

It's nearly impossible to not care about our children's health and body size, especially in a culture that is constantly sending us messages about the right and wrong ways to raise our kids around food and their bodies. Everywhere we go, we see and hear the message that we must save our children from food and fatness. This is where the problem begins. We have lost sight of the benefits of having a healthy relationship with food.

Can you recall the first memory you have of feeling bad about your body? Or a memory of when you realized we have a cultural obsession with dieting, bodies, and thinness? A question that I (Amee) often ask my clients is how old they were the first time they realized their body wasn't acceptable. The answer is almost always before puberty, and too often even younger than the age of ten. For many of us, our earliest memories about our weight and bodies are shameful experiences of feeling teased, unaccepted, or judged. For every person the story is different, and yet so many of us have experienced a common theme: the loss of body confidence and the development of an unhealthy relationship with food.

Focusing on weight and appearance, as well as feeling the responsibility to restrict and regulate everything kids eat—all under the guise of health and "obesity prevention"—is backfiring. It's impacting our children's natural ability to self-regulate.

Self-regulation is the backbone of Intuitive Eating. For the most part, humans are born with the ability to self-regulate with food—we are designed to stay in balance and know what and how much to eat. There is a miraculous and intricate system of hormones, nerves, and neurochemicals that create this ability. Control, pressure, and restriction all dilute our children's ability to hear and trust their body signals.

There is a great deal of research looking at the impact that overcontrol of and attention to weight from parents has on children and teens, and you don't even have to know the science to see the result of this. Kids, teens, and adults are facing an epidemic of disordered eating and body shame that have lasting consequences on self-esteem, health behaviors, and both physical and mental health.

Almost everyone in today's world learns early in life that what and how much we eat are things to carefully monitor if we want to attain a body that is acceptable, healthy, and lovable. On the other hand, if you weren't exposed to weight worries, a dieting family, or food restriction of any kind as a child, you might not know it, but you actually experienced a protective environment against body dissatisfaction and disordered eating.

For generations, dieting practices in Western cultures have been growing to the point where we now are so immersed in dieting that it's socially normal. It's almost impossible to walk into a social space and not hear someone moralizing food, discussing their weight or their current diet interest. We believe certain parenting choices boil down to making informed decisions and feel strongly that you deserve to be accurately informed about how feeding practices and Intuitive Eating can help you and your family.

Intuitive Eating—a way of eating without dieting—is countercultural, yet the research is convincing. It is the way to live to avoid the mental harm and physical health risks dieting causes. The long-term ramifications that dieting, weight shame, and disordered eating have on our physical, emotional, and mental well-being are severe. One of the biggest nutrition concerns facing children and young people today is that their natural Intuitive Eating ability is being stolen from them.

Maybe you yourself have endured a struggle with food, and you would give anything to rescue your child from having to live through that same experience. Or maybe you haven't suffered with food or body issues a day in your life, but instead you're beginning to notice something worrisome about your child's behavior and you're looking for guidance.

THE RESEARCHED AND STUDIED TRUTH

Perhaps you picked up this book because you've heard of Intuitive Eating, maybe you're at your wits' end over food battles in your household, or maybe you just like the concept. Whatever the reason, we are glad you're here. The 3 Keys you'll learn about were developed using our own trial and error coupled with the ever-growing amount of research that has been done on Intuitive Eating, along with psychology-based research. Some of what you'll learn will feel very contrary to the beliefs and messages we hear day in and day out about kids' bodies, nutrition, and feeding. We encourage you to stay open-minded and thoughtful about challenging what you learn about diet culture throughout this book.

We live inside diet culture. This may be the first time you're noticing diet culture and how it may have affected you. Now that you see this, notice how you may have an urge to make excuses for, or even defend, diet culture. Here is a great definition of diet culture that can help you unpack your emotions around the concept:

Christy Harrison, dietitian and author of *Anti-Diet*, defines diet culture:[1]

Diet culture is a system of beliefs that:

Worships thinness and equates it to health and moral virtue, which means you can spend your whole life thinking you're irreparably broken just because you don't look like the impossibly thin "ideal."

Promotes weight loss as a means of attaining higher status, which means you feel compelled to spend a massive amount of time, energy, and money trying to shrink your body, even though the research is very clear that almost no one can sustain intentional weight loss for more than a few years.

Demonizes certain ways of eating while elevating others, which means you're forced to be hyper-vigilant about your eating, ashamed of making certain food choices, and distracted from your pleasure, your purpose, and your power.

Oppresses people who don't match up with its supposed picture of "health," which disproportionately harms women, femmes, trans folks, people in larger bodies, people of color, and people with disabilities, damaging both their mental and physical health.

Back to diet culture's intentions—the more you think you're not attractive enough or not healthy enough, the more you will pursue fixing all your flaws and the more money you will spend. Profits rise for every company invested in your low self-esteem. When you don't decide to opt out of diet culture, or when your survival, your job, or your safety in your domestic relationship requires you to pursue dieting, you're forced to uphold diet culture's standards. You were not born believing in diet culture.

Diet culture is incredibly successful at making people believe their body isn't good enough and that the solution is more dieting. In fact, it might be the only way it's actually successful. It sells the lie that looking a certain way leads to a happy life. Yes, thin privilege has some very real advantages, but that's because our society doesn't treat all bodies equally. Not because you're inherently happier, better, or more successful in a thinner body. That's the lie.

Diet culture has one more trick up its sleeve: when parents adopt a diet mentality, there is a guaranteed next generation filling the pipeline of future customers. Yes, this is intentional, and we're sorry you didn't know this sooner. But it's not too late.

HIGHER WEIGHT DOESN'T MEAN HIGHER RISK OF DEATH

Whoa, whoa. That's a big statement. We're almost afraid that the lawyer for "diet culture" will walk in our door and slap a libel lawsuit on the table. (That won't happen, obviously, but it does feel like a statement that could almost be considered treasonous.)

What is commonly understood to be true is the myth that there is a direct linear relationship between weight and risk of death. (A direct linear relationship is like the distance traveled over time while on a walk. The longer you walk, the more distance you cover. Increase one value, and you see an increase in the other.)

When a person visits their doctor, and their weight automatically is described to them as a disease, with a diagnosis of "obesity," they come to the implied conclusion, *I have become too heavy, and it's going to kill me if I don't fix it.*

We also do the same thing with kids. If their weight climbs, we think something must be wrong, and we need to "fix it." If they become thinner, we attribute it to healthy choices, as a good thing—until we discover they are dieting "too much" and we tell them they have to eat more. In our society, you're supposed to constantly strive for thinness, but don't get too thin that you have a problem—or suddenly your disordered calorie counting calls for an intervention, while everyone else around you continue to count calories.

This misunderstanding that weight directly contributes to increased risk of death is one of the more harmful beliefs perpetuated by diet culture. It creates a feeling of shame for people who live in higher-weight bodies. We think if the scale goes up it must mean we are that many pounds closer to death, and we are that many pounds further from health, self-control, and worthiness.

The true relationship between weight and mortality isn't linear; in fact, it's U-shaped. The highest risk of death is for those with very low BMI (body mass index), and the second highest risk of mortality is for those in the upper range of high BMI, >50. In one key study, known as the ALLHAT—Antihypertensive and Lipid-Lowering Treatment to Prevent Heart Attack Trial—researchers examined data on more than 32,800 adults over the age of fifty-five, and followed them from baseline over eight years, examining all causes of mortality. The data shows that the *lowest-risk* BMI category of death from any cause, for the nearly 33,000 individuals, was within the obese weight range—as you can see in the following graph. Increased risk for death doesn't rise until BMI ranges above about 50, yet the underweight and normal-weight BMI ranges show significant increased risk. Does this mean that we need to be telling someone with a BMI of 22 to intentionally gain weight to reduce risk of death? No. What it does tell us is that body weight isn't a major factor contributing to mortality for the majority of people who have a BMI in the overweight or obese ranges. Other factors also contribute to disease and death, such as lifestyle, trauma, environment, genetics, and fitness, to name a few.

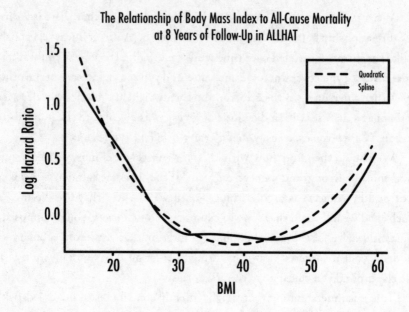

The Relationship of Body Mass Index to All-Cause Mortality
at 8 Years of Follow-Up in ALLHAT

FITNESS, NOT FATNESS, CAN IMPACT MORTALITY

Our societal obsession with thinness is so mainstream that hardly anyone questions the blanket recommendation that striving to be in a "normal" BMI range is healthiest. For many people, reaching a BMI of under 25 requires consistent and stringent food and exercise control and restriction. We know there are negative side effects to undereating, yet they're largely not disclosed, and studies actually show that not only is it unrealistic for most people to strive for the "normal" BMI range—it's actually less likely to be healthy for their body. A large multi-study analysis published in 2014 looked at data from more than 90,000 individuals and determined that *risk of death is dependent on cardiorespiratory fitness, not weight or BMI.* Even when researchers specifically assessed only the "unfit" individuals, the science showed that being overweight was actually a protective factor against all-cause mortality, not something that is harmful.[2]

BODY DIVERSITY IS NATURALLY OCCURRING

There is robust evidence that size isn't completely within a person's control.[3] Many different factors influence a person's weight. They can include dieting or restriction for intentional weight loss and exercise with the goal of weight change. Although these factors can initially result in weight loss, it's unlikely to last and more likely to lead to weight cycling (losing and regaining) or yo-yo dieting. Contrary to the popular belief that weight can easily be controlled through diet and exercise, the most impactful factors on body weight are things like genetics, environment, whether you have dieted in the past, weight cycling, and stigma.

No matter what parents do, there will always be people, from newborn babies to our oldest family members, who exist across a range of sizes and shapes. Our genetics largely determine this. Some kids are naturally thin, some are naturally larger. Some are born as larger babies and grow to become thin and lean, while smaller babies on the growth chart can gain weight in a future growth phase and become larger-bodied teens or adults. There's nothing inherently wrong or unhealthy about any of this. In our current status quo ideals for children and food, kids who are naturally thin are less likely to be exposed to dieting early on, protecting them from weight stigma and protecting their relationship with food. This plays a role in preventing weight gain and weight cycling that results directly from dieting, while larger-bodied children—no matter what the reason for their body size—are often subjected to food restriction, launching them into a lifetime of disordered eating and shame. No child deserves that.

If body diversity is real, then why do we keep believing that dieting and restriction are effective? Why are dietitians and medical professionals still telling people to lose weight? Culturally, we (including medical and health professionals) are all introduced and conditioned to the beliefs of diet culture early on in our lives. It comes from messages like: *Don't eat too much, Don't gain weight, Look like the pictures you see of celebrities,* and, even more common (and deceiving) in recent years due to the popularity of social media, *Be as beautiful, successful, and high-achieving as "real-life" influencers.* **We have all essentially been duped into believing thinness—and all the rewards associated with it—are achievable for anyone if you just try hard enough.** The inverse message is that if you aren't thin enough, you haven't tried hard enough. The truth is much simpler: body diversity does and should exist. Due to genetic diversity, we know that not all bodies are designed to be thin or to have a "normal" BMI. Everyone could exercise and eat the same every day of their life and body diversity would still exist. Just because someone lives in a larger body than is deemed acceptable doesn't mean they are sick, lazy, going to have a particular chronic disease, or have "let themselves go." Some people are thin, some people are fat—and many people are being hurt by weight stigma associated with the thin ideal.

We will mention the impact of how doctors and health professionals who encourage a weight-centered approach to health harm us all. With that, we want to emphasize that this isn't aimed at all doctors. Doctors aren't a monolith; they are individuals who practice from a variety of approaches and beliefs. We know there are amazing pediatricians out there who are already aware that scales, restriction, and weight management aren't helpful or healthy for kids in any body size. We appreciate you and we will continue to need your help and support. To all the doctors out there who are already informed about what we strive to share in this book: thank you for being absolutely essential players in the field and for helping to prevent harm. To the doctors who currently practice from a weight-centered approach, we invite you to open your minds and see the bigger picture beyond weight and "childhood obesity." Understand the history and context of BMI, and consider how what you say and what happens in your exam rooms may impact a young person for the rest of their life. You're in a position of incredible power, and we need your help.

OUR FIRST LOOK AT THE 3 KEYS

Parents can feel empowered to go against the grain of diet culture and ultimately do what is best for their families using the **3 Keys for How to Raise an Intuitive Eater**:

1. **Provide unconditional love and support for your child's body.**
2. **Implement a flexible and reliable feeding routine.**
3. **Develop and use your Intuitive Eating voice.**

The 3 Keys are based on what research (to date) concludes about feeding and food psychology, eating disorder prevention, and the factors that play into developing a healthy relationship with food and body. Food is something we interact with multiple times a day, every single day of our lives, and is one of our most fundamental needs for survival. Our bodies are what we carry with us each day of our lives, and the way we relate to our bodies has enormous potential to shape our life experiences. We must nourish our bodies.

The 3 Keys will teach you what you can do daily to fulfill your role, starting with how you can ensure you're providing unconditional love and respect for your child's here-and-now body. Next is guidance about how to create a flexible feeding routine; making decisions about what food is provided, while involving your child in a way that is developmentally appropriate and helps them build curiosity and interest in their food and appetite. We will dive into the essential truth that hunger is sometimes about more than an empty stomach. Learning to develop and use

3 Keys:
How to Raise an Intuitive Eater

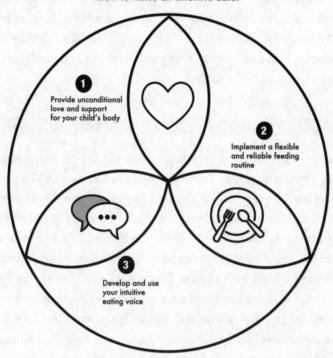

your Intuitive Eating voice is the third key. Key 3 teaches you about the power of using your voice, not only in how you talk to your child, but in how you talk to yourself. The 3 Keys combined will support you in embracing body diversity, size acceptance, and emotional attunement, and in demystifying bodies. These are all important ways we provide support for kids while they live in a changing and developing body and build resilience against diet culture and weight stigma. This balance between providing flexible structure while allowing space and honoring diversity is what we need to do in order to allow kids to develop their own limits, opinions, and trust. We have another example of when we have found this balance of structure and autonomy: learning to walk.

Eating and walking are both internally driven processes—you don't have to teach a child they should try to walk, and the same is true with eating.

When kids are learning to walk, we want them to explore. We don't have a rule book because parents are trusted to keep their children safe. We want our wobblers to try those steps on different surfaces and to learn to trust their little legs and feet. We use positive and necessary control to set boundaries and not allow them to run into the street. With our guidance, they will eventually know that running into the street without looking isn't safe and we will trust them to stay on the sidewalk. We do this again and again in parenting. It's instinctual to provide boundaries and show them where danger or consequences exist, while still allowing them the space to learn their own limits and to watch where they're stepping. Applying the same principle to feeding is a similar concept.

A FLEXIBLE ROUTINE IS A LEADING INGREDIENT

This is critical—there are going to be times when you feel like you're supposed to "follow rules" about structure and timing of meals and snacks. *That's a very normal thought—structure is important—but keep reading.* This goes back to wanting a set of rules—and what Intuitive Eating for kids really is, is letting the 3 Keys guide you while you make the decisions. Diet mentality is rigid, full of rules, while Intuitive Eating is flexible. Rigid rules are the opposite of flexibility. For the most part we need to embrace flexibility, even when it goes against everything we think we know. Each day there could be unanticipated ways that eating opportunities show up, and with the 3 Keys, you can feel capable of making a choice that *feels right to you*, armed with information about tuning in to the hunger your child may be expressing, mindful behavior changes, the psychology behind Intuitive Eating, the fallout from negative control or pressure around food, and the science of nutrition. We didn't want to come up with rigid rules that when broken could leave you feeling guilty. *We want to set you free—break away from rules!* You're already under so much pressure from diet culture, medical advice, school nutrition parameters, other parents, and yes, even from yourself. Intuitive Eating at its core is about setting you free to trust yourself, to tune in, and to have choices. With this freedom comes a clear path to hearing and trusting your and your child's body's signals, along with their needs and desires. We wanted to follow in the spirit of Intuitive Eating and really help parents be able to do this for their children.

Before we dive into the 3 Keys, we have to talk about diet culture and how we, as parents and caregivers, allow it to take up space in our minds and lives. This is known as modeling. Modeling is the most effective way to teach our kids almost everything. Kids learn from what we do, not what we tell them to do. Give yourself the chance to fully unpack your own history, so that you can best provide the guidance your child needs when it comes to Intuitive Eating. Remember that being vulnerable is hard.

We're sure you already know your kid is basically a sponge soaking up everything they see you do and say. There is so much messaging flooding their brain about bodies. From the beginning, our kids are conditioned to the societal standard that thinner is preferred. (We aren't blaming you . . . Let's say that again: we aren't blaming parents!) This may or may not be an intention of yours, but it's critical to see it for what it is: fatphobia and weight stigma. Fear of fat is presented to kids in many forms, from the way fat cartoon characters are rarely portrayed as the main character but usually as the "bad guy" or the "funny one," to the comments adults around them make. How often are your kids hearing *You look great! Have you lost weight?* Or: *I'm trying to lose this belly.* Or: *That's a terrible picture—I look so fat.* Or how about: *I'm so bad for eating this* when it's time for birthday cake. We have all been conditioned to overthink our weight, judge bodies, and assume things based on stereotypes and media messaging.

Not only are we overdue to release our kids from these harmful body expectations, but we deserve to do the same for ourselves. We—including us (Sumner and Amee), you, and everyone else raising children—are human and unique. We have big bodies, small bodies, wrinkly, dimply, soft, and firm bodies. We experience varying degrees of what our culture defines as "health." We all desire to create a social and cultural landscape that can be welcoming and appreciative of our children's wonderful bodies. We love every square inch of our children. It's time we love ourselves the same way.

In digging deep into this research, some recurring themes that can protect a child from losing their Intuitive Eating ability have stood out to us. The themes we've identified and used to create the 3 Keys are:

- **MODELING:** Model the behavior you want for your children.
- **AVOIDING NEGATIVE PARENTAL CONTROL:** Maintain trust in your child's body and avoid inappropriate negative control of their eating (you'll learn more about the term "negative control" in part 2).
- **TUNING IN TO EMOTIONAL NEEDS:** Provide and foster emotional attunement and agility.
- **BODY RESPECT:** Create an environment at home that is respectful toward all body types, weights, skin colors, ethnicities, ages, ability levels, gender and sexual identities, and more.

These are all complex concepts on their own, so we will be fully diving into these in later chapters.

Our culture dictates that we need to be familiar with the "problem" of our children's weight and their appearance. Terms like BMI, belly fat, "overweight," and "childhood obesity" have become everyday words when we talk about kids and health. However, the real facts are: you can't see health, and weight actually doesn't dictate health. Why is this so important? Because people of every age are struggling to maintain a healthy relationship with food and their bodies as a result of our culture's obsession with weight and appearance.

So, what's the big deal if a child doesn't have a positive relationship with their body or food? Aren't their growth, development, and weight most important to consider with regard to nutrition? Well, no.

The problem that has been developing over the past few decades, particularly with respect to the response to the "childhood obesity epidemic," is that the more we focus on kids' weight and body size, the worse the impact actually is on their overall health. Overemphasizing appearance—whether it comes from our family or from the society we live in—directly impacts how a person eats. Over one-half of adolescent girls are on a diet or attempting weight loss, and more than one-third of adolescent boys are engaging in similar behaviors. When a person is five to eighteen times more likely to develop an eating disorder after dieting, we have to take those numbers seriously.[4] Some develop subclinical disordered eating, eating disorders, or weight cycle throughout their entire life.

Here is some perspective about what the big fuss is with dieting:

- Fifty percent of girls and thirty percent of boys ages six to eight want to be thinner.[5]
- At least one out of four "normal dieters" progress to a clinical eating disorder, and 35 percent progress to pathological dieting.[6]
- Binge eating disorder (BED), although not as well known as anorexia and bulimia, is by far the most common eating disorder.[7]
- More than 74 percent of women between the ages of twenty-five and forty-five reported that their concerns about shape and weight interfered with their happiness.[8]
- Nearly 90 percent of parents of five-year-olds have actively dieted within the last year in the United States.[9]
- Prevalence of eating disorders is high: 2.7 percent of adolescents (ages thirteen to eighteen) will experience an eating disorder,[10] with many more struggling into adulthood and just as many (or more) who will never receive a formal diagnosis.

- Anorexia nervosa is the second most deadly of all mental illnesses (behind opioid addictions) because of health risks and high rates of suicide.[11]
- One in five deaths of people suffering from anorexia is by suicide.
- The mortality rate associated with anorexia nervosa is twelve times higher than the death rate of *all* causes of death for females fifteen to twenty-four years old.
- Only one in ten people with eating disorders will receive treatment.

Throughout the book, when we talk about eating disorders, we are referring to anorexia nervosa (AN), bulimia nervosa (BN), binge eating disorder (BED), and other specified feeding and eating disorders (OS-FED), which may include a combination of signs and symptoms of the first three. We aren't specifically referencing avoidant/restrictive food intake disorder (ARFID). ARFID, also referred to as "extreme picky eating," selective eating disorder (SED), or pediatric feeding disorder (PFD), is categorically different from the other eating disorders we are referring to. Many kids with ARFID require thoughtful integration of structure beyond the 3 Keys model and will benefit from individualized treatment with a specialist.

We could easily go on. Others who don't seek or receive help for disordered eating concerns will experience depression or anxiety tied to their appearance. Many people will spend years diverting their attention, thoughts, and energy to food and exercise—something so impactful, we may never know the depth of the damage. A huge concern is that the majority of people who suffer from subclinical disordered eating (meaning they experience significant interruptions in life, but never receive a diagnosis), despite the fact that it may be wreaking havoc on their life and relationships, don't know why they are suffering because this is so rarely discussed.

Many parents tell us they would never recommend dieting, weight loss, or food restriction for their child, yet they fail to see that their own dieting practices, body dissatisfaction, and our cultural dialogue all contribute to how kids come to think about food and bodies. Kids do not need to be put on a diet in order to develop diet mentality or body dissatisfaction. We believe that the vast majority of parents would never want to do anything to cause harm to their child, and that if they knew the impact some of their behaviors are having on their child, they would change their behavior.

MENTAL HEALTH IS HEALTH

The state of someone's mental health is not something you can see by looking at a person or by assessing their weight. However, the belief that health is something we can see or measure, by BMI or appearance, is now mainstream. You might see a person of a certain size and immediately make assumptions about their health and behaviors. A thin person must be doing "all the right things," and a larger person might be seen as "lazy." That's called weight bias, and it's something we are conditioned to by our culture, not something we choose.

Weight bias is derived from the fact that people have been dieting for generations and it has infiltrated medical care, fitness, wellness, and even school curriculums. The complex history of weight bias and fatphobia actually dates back centuries. Thankfully, over the past thirty years or so, the medical and nutrition science fields have started to realize how harmful dieting is and the true toll it takes on our health. There is a slowly building cultural shift away from dieting—finally!

PARENTAL PRESSURE

It's never a parent's fault for feeling uncertainty or worry over their child's eating. As we mentioned earlier, the metaphorical microscope that's been placed on kids' weight and shape has dramatically increased parental anxiety over the last thirty or so years, and significantly more so since the early 2000s when the "childhood obesity epidemic" began to be discussed in public spaces. Along with fears of kids becoming "too big," or being "too small," are fears around kids eating too much of "the wrong thing"—fast food, sugary foods, processed foods, nonorganic foods, additives—the list goes on and on. When you zoom out just a touch further, you can easily see the immense pressure on parents to feed their kids perfectly. Not only is this pressure stressful and classist (few can afford to provide all the "right" meals, all the time), it has a very clear negative spiral-down effect on kids that reflects the typical dieting cycle adults often experience. The parental and cultural influence eventually creates the internalized beliefs of a child, and then eventually becomes the child's own diet cycle.

A typical diet cycle is quite predictable, and experienced by the majority of people who report dieting in their life. It goes like this:

1. Intention to lose weight or to improve health

2. Deprivation of amount of food or certain types of food

3. Short-term "honeymoon phase" where you may feel good or lose weight

4. Cravings build, urges to "cheat" or binge

5. Feelings of guilt, shame, or failure along with physical discomfort from overeating

6. Begin a new diet. And the cycle continues. A child can be set into motion on their own diet cycle very early in life.

Remember, you aren't to blame for how you may have been feeding or controlling your kids' eating. You were influenced and taught to do this, and you've only been doing your best with what you knew. Here's our first practice in self-compassion.

WEIGHT STIGMA VS. BODY RESPECT

Many studies claim to prove that higher-weight children have lower self-esteem, concluding that weight is to blame for low self-esteem, and therefore the solution is to seek weight loss. These studies fail to control for how weight stigma (discrimination, bullying, shaming), dieting, and disordered eating impact a person's self-esteem.[12]

What is weight stigma? It's the assumptions we make about a person based on their weight, usually with negative associations. It's also the social rejection that a person faces based on their body size. All of the effects of weight stigma can be either overt or implicit. Intentional or unintentional. The important thing to remember is that impact is more important than intent. What we (as parents and humans) intended to happen doesn't negate the effect we actually had. For example, often when comments about weight or a suggestion to diet are made by a healthcare provider or loved one, they are an attempt to help. Despite this positive intention, the impact is almost always harm, by way of increased feelings of unworthiness or shame that people experience from weight stigma in a culture that values thinness as much as ours does. Most people who experience weight stigma don't experience it in an actual scientific setting as kids in weight-loss trials do. It's day-to-day microaggressions, like not having tables that you can sit comfortably in, not finding clothes that fit, asserting assumptions about how someone eats or moves without asking, and comments that seem harmless, or even helpful, but aren't. It's existing in a world that clearly thinks you need to change your body because it isn't seen as being "good enough." As a result, kids—and adults—who live in larger bodies often experience more negative stress related to size, eating, and appearance than their thinner peers. **Weight stigma is the discrimination, negative stereotyping, and prejudice that people who are thought of as carrying excess weight face in our society.** We are taught that the way to reduce weight stigma is to reduce our body size and therefore our likelihood of experiencing it, instead of trying to eliminate weight stigma. The sad truth is weight stigma isn't just reserved for shaming people in bigger bodies. It has its hands in every pot.

Weight stigma, when studied, has been found to be more detrimental to health than having a higher-than-average BMI.[13,14,15] Those who experience weight discrimination have double the risk of having ten-year high allostatic load[16]—a measure of the negative cumulative wear and tear on the body from chronic stress, including negative effects on the cardiovascular system, immune system, and metabolic system.[17] All of the attention on saving kids from "becoming too fat" has backfired, spurred an intense fear of fat for kids of all sizes, and caused us to lose sight of the value of a child's relationship with food and their body. In a study about the way adolescents behave around food when they perceive their weight as healthy, it was found that when both boys and girls perceived their weight as healthy (meaning they just assumed they were considered healthy regardless of what others thought or what they weighed), they were less likely to engage in risky restrictive dieting behaviors and less likely to start purging or using drugs for body-centered results (performance-enhancing drugs for boys and diet pills or laxatives for girls. These gender-specific drug labels were created by the study designers.). When these kids assumed they were healthy, they engaged in healthier behavior and were able to have a healthier relationship with their body and food. They were actually healthier overall simply because they didn't have internalized weight stigma! Rebecca Puhl, a researcher who has done multiple studies on both the prevalence of weight stigma and its effects, has learned that not only is weight stigma everywhere—from the doctor's office to school to employers—it's likely to cause multiple adverse health effects. Quite possibly the very health conditions we are trying to help our kids avoid. In these studies, she found evidence that even doctors entering the field felt negatively about those in "overweight" or "obese" bodies to the point where they were less likely to perform routine exams on them. Many people who live in fat bodies are afraid to ask for these procedures due to past experiences or fears that their doctor does indeed feel disgusted by them. The end result? Less preventative medical care for those in fat bodies. We know for a fact that this causes negative health outcomes—that's why in the early 2000s there was a public health initiative to prevent heart attacks in men by encouraging them to go to the doctor more. What happens when it feels unsafe to go to the doctor? When nurses report that it's repulsive to touch an "obese" body? We create risk.

*A note on language: We use words like "fat" in this context—and throughout the book—as a reclaimed descriptor. It isn't intended as a slur or in a derogatory way. *

LEARNING FROM OUR OWN PAST

Go back to those early memories of first feeling bad about your body. (Remember, if you didn't ever experience this, you were protected!) Think about how different it would feel as a child or a young person if adults around you said things like:

Do you have a safe place to go play outside after school?
Are you getting enough to eat when you need it?
How can I help you take care of your precious and incredible body?
How much time do you spend worrying about your appearance or body size?

Instead of statements like those above, we are teaching kids that there are "healthy bodies" and "unhealthy bodies" based on size, as if fear were a motivator for self-care. We are teaching them what their body "should" be like instead of respecting their current body and prioritizing mental health. We are enforcing pressure, control, and limits over what they eat in a way that triggers a healthy ego response to do just the opposite when we're not around. What we say, how we say it, and how we talk about bodies and food can make the biggest difference for your child's future relationship with their body and with food.

WHY WE NEED TO SAY
"NO" TO THE STATUS QUO

Weight stigma and diet culture are so deeply ingrained in our culture that we don't even need to be explicitly taught them. We live with the results of this conditioning daily. Kids today are learning these lessons from caregivers, educators, advertisements, and everywhere else. We are all taught that certain bodies are better than others and that certain foods are better to eat than others. We are taught that the problem is us and our body. But the real problem, the one that is so deeply buried we can't even see it, is the mistrust that starts to grow in children's minds. As early as five years of age, perhaps earlier, kids have stopped trusting their body cues, and instead believe that bodies—specifically body weight—is something to be controlled, molded, and managed. Mistrust has a steep cost: the physical and mental health of our kids. This happens when we fail to put their relationship with food and their bodies at the forefront. This is happening to kids in all body shapes and sizes, of all races and ethnicities, and across socioeconomic groups.

The status quo is diet culture. The status quo is focusing on "healthy eating"—not how you care for your body, or how comfortable you are in your body. No, the real things that actually influence our life experiences the most—the relationship we have with ourselves—are left out of the picture and have been replaced by a focus on weight targets, BMI, calorie counting, and "good" and "bad" ways of eating. Along with diet culture, parents are unintentionally driving kids away from caring, compassionate relationships with their own bodies—at a huge cost.

We believe the problem is that our culture—meaning mainstream Western culture—has lost sight of how important it is for children to maintain a healthy relationship with food and their bodies. This isn't to suggest that nutrition isn't important, but the evidence shows that the relationship you have with your body, food, and the way in which your body is treated by society is just as important as what you eat, if not more important.

There is a very instinctual trust with our bodies that we are born with, but many adults don't know that experience when we speak about it—it's far too faded to grasp anymore. That trust is easily broken in this culture. It can be broken by many things, all of which are traumatic for our body. One way it can be damaged is related to how we are fed and how our bodies are perceived in the world. When that trust is broken, whether it's because an early caregiver can't or won't feed an infant enough milk or formula, or because a young person repeatedly hears they need to do something to control their size, shape, or appearance—a part of us is lost. That part is the space that genuinely believes we are good for this world, that we have something important to contribute, that we are lovable and worthy of having our needs met, and that the people we need the most to take care of us will meet those needs. When we lose that part, we doubt our worth. This becomes internalized over time until we stop questioning it, and it becomes our own inner critic.

The status quo is telling kids what to eat, moralizing food (making it "good" or "bad"), and restricting access to certain foods that are considered "junk." It's teaching kids to be afraid of being fat or even of having a body that doesn't measure up to mainstream beauty ideals, of being not good enough. It's also assuming a child needs to be coerced or pressured to eat more, to finish their plate or their vegetables. It pushes all these things in the name of health, in the name of fitting in, in the name of beauty. It has long-term, detrimental impacts that many parents aren't aware of. The status quo is such because no one talks about those detrimental impacts, but we are here to talk about them now.

The advice that is given most often is: "restrict." Our culture recognizes "junk" foods as a food group to avoid as much as possible. We have moralized foods and encouraged parents to exert control over their children's diets. We've been told that without control, kids will never choose the "healthy" options. It also means pushing "moderation" as the goal. You've probably heard all of this from parent friends—or even recommended by doctors. Since the 1980s, an extreme focus on body weight and BMI has become standard among pediatricians, parents, and even within schools. There is growing scientific evidence about the risks of any level of dieting—even when it's not called dieting—and the distrust it begins to cultivate within our children. When parents attempt to assert control over the food choices that children make, we risk creating trauma that severs that innate trust kids have in their bodies. When that is broken, they start to lose the natural ability to choose the types and amounts of food that they need for satisfaction, growth, and development. They lose the Intuitive Eating skills they were born with. When parents and other influential adults put too much stock in weight, shape, and health, the kids will begin to mirror those same beliefs. This can quickly develop into body dissatisfaction, which can lead to the dangerous path toward disordered eating behaviors.

You may feel like thinness, healthy eating, not being fat, or some other wellness- or appearance-based goals are some of the most important things in life. You aren't alone. That's how we're conditioned. Thin people are successful, happy, good. Health and wellness are requirements. But these aren't the most important things.

We do, however, know that a change in that kind of thinking can take time. We are pushing against things you have known for so long and many other messages that exist in our world. So we can't and won't blame you, shame you, or judge you for thinking that controlling weight and food for your kids is something you have to do. **Right now, we just want you to hold on to the possibility that your child's relationship with food could be more important for their long-term health and happiness than anything else about how they eat.**

Remember: your child's health *includes* mental health. Mental and physical health are inextricably connected. Physical health is drastically impacted by weight stigma, shame, and disordered eating. You could feed your child the "healthiest," "cleanest," lowest-sugar diet in the world, but if they aren't mentally well, don't trust their bodies, don't feel calm or at ease with food—they aren't likely to feel as confident, capable, or well in their body or in the world around them as they would with a secure and positive relationship with food and body.

It can be uncomfortable for any parent to recognize that this status quo has potentially dangerous side effects. You don't have to dive into this chapter or the next feeling like this is the perfect solution and you're completely ready to try helping your kid grow up as an Intuitive Eater. You might still be questioning all of this. There is space for compassion and imperfection here and always.

THE STATUS QUO: FOLLOWING DIET CULTURE'S LEAD AND ASSERTING PARENTAL CONTROL

We know (from being parents ourselves, and also from having worked with many families in our nutrition counseling practices) that parents want their kids to eat healthfully for a very good reason—they love their kids, they want them to feel good and live long and healthy lives. Every parent has the right to do what they think is best for their child.

Remember: have self-compassion and a mindset focused on doing better moving forward—not beating yourself up for the past! We are both parents; we know the struggle is real. Even we struggle to shake off all the diet mentality and internalized fatphobia all the time.

MAYBE YOU'VE NEVER QUESTIONED ANY OF THIS

It's completely normal for many parents to not even question some of the most widely accepted and recommended approaches to raising "healthy" eaters. These include: pressuring kids to taste, eat, or finish "healthy" foods; using food as a way to control a child's behavior (such as for punishment or reward for certain behaviors); controlling eating with pressure and portion size limits; restricting access to certain foods (e.g., hiding the candy); and even using nutrition and health education to try to coerce kids into making healthy choices.

Here's the rub: all of the above have been taught to you by diet culture. The food rules, the fear of weight gain, the pressure to eat certain foods and avoid others. All of it.

Diet culture has been around for centuries, so much of what you think might have been passed down from your own parents and grandparents. This makes it really hard to recognize that all this is from powerful external forces, not just your own parents.

Remember how we talked about the sneaky, silent ways dieting sneaks into, well, diets? Well, it's just as sneaky when it comes to your mind. Dieting is so pervasive, you've been conditioned to believe it's *your idea* that you need to be a certain size or weight. People of all sizes and backgrounds get defensive when they are confronted by someone (like we are doing now) who questions the intent of their dieting. If you feel defensive of your need to diet, it's because you may feel like discrediting dieting is discrediting your own ideas ... That's how powerful diet culture is.

ENGINEERED CONSENT

This sneaky, pervasive conditioning isn't unique to dieting, either. In her book *Quit Like a Woman: The Radical Choice to Not Drink in a Culture Obsessed with Alcohol,* Holly Whitaker defines "engineered consent," a term coined by Edward Bernays sometime around the late 1920s. She describes how Bernays was brought in to work with the tobacco industry in 1929 to determine a marketing strategy for getting more women to smoke more cigarettes, for, not surprisingly, more profits. The industry had recognized they had an untapped opportunity in American women, who were only smoking indoors, not outside—as it was not socially acceptable because of feminine standards at the time. Bernays understood that cigarette marketing could use the power of social influence to manipulate people into thinking they were maintaining control over their own choices. So Big Tobacco used the women's liberation movement as a launchpad for sales. Cigarette ads began depicting women smoking outdoors, "inviting women across the nation to smoke a Torch of Freedom in public as a fuck-you to the patriarchy and a nod to their increasing liberation."[1] Well, it worked. This strategically engineered sales ploy by a group of men resulted in rates of women who smoked to climb over the following four decades. Women believed they were making a choice to act out against the patriarchy, but in reality, they were being manipulated into believing that. All in order to line the pockets of wealthy men who didn't care about their liberation, their health, or their movement.

Diet culture and Big Tobacco have something huge in common. Manipulation by diet culture is a story that has been spun again and again. It's the same in the tobacco industry and the alcohol industry. We are willing to argue that the influence the diet industry has created is just as present, insidious, and dangerous, from the monetary gains the industry experiences with dieting to the physical and mental health risks that are ever-present. The worse we feel about ourselves, the more money we will spend trying to fix those flaws. The US weight-loss and diet-control market alone is a $72 *billion* industry. This doesn't include the fitness and beauty industries, which are inextricably linked to the diet industry in terms of how they work together to degrade our self-esteem, self-worth, and body respect. Seventy-two billion dollars' worth of dieting and weight-loss products. This isn't all about health, folks.

Diet culture has used engineered consent in a way to first make us believe that we are taking back the power to control our own health and weight, and then to use that against us so that we think we are "choosing" that our weight has to be lower, or our diet has to be "cleaner." Once we achieve these things, we can finally achieve what we deserve: success, love, attention, younger looks, strength, and desirability. The diet industry has done an exceptional job at controlling how we feel about ourselves. The recent evolution of marketing to now include social media influencers has only strengthened the hold the diet industry has over us all—including the health and medical field. This goes for people of all genders and ages, not just young women.

THE WHITE MEN BEHIND YOUR DIET MINDSET

We keep talking about men and the patriarchy. Let's get more specific: *the white men behind your diet are making more money.* Sabrina Strings, author of *Fearing the Black Body*, details the history of how the idea that thin is attractive and healthy actually stems from the onset of the slave trade in the fifteenth century. White-supremacist thinking taught people to think and believe that white bodies were better than Black bodies, and because Black women were often, but not always, genetically built larger than white women, size came to be associated with moral status—and whiteness. White European societies that became US colonies elevated and served the patriarchy and capitalism and, therefore, the mindset that some bodies (white bodies) were "closer to God." This became more mainstream during the early decades of US history alongside slavery, genocide, and the removal of Indigenous people from their land. You might find it interesting to know that every mainstream diet trend we've ever seen over the last one hundred years was developed—at least partially—by a white male.[2]

Why are the white cultural beliefs what dictate mainstream Western cultural thinking, appearance standards, medicine, and pop culture? That answer is simple: systemic racism and white supremacy are what has controlled society in the United States, Europe, and colonized nations for hundreds of years. The abolition of slavery didn't end anti-Black and racist beliefs. In fact, they are alive and well today in 2021—and diet culture is still one of the "most potent political sedatives"[3] alive and well today. Think about how much a diet mindset keeps people—particularly women and and sexual and gender minority populations—distracted, powerless, anxious, and busy.

The status quo includes widely accepted (it is, after all, five hundred years' worth of passed-down beliefs that have infiltrated society) and normalized practices that Western culture has encouraged for parents. This is often delivered via mass media and directly from health professionals themselves who have been misled by the diet industry. Despite all the emphasis on "healthy eating" and preventing "childhood obesity," rates of eating disorders and disordered eating in youth continue to climb. While everyone from the highest rung of government to your kindergarten teacher is trying to combat "childhood obesity," rampant eating disorders are hardly acknowledged. A critical look at the normalized approach to feeding kids points out how what we, as a society, are currently doing is causing our kids a lot of harm and contributing to disordered eating prevalence.

Our culture's normalized approach to feeding kids—the status quo—includes two main contributing influences: the use of negative parental control and diet culture.

1. NEGATIVE PARENTAL CONTROL (two main forms)

- **Pressuring kids to eat "healthy" foods:** Either by rewarding eating or punishment for not eating. Pressuring can also be prompting (*Don't you want to have some salad?*) or using nutritional guidance (*You should really have some vegetables, they're good for you*). Importantly, pressure can be perceived and felt differently by kids with different temperaments.
- **Restricting "unhealthy" foods:** Not keeping certain food groups or types of food in the house. Hiding sweet foods or "junk" food. Placing limits on portion sizes on some foods but not others.

2. DIET CULTURE

- Diet mentality, including attitudes about bodies in general, fatphobia, promoting thin as best, assuming all kids should be somewhere near the fiftieth percentile on a growth chart, and the use of diet talk and weight talk in the home. This also includes many health beliefs about certain foods—especially when it involves restricting or removing them.

Now, let's break down the evidence around parental control and what we know about diet culture to help you understand how these things impact your child's behavior and their relationship with food.

NEGATIVE PARENTAL CONTROL

"Parental control" is an interesting term. Yes, our goal is often to be in control. When we talk about *negative parental control* in this book, we are specifically referring to the ways we try to control the way our children eat. This includes: (1) using negative or positive pressure to get a child to eat certain foods, and (2) restricting access to certain foods, most commonly "unhealthy" or "junk" foods. Some of the ways parents use pressure are so normalized, we don't intend to be pressuring at all, particularly with how we praise young children or early eaters advancing from milk to solid foods: *Yay, Cecilia ate avocado!* This starts very early. The problem is, praise is one of the first ways we condition kids to eat *to please us*. When we do this, it teaches them to eat for external reasons, rather than for their natural internal drive to eat because it tastes good and is inherently nourishing. Prompting is another way we pressure without knowing it: *Make sure to have some carrots with your pizza.* They actually don't need external pressure to eat at all. They just need an environment that fosters a sense of warmth, safety, and relaxed eating with enough tasty food consistently provided. If you question this—*My kids would never eat a vegetable unless I pressured them to*—you might find kids don't eat dry, plain carrots, but may love them when introduced with a dip or cooked and seasoned with oil and salt. There are also many kids who don't prefer a lot of vegetables in any way you've prepared them, and in that case, pressure is still not the way to make them eat the vegetables.

EXAMPLES OF THE TWO TYPES OF NEGATIVE CONTROL

PRESSURE

POSITIVE PRESSURE
I'm so proud of you, you ate your broccoli! (praise)
Great job on finishing your dinner, now you can have dessert. (reward)

NEGATIVE PRESSURE

If you don't finish your oatmeal, you can't have any iPad time today.
There will be no ice cream for you if you don't do what I tell you right now.

RESTRICTION

You can only have one cookie. After that you need to choose something healthy.
We don't allow white flour in our house, everything has to be whole wheat.
Don't have too many chips. Why don't you have an apple instead?
Not allowing sweet foods like ice cream, cookies, and candy in the house on a
   regular basis.

When parents exert negative control, food becomes currency between you and your child. It's used to encourage and reward some behaviors such as being quiet, eating vegetables, or following directions. It's also used as a punishment: dessert may be withheld if rules are broken or behavior is out of line.

LET'S TALK ABOUT PRESSURE

The general belief (that status quo) is that you need to urge your child to eat their salad, broccoli, or apple slices. You may feel you have to enforce a consequence if they don't eat what you tell them to eat. The illusion this approach upholds is that if you make your child eat what they're told they will get used to it and then choose to eat that broccoli on their own. (Spoiler alert: this rarely works.) Parents are often also unconsciously highly motivated to raise a "good" eater so they feel better about their own parenting ability. Intuitive Eating teaches us the opposite: our best shot at raising a child who eats a variety of nourishing foods is to make mealtime pleasant and to steer clear of diet culture and pressure. We can't talk about this without acknowledging that it's highly likely you were raised under some pressure to eat certain foods, and your parents (even your grandparents and great-grandparents) were likely also raised this way, and Intuitive Eating feels out of reach.

Generations of food beliefs and rules may have created a habit that you didn't even realize you had—pressuring your child to eat something because it's "healthy." When you're successful at this, you feel better because you're "teaching good eating habits" and doing what other parents are doing (or are so desperately trying to do), so it must be the right thing. This might work in the short term, but when we look at the long-term impact, the results are less than promising.

Even when our kids aren't picky eaters, we feel pressure to get their eating to be "better" and "healthier." This pressure we feel from society and from the status quo is passed on to our kids. They feel the pressure from us to eat "better" and "healthier." This pressure may get our kids to finish their bell peppers, or to believe that cookies are inherently unhealthy, but they are losing the ability to trust their own hunger. Studies show that kids who experience more parental pressure to eat in childhood have lower Intuitive Eating scores as adults, which means they are less likely to be Intuitive Eaters and are associated with increased risk for eating disorders.[4] So, contrary to our fears that our child will never eat "well," kids who are "picky eaters" do not necessarily show low Intuitive Eating scores when they are adults. Many people who are "picky" early in life naturally grow to become more adventurous and open to a wider variety of foods later in life. The reaction to put pressure on kids to eat "healthy" foods—or a rich-enough variety of foods—can create a rupture in their relationship to food.[5] Now, one of the common arguments against Intuitive Eating is the idea that kids need to be given restrictive guidance and limits on "unhealthy" food and that verbal praise is effective in preventing "unhealthy" eating.[6] The concern with this data is that it looked for *types of foods consumed* (i.e., fruits and vegetables), not how these parenting styles impacted their child's *relationship with food and body*. Parental control can work in the short term to get a child to eat; however, it's the long-term impacts and risk of disordered eating that also have a significant impact on your child's well-being.

I (Amee) wasn't raised as an Intuitive Eater—I was raised as a dieter by dieters. As a result of this, and my own time not being an Intuitive Eater, I had no idea how to raise an Intuitive Eater. I still get nervous when my kid hasn't had a vegetable recently. The pressure and fear I feel as a parent are very real. I know there have been plenty of times when my partner and I ventured into "pressuring" our child to eat certain foods, and . . . it never worked. All of us would leave the table frustrated and unsatisfied. The more we pushed, the more she pushed back. I have spent a lot of time reminding myself (and my partner) that it isn't helping any of us to fight, to put pressure on food. It takes a lot of constant self-compassion, but so does all of parenting.

REWARDING AND PUNISHING WITH FOOD IS A FORM OF PRESSURE

It's five o'clock. I'm (Sumner) in the grocery store with my children. If I could ask for just one thing in the moment, it would be twenty minutes to get what's on my list, get through the checkout, and arrive home peacefully without them having a meltdown. The reality is, young kids live out loud. They have big emotions, lots of energy, and big responses to disappointment. Sometimes the easiest way to get through the store in one piece is by offering a reward—most easily in the form of food. This is something I have done more than I care to admit. I have compassion for myself when it happens and I try to avoid it.

I try to be mindful of what message it sends my children. I try to keep food neutral, and stay present even in the yuckiest of moments, when they are scream-ing or having a meltdown and I just want to run away. I remind myself that they can trust their bodies, and when they're having a hard time at the store, part of my parenting values is that I want to help them build skills to work through their emotions instead of reacting with food to bribe or reward, or stop whatever it is they're doing that's hard for me to tolerate. As parents we can help bring them back to a better spot, not gloss over the tiredness or the frustration with a treat. Kids need to learn how to be patient and tolerate distress so that they can success-fully achieve these skills for life. Using food skips right over the hard stuff, puts certain foods on a pedestal, and creates the association for them that when they're upset they need food to soothe. Intuitive Eating teaches us that honoring our emotions with acceptance and kindness, not jumping to use food, is really helpful and allows food to just be something we have permission to eat when we really want it, when we're hungry for it, or when we desire it.

We know what you're thinking: *You want me to stop using food to bribe "good" behavior or punish "poor" behavior?! You've got to be out of your mind!*

We know. We hear you. But here's why we suggest not using food in these ways: when food is used as a reward, we change the meaning of the food and give it more power.

In many cases, this looks like dangling the idea of a tasty dessert over your child's head in order to get them to eat their veggies or their dinner. This com-pletely normalized and common approach sends a loud and clear message: The dessert food is special, you have to earn it, you can't just have it because you want it. This way you won't be unhealthy and you can have this "bad for you" thing that is so pleasurable and yummy, but only if you eat other things first even if you don't have room for it because you're full from dinner.

What happens after repeating this scenario over and over again is that it makes the reward foods very powerful. Similar to the effects of restriction, re-warding with food makes these foods the very foods your kids will prefer and choose when you're not around. In the short term, they may eat their broccoli in order to get the ice cream. But in the long term, they'll run the other way from the broccoli unless they truly enjoy it.[7] When we use food to change behavior, it detaches food from its primary role, which is to satisfy hunger.

HOW RESTRICTION REALLY PLAYS OUT

So, what is the most predictable reaction for a child when food restriction is actively happening? Eating more. Restriction will often be followed by eating more of the restricted food, particularly when you, the parent or caregiver, aren't around. Restrictive feeding practices are associated with:

- Eating in the absence of hunger (eating to cope with emotions)
- Negative attitudes toward one's body (body dissatisfaction)
- Restrained eating (restrictive eating disorders)
- Disinhibition—a sense of loss of control around food (binge eating)
- Weight gain outside of normal growth and development

One study looked at 112 pairs of parents and children in England.[8] The children whose parents exerted more control at home were found to feel worse about their bodies. This could be a combination of believing that their parents feel there is something wrong with their body, which is why they're not allowed to eat what they want, and feeling disconnected from their Intuitive Eating cues. Overeating often feels uncomfortable, and, even for a child, is associated with shame, feeling out of control, and like they're doing something wrong. Restriction quickly and significantly alters a child's Intuitive Eating ability and they begin to view their natural appetite and desires as bad or not to be trusted. Children believe *If I'm eating bad, that must mean I'm bad.* They also want to please you and do the right thing. It's an incredibly difficult place to be for a child, being torn between making your parents proud, and loud, unsatisfied food cravings. Most likely, any rigid food rules or restriction that may be happening in your home are causing not just stress for your child, but you as well. Let's not make our children have to choose. Their health *doesn't* depend on it.

You may believe the right thing to do is to keep certain foods out of reach, not allow them in the house (commonly recommended by health professionals, including some doctors and dietitians), or to place constraints on when and how much can be consumed. These behaviors are all various forms of *food restriction*. This shows up in all kinds of ways, both out of the house and in. For example, do you not keep sweetened cereal, candy, cookies, or ice cream in the house because you think you or your kids will just eat more of it if it's there? (Or maybe you don't keep them in the house due to your own relationship with those foods.) You may feel you have to limit those foods or you won't be setting the right example, or you're hurting their health if there are a variety of choices. Although it makes logical sense—*If the foods aren't there, no one will eat them*—the real effects of these practices are important to be aware of.

RESTRICTING ACCESS TO CERTAIN FOODS MAKES THE RESTRICTED FOOD MORE ATTRACTIVE

Studies show that restrictive feeding practices have two worrisome outcomes on kids:

1. They increase their preference for the restricted food over other foods that are freely available—so you're creating a stronger desire for the very food you're intending for them to avoid.

2. When your child is exposed to the restricted food, they will have a heightened response to the taste and pleasure of it as a result of the restriction, triggering a drive to eat more of it.[9,10] Then, if the pattern continues, this can feel like confirmation to a parent that you need to further "control" their eating, and young people learn to associate those foods *with that drive to eat* and as they grow older develop the belief that *I can't control myself with those foods*.

A core construct of Intuitive Eating is trusting your body and having unconditional permission to eat. Yes, **unconditional permission to eat**. Permission is the opposite of restriction. Permission doesn't mean you never say "no" to a child's food requests. A routine, especially for young kids, but really for most of us into adulthood, is important for self-regulation (knowing when to stop eating when you've had enough) and allows for showing up to the table comfortably hungry with the ability to respond to satiety cues. With Intuitive Eating, you'll be allowing your child to eat in accordance with what feels good to them based on what foods are prepared or available, in amounts that leave them feeling satisfied and energized, and even sometimes eating more than feels comfortable, which is an essential learning opportunity. Diet culture sees having more to eat than is comfortable, or being overfull, as a "mistake." We are taught to feel bad or guilty when this happens, although it's not always explicit. Children learn this through hearing how adults react to feeling their fullness (*I'm so "bad" for eating so much pie! I'm stuffed!*) or they are punished or shamed for eating a large amount (*Wow, I can't believe you ate all that ice cream. Next time you're only having a kiddie scoop*). In truth, having too much food, getting a tummy ache, and learning how that feels without being shamed or punished is an important learning experience for a child. It gives them the opportunity to learn how they might want to do something differently next time without you having to say anything at all (like falling and scraping their knees helps them learn to watch where they're going). Diet culture has made parents terrified of allowing for "natural consequences," like feeling a tummy ache, to take place.

There are some kids who don't experience restriction or pressure to eat even when living in a house where one or more family members are dieting or concerned about weight. Often, these kids who are given such permission and freedom are an "average" size or naturally thin. However, if (or more likely, when) they reach an age, like pre-puberty, where weight gain starts to happen, that permission is often removed or restrained.

In a 2003 study of nearly two hundred girls between the ages of five and nine and their parents in the United States, researchers assessed how the use of restriction placed on daughters by their parents at age four impacted their eating behavior by the time they were nine (particularly on overeating and eating when not hungry). What they found was that the parents who perceived their daughter's weight to be too high were the parents who exerted the most restriction and negative control over their child's eating. By age seven, the girls who were experiencing restriction at home had a significant increase in eating in the absence of hunger compared to the girls who experienced a low level of restriction at home. They found that higher-weight girls who also experienced restriction demonstrated the highest scores of eating when they weren't hungry—they were eating more often for other reasons. Parents of children who live in larger bodies are more likely to be influenced by public health messages and doctors to use restriction at home as a way of limiting their child's caloric intake. However, we see that this has a significant and lasting impact on eating behavior that ultimately can cause a child to eat more food than they would have had they been encouraged and allowed to trust their body. **The bottom line: restriction has the opposite effect that you're led to believe it has!** It leads to patterns of eating for reasons other than hunger. No matter your child's weight, restriction isn't helpful, as it has the paradoxical effect of triggering overeating in children.[11]

DIET CULTURE HAS MADE ITS
WAY INTO OUR SCHOOLS

The status quo tells us that we need to teach kids early on about nutrition, as if the more they know about food in kindergarten, the healthier they'll turn out (not true). We have nationally mandated standards to teach nutrition lessons, about "healthy" foods and "unhealthy" foods, about why the "yummy" foods are actually more off-limits, and we need to do this in order to ensure that we have kids who eat vegetables and "never have problems with their weight." It's incredibly common to hear of families who have been told by their pediatrician before their child is even in preschool that they need to "watch their weight." Some schools use BMI and weight monitoring and send home a BMI report card. This again reinforces the message, often continued throughout childhood, that parents need to make sure their child's weight is "managed." Studies examining the effectiveness or usefulness of such report cards have not shown a positive impact.[12] There are serious and life-threatening unintended consequences from the resulting weight stigmatization kids experience from being weighed at school. Unhealthy weight control behaviors and practices among kids at various sizes can be triggered from school-based weight stigmatizing experiences.[13] Further, medical experts know that BMI categories provide limited utility and there isn't strong evidence to support the categorization, yet it continues to be used. Around the onset of puberty, parents and kids frequently get the message that their child is gaining too much weight and should be doing more to prevent "obesity" in a "healthy way," of course. It's been indoctrinated into the minds of parents that their child's weight and health is in their hands. Parents are pressured from many directions to extend control over their child's eating and weight.

MESSAGING ABOUT FOOD IS EVERYWHERE

We are constantly barraged with reminders about weight gain and why we should fear it. Parents respond to this (almost automatically) by assuming the best course of action is to restrict their child's access to foods that are labeled as "unhealthy" or "bad." (These terms cover any and all foods that for whatever reason you believe your child should not have: cookies, candy, juice, soda, chips, sugary cereal . . .) At the same time, you're thinking your child should not have these foods, or should have only limited amounts of them because of the messaging you're getting from diet culture, while your child is seeing commercials that sell the idea that these foods are fun, will make them happy, and that parents who give these foods to their kids must really love them. (Take a closer look at commercials, marketing, and packaging—you'll see what we mean.) This is just one example of how kids are receiving mixed messaging around food. Another example is the way they observe you eating and talking about food. Your child may hear you tell everyone at a birthday party that you can't have cake "because you're cutting out sugar," and yet a moment later someone is serving them up a piece of that very same cake. For a child, that is confusing—*Why does Mom not want to eat the cake when it's so yummy? And why would grown-ups say it's okay to have this to celebrate someone's birthday if it's so bad?* And: *If I want to be like Mom, maybe I shouldn't have any cake either.*

We often work with kids and families who have siblings that are genetically built differently, and who may have very different eating tendencies. Parents can react to the weight or appearance of a larger-bodied child with food rules, shame, or pressure to eat "healthier" foods while they allow a smaller-bodied child to eat naturally, without concern or intervention, no matter how they are eating. We understand parents in these scenarios are often intending to help their child maintain a "healthy weight"; however, thanks to diet culture, parents are hesitant to want to accept that their child's current larger body size may be healthier for them than attempting to lose weight will ever be. Parents are often unaware of how they've been influenced by diet culture. Generally, parents are repeatedly given the message that weight gain is bad and can be "managed." In the case of multiple siblings of different sizes, the child or sibling who faces judgment, and sometimes overt criticism, begins to internalize the messages, creating deep body mistrust and shame. Potential sources of criticism could be from parents, doctors, siblings, coaches, social media, peers, or anyone else in a child's life who begins to comment on their body size or weight changes. External pressure: *Don't eat too much* begins to set in and leads to internal pressure, *I shouldn't eat too much*. **Judgment about their appearance from someone else is often when kids first start to notice that their body is more than just a body that helps them play and live. It's something other people judge and manipulate. Their appearance becomes a measure of how much love and respect they will receive from those around them, be it from their parents, siblings, or someone else.**

YOUR FEARS ABOUT YOUR CHILD'S WEIGHT
ARE FELT BY YOUR CHILD

How did it feel the first time you heard your child say something negative about their own body? Did your heart break? Did you think in shock, *Where did they learn to say that?* Did you want to yell, *There's nothing wrong with your body! Don't listen to anyone who tells you otherwise.* For some parents, this moment is our worst nightmare coming true. For others, it's a moment you expected all along. It's what you have come to view as normal.

Studies mirror the aforementioned pattern, indicating that it's a common experience. Parents who aren't concerned about their child's weight are less likely to exert parental control or pressure over eating, and parents who are more likely to apply pressure are the parents who are concerned about their child's weight being "too high." The result of this dynamic often seen in the research is that children who experienced more parental pressure to eat a certain way or were deprived of food are more likely to show signs of food avoidance (self-induced dieting) and are more likely to experience weight cycling later in life—a predictable and common outcome of repeated dieting. Your fears regarding your child's weight—which are reinforced by the status quo—are felt by your child and impact their relationship with food and their body.

WEIGHT CHANGES ARE COMPLEX

The truth is that no one food causes weight gain. Weight gain is a complex result of eating more, neurochemical signaling to build tissue and store fat, and is often hormonally initiated as a healthy part of growth and development or an adaptive response to inconsistent energy availability (dieting). It's only weight stigma and fatphobia that have labeled weight gain as an unquestionably bad thing. Kids may gain weight if they become disconnected from their natural hunger and satiety signals and eat food just because it's available or when attempting to disconnect from uncomfortable or painful experiences. This could result as a response to not having had access to enough food, or coping with stress, unmet needs, and other emotions. Kids also gain weight simply because that is the growth trajectory for their unique body according to their genetic blueprint, or a combination of all of the above. It's rarely clear if weight gain is happening because of "natural and genetically determined" reasons or if it's a side effect of eating in the absence of hunger, or both, among other possibilities. Whatever the reason, using control, shame, or dieting practices with kids will backfire and create an entirely new set of risks. Worst of all, they feel really bad about themselves. But they really feel bad about themselves because they are treated differently, feel like they may be disappointing you, feel unattractive, or feel the stress of being in a bigger body in a society that is extremely judgmental.

FOCUS ON WEIGHT TAKES KIDS FURTHER FROM HEALTH

No matter their actual weight, if kids and young adults perceive their weight to be too high, they are significantly more likely to:

- Skip breakfast
- Diet for weight control
- Have lower self-esteem
- Fast
- Vomit after meals
- Take laxatives
- Binge eat
- Eat in the absence of hunger
- Have high depressive symptoms
- Experience more weight gain over time as a result of dieting
- Gain more weight over time compared to peers who perceive their weight as healthy

Those who perceive their weight to be healthy, no matter what their weight is, are less likely to:

- Diet
- Overeat or binge eat
- Experience loss of control when eating
- Use risky weight control behaviors like diet pills, vomiting, and laxatives
- Experience depression

And they are more likely to:

- Maintain relatively stable growth and development, including predicted weight gain into adulthood
- Exercise
- Have higher self-esteem
- Have lower rates of disordered eating and eating disorders[14]

WHAT ABOUT BMI?

BMI is the most widely utilized way of "diagnosing" a person's weight status and, for many medical providers, is attached to a health status. However, the true history behind BMI may surprise you—it was never intended to be a way of measuring individual body fat or build, or as a way of assessing health.

Despite this history and the fact that it's been discussed for years that BMI isn't a useful measure, it's still commonly used in medical practice. It's even used as an official medical diagnosis, even though it was highly recommended by the American Medical Association's own research committee that it should not be used as such.[15] In fact, we're confident that if most medical doctors were fully informed about the history of BMI, it would not have risen to become such a significant measure used today. Unfortunately, we are stuck in a cycle of medical education now. All healthcare practitioners are taught the same things again and again about BMI—so the belief system continues.

WELL-BEING OVER WEIGHT

So, if we are suggesting that the status quo isn't the answer—what is? Well, what about **well-being**? We want to start to look at health from a holistic view. Let's look at the whole life experience.

WHAT IS WELL-BEING?

Well-being is the overall health of a person—including their state of mind. Everything from stress levels to mental health, physical health, socioeconomic status, and racial pressure contribute to well-being. We don't have control over everything that impacts our well-being. It's problematic that we've narrowed our cultural definition of health down to the body alone. But there is so much more to it. To start, having flexible definitions of health and well-being are key, because there are people—including those with chronic illnesses—who will never meet a generic definition of healthy. But every single person can have their own definition of what well-being and health means to them, and have goals in life that can optimize the joy they experience, the meaning and impact of their life, and recognize the things they do have control over and the things they don't.

BODY DISSATISFACTION:
A NORMALIZED FRIEND, BUT TRULY A FOE

It feels awful to live with constant thoughts of evaluating your appearance and body dissatisfaction. As awful as it feels, that inner critic becomes a constant companion, the friend that gives you "tough love." You might think, *Without my narrative of body dissatisfaction, how would I keep myself in check, get enough exercise, or limit sweets?* We are told we need to rely on our inner critic to control ourselves. If you suffer from it, body dissatisfaction can feel like a trusted friend (you may be thinking: Doesn't everyone feel negatively toward their body?), but truthfully, it's a harsh enemy, silencing your inner Intuitive Eater.

We mentioned how body dissatisfaction can quickly set in when a young person is exposed to peers who are body comparing, taught about ideal body size, weight, or shape, or when they are taught the myth that size equates to health status. The risks to your child's physical and mental health from body dissatisfaction go beyond tampering with their confidence or self-esteem and the potential for lifelong weight cycling. The effects can be even more far-reaching.

Body dissatisfaction—that evil inner foe—sadly predicts disordered eating and significantly increases your child's risk for becoming a smoker, self-harming, using drugs, and engaging in heavy drinking. A 2018 study out of Canada found that among teens, dieting at fourteen years old predicted smoking behaviors just two years later, and many studies have found that disordered eating predicts drug use. A 2019 study conducted on British adolescents found not only that dieting and body dissatisfaction predicted the presence of risky health behaviors in early adulthood, but also that every increased unit of body dissatisfaction (a measure used in this study) among female teens led to 41 percent increased odds of being a high-risk drinker by the age of twenty-one.[16] (This is adding evidence to a previous study showing a positive association between poor body image and binge drinking.[17])

So, what is it that we're seeing in all this research on kids and teens who diet and increasingly do not like their bodies? Self-care and self-respect go out the window.

How your child views, cares for, and respects their body has everything to do with their well-being for the rest of their life. Caring for and respecting your body doesn't have to be about maintaining any particular weight or BMI. In fact, we aren't referring to weight at all. Many parents attempt to help their child lose weight in a "healthy way," with intentions of just that: improved health. We believe parents do this because they truly believe it's a supportive, loving thing to do. This comes back to wanting to protect your child from pain, from being different, from being unhealthy. Most parents want to give their kids the world, and weight control is what we have been told is the most-needed solution. It's not. **Your child can be healthy and well in their natural body, and their size isn't an indicator of their health or happiness.**

What we are about to say is hard to believe (and hard to say), but it's true. **The medical system is inherently and systemically wrong about weight and health.** This isn't something that is widely known—because saying that our medical system and our doctors are wrong is frightening. We, as registered dietitians, were trained in the same medical system and learned the same fallacies. That is the systemic issue: there is a loop of teaching incoming healthcare students the same, problematic information. This is also the case with racism, misogyny, transphobia, and other systemic issues. Professors who know and deeply believe in a weight-equals-health paradigm teach new incoming students. *But the evidence that dieting predicts weight gain and disordered eating, and that weight loss isn't critical for improving health, is very strong.*

What we do see in the research to date is that attempting weight loss is highly likely to be harmful—it predicts weight cycling, and causes more health problems than it solves. If the entire healthcare system exists with these intrinsic flaws that originate in the messaging, how is everyone else supposed to believe us?

An important question that we can all ask is: How are "childhood obesity" initiatives working out? They aren't. Rates of eating disorders are climbing and kids aren't losing weight. A team member working to find a solution to "childhood obesity" with a coalition from Duke University, Wake Forest University, and others stated in a 2019 article, "Despite intense focus on reducing the U.S. childhood obesity epidemic over the past two decades, our progress remains unclear."[18] Even the researchers themselves aren't able to admit yet that intentional weight-control attempts not only don't create healthful weight loss, they contribute to increased weight and disordered eating. NBC News published an article in 2018 about childhood obesity. In it, the author notes that pushes to diet and public health initiatives aimed at "solving" the problem have been ineffective. If it's common knowledge that it's ineffective, why are we still attempting the same things?

It's not your fault for believing that you're responsible for your child's weight and therefore for their health. You're hearing this from all angles, including trusted people such as friends, family, and doctors. But this information is given like a medication you take without knowing the side effects, often without anyone being told the risks. That's why it's so easy to go through life never having heard this information before. But the side effects are real and they are impacting millions of children and adults today. The reality is that we have been avoiding the truth. People—parents—like us are appalled and just plain sad that this isn't common knowledge, that the status quo is still the status quo. If you read stories and books written by parents who have lived through the journey of eating disorder recovery alongside their child, you will hear one consistent thread over and over: *Never put your kid on a diet.*

We will start with Olivia's story (content warning for eating disorder behaviors):

OLIVIA'S STORY

Olivia describes her story as normal, yet traumatic. She developed values and interests in things like music, poetry, and reading, while she silently also developed an obsession with restricting calories, overexercising, binging and purging, and abusing laxatives. She did well in school and appeared fine, yet inside she was sick. Weight shaming and her developing eating disorder kept her isolated from forming meaningful, trusting friendships. Olivia is a woman of color, a spoken word poet, and a graduate of Brown University. Her early memories of school paint the picture of where her eating disorder first started. She learned about good and bad foods, avoiding sweets, the importance of working out, and how to cut calories. After-school sports taught her she could never exercise too much and she often felt what her body could do was compared with her much thinner peers. The words "eating disorder" were never mentioned, only "obesity epidemic," and she quickly learned to prioritize one goal: To not become fat.

"I felt like I was addicted to food from a young age because I thought about it so much, like there was something seriously wrong with me. I would look forward to any chance to be alone and finally eat, after long days of restricting and always trying to lose weight."

Olivia became hyperconscious of her body, and felt that every missed goal and less-than-perfect grade was a result of her weight. In middle school she tried to ignore what others said and hid her body with baggy clothes to protect herself from criticism and attention. She began to isolate herself even more, and her eating disorder felt like her only companion. As her eating disorder developed, it offered her some relief and hope that she could earn some attention by giving her a way to try to change her body so that others could finally appreciate her. She had internalized every anti-fat message over the years, all of which she felt were directed at her naturally larger body.

Olivia's body never should have been presented as a problem.

By high school, she had fully developed a life-threatening eating disorder, although stereotypes about who gets one successfully kept her illness off everyone's radar. In high school her peers were all restricting. Coaches often made inappropriate comments about their own diets and people's weight, and even shamed students for what they were eating. She was told, "You could be so pretty if you lost some weight."

Eating disorders aren't something you outgrow; they are ageless. Olivia's eating disorder flourished further in her college years, as her life continued to get smaller with a focus on perfectionism, pleasing others, getting stellar grades, and of course striving to find a way to make her body smaller.

When she finally hit rock bottom and wanted help, her parents had only been educated on the "obesity epidemic"; no one had ever told them this could happen to their "average weight, lower-middle class, honor roll student." They had never once encouraged her to diet. They had assumed eating disorders happen only to thin, rich white girls. They didn't know the warning signs. It can take years for families to pay off debts from treatment. Eating disorder treatment has taken over nearly a decade of Olivia's life. Sadly, she missed semesters of college and spent breaks from school in treatment centers.

An eating disorder isn't a modest hindrance, it can be deadly and debilitating, but most people will never receive treatment.

By educating parents, caregivers, schools and teachers, pediatricians, coaches, grandparents, and anyone and everyone who plays a role in raising kids about the value of fostering a healthy relationship with food and body, we will save lives and we will help prevent more kids from going down the same path of declining mental and physical health that Olivia did.

EATING DISORDERS ARE DEADLY

You might think, *An eating disorder? Oh, that would never happen to my child.* We often hear in our offices when meeting with parents: "My son/daughter has the 'opposite' problem of an eating disorder—if anything, they eat *too much*." Or: "My son is just really focused on his goal of being a champion wrestler, he doesn't have an eating disorder."

Eating disorders don't have a "look" or one set of symptoms, and often the kids who are judged as "eating too much" struggle just as deeply if not more so than those with typical signs of malnutrition from anorexia. The stereotypes about who gets eating disorders, what they actually are, and their signs create a lot of misinformation for parents. In fact, the majority of disordered eating cases aren't among people who are "underweight."

EXPERIENCES IN OUR BODIES ARE ABOUT MORE THAN SIZE

Disordered eating and body image distress aren't always about diet culture, weight, fatphobia, or appearance *explicitly*; they can develop out of the need to cope with living in a world that doesn't validate you, doesn't reflect your identity, or doesn't understand you. These experiences are traumatic, particularly when we are young.

(A person's identity is a combination of race, ethnicity, gender, culture, size, religion, sexuality, ability, age, socioeconomic status, spirituality, immigration status, and many more potential contributing factors.)

It's not a person's body that is the problem, it's the stigma that society places on certain bodies. It creates systemic limitations to the accessibility of Intuitive Eating. For example, being a woman, transgender or nonbinary, an immigrant, Black or Indigenous person of color (BIPOC), queer, disabled, fat or higher weight, non-Christian, a trauma survivor, food insecure, older, or a person with any other marginalized identity can disrupt positive embodiment. There is nuance in the privilege and marginalization that results from the intersections of these identities (intersectionality). Intersectionality is a political framework first introduced by professor and scholar Kimberlé Williams Crenshaw.[19] The importance of understanding intersectionality and its impact on embodiment cannot be overstated—it's *inseparable* from conversations around eating disorders, mental health, physical health, and body image.

People who identify as any of the above—or exist at the intersection of multiple different marginalized identities—are more likely to be harmed by the culture we live in *just by existing*. In our current social and cultural climate, not everyone is equally supported by society in having a healthy relationship with food and body, and some are outright oppressed. If we really want to focus on well-being, we cannot simply ask individuals to heal and make the changes needed—although that may help them. We need to be working on societal and systemic changes to reduce the oppressions that interrupt positive embodied experiences for all. This is why, in the words of Gloria Lucas, creator of Nalgona Positivity Pride, *eating disorders are a social justice issue*. **Choosing to take part in diet culture can be a place of safety for those who are living in marginalized bodies—this will continue to be a route to acceptability as long as our society is demanding conformity to privileged standards (white, thin, cis, straight, conventionally attractive, and so on).**

> *The way we imagine discrimination or disempowerment often is more complicated for people who are subjected to multiple forms of exclusion. The good news is that intersectionality provides us a way to see it.*
> —KIMBERLÉ WILLIAMS CRENSHAW

The identities your child holds, both independently and interactively, will inform the relationship they have with their body and the experiences they have in their body in relation to the world around them.[20] There is only preliminary research around eating disorders and how having multiple marginalized identities impacts a person's relationship with food and with their body—*but we know the impact is real and it's significant*.

As your child's greatest supporter, you may recognize concerning behaviors, such as restriction, purging, overexercise, or binge eating, that may be overlooked or missed by a medical provider.

EATING DISORDER STATISTICS—BIPOC
(BLACK, INDIGENOUS, PEOPLE OF COLOR)

- BIPOC are significantly less likely than white people to have been asked by a doctor about eating disorder symptoms.[21]
- BIPOC with eating disorders are half as likely to be diagnosed or to receive treatment.[22]
- Black people are less likely to be diagnosed with anorexia than white people but may experience the condition for a longer period of time.[23]
- Black teenagers are 50 percent more likely than white teenagers to exhibit bulimic behavior, such as binge eating and purging.[24]
- Hispanic people are significantly more likely to suffer from bulimia nervosa than their non-Hispanic peers.[25]

EATING DISORDER STATISTICS—LGBTQ+

- Gay men are seven times more likely to report binge eating and twelve times more likely to report purging than heterosexual men.[26]
- Gay and bisexual boys are significantly more likely to fast, vomit, or take laxatives or diet pills to control their weight.[27]
- Transgender college students report experiencing disordered eating at approximately four times the rate of their cisgender classmates.[28]
- Thirty-two percent of transgender people report using their eating disorder to modify their body without hormones.[29]
- Gender dysphoria and body dissatisfaction in transgender people is often cited as a key link to eating disorders.[30]

EATING DISORDER STATISTICS—NEURODIVERGENCE
AND DISABILITY

- Women with physical disabilities are more likely to develop eating disorders.[31]
- There are associations between autism, ADHD, and eating disorders among young people as well as adults.[32]
- More than 90 percent of developmentally disabled people experience sexual abuse in their lives, and there is a significant association between surviving sexual abuse and developing an eating disorder.[33]

- Disabled people are much more likely to experience medical trauma in their life, which is a risk factor for PTSD, disassociation, and avoidance. For this and other reasons, many disabled people have high levels of disconnection from their bodies.

YOUR CHILD, GENDER, and SEXUALITY

Feeling a need to conform to a new culture or fit into a community or peer group where you're different can be extremely isolating and stressful for a child, be it related to race, ethnicity, religion, ability, or any other identity. These are experiences that kids are often dealing with on their own, without having the words to share what they need from you, yet these are the very experiences that are too often disregarded by the adults around them. There also may be shame, confusion, fear, or uncertainty about the way they self-identify if it differs from the identity they may have had since birth, such as not identifying as a boy or a girl, but having lived a life with she/her or he/him pronouns.

In addition to race, immigration status, ability, body size, and other identities, one's identity can include their gender identity (their inner concept of what gender they are along a spectrum of male to female and a range of diverse gender identities in between), gender expression (their outward gender appearance characteristics), and sexuality.

Prevalence of body dissatisfaction and eating disorders are significantly higher among sexual and gender minorities (SGM). SGM is a term that encompasses, but isn't limited to, individuals who identify as lesbian, gay, bisexual, asexual, transgender, Two-Spirit, queer, and/or intersex.[34] In fact, one large study including more than 289,000 people with 479 transgender participants found 1.85 percent of cisgender heterosexual women and 0.55 percent of cisgender heterosexual male participants had been diagnosed with an eating disorder in the last year, while that number was 16 percent among trans participants.[35] Parents and family members may be important allies for a child or young adult who is trans, gender nonconforming, or gender questioning. Children in middle and late childhood, heading into adolescence, may become more aware of their gender identity, or may have increasing interest and agency in showing on the outside who they are on the inside. It's vital for parents and others around these young people to understand how we can best support and validate each individual child's identity as a critical and *essential* way to provide unconditional love and support for their body.

For most kids, their identity may have been acquired through *what they have been told about their identity*, the way their parents and their community view them. If your child sees their identity one way, yet others insist their identity is something else, or hold high expectations for them to be someone who they aren't, it can result in mental health disturbance (including eating disorders) and disconnection from relationships. One of the most critical things we can do for our kids is show them that we trust their body in every way—so *they* can trust their body in every way. We can't be selective about what we trust and what we don't. By loving and trusting them unconditionally, they have more space to experience the same connection with themselves. There are resources listed in the back of this book regarding how you can be your child's ally.

(We'll talk more about eating disorders in chapter 12. There, you'll find information on signs and symptoms as well as types of eating disorders. If you're reading this and you already think your child may have signs of an eating disorder, we encourage you to reach out to a Health at Every Size™–informed eating disorder specialist, either a doctor, therapist, psychologist, psychiatrist, or registered dietitian for assessment and help. At the back of this book, you will find a list of websites that can help you find a treatment provider.)

We can learn a lot from Olivia's story and the countless others like her who experience an eating disorder starting at a young age. Often, neither these kids nor their parents are given the support, acknowledgment, or access to treatment they need due to eating disorder stereotypes, weight stigma, and financial barriers. These kids internalize their behaviors, develop deep body shame and dissatisfaction, and self-blame rather than blaming the culture. Additionally, you—and parents everywhere—aren't given the tools to stand up to harmful policies or weight discrimination, or the skills to be aware of what is inappropriate and fear-based. Fear-based nutrition education is thinking that if we educate young kids better and earlier, we can scare them into doing everything they need to do to avoid becoming too fat. This education can start as young as preschool. Not only is it not developmentally appropriate education, it teaches kids to be afraid of the things that nourish them, often with very little parental consent. It's education like this that has been developed in response to fears about the "childhood obesity epidemic." In reality, not only are young kids not responsible for their food choices (their parents and caregivers are), this just begins the cycle of creating an unhealthy preoccupation with body size, weight, and stress about eating "healthy enough," which doesn't belong on the shoulders of a child.

As you read in Olivia's story, we know this kind of fear-based education is common, and it can be incredibly harmful. We must do better and we can do better to protect our kids.

THE AWARENESS GAP

You may be asking yourself why we are so concerned with eating disorders. It's a fair question. Our concern is caused by the *awareness gap*. Eating disorders are undertreated and underreported, and the impacts of these deadly illnesses are far-reaching, yet *very few people talk about them*. One of the most recent studies investigating the estimated lifetime prevalence of eating disorders found that **nearly one in seven male individuals and one in five female individuals will experience an eating disorder by the age of forty**.[36] This is a shocker to a lot of people. Statistically, everyone knows someone whose life has been dramatically altered by an eating disorder, yet rarely is it talked about as a big problem we need to be protecting our kids from. Why is that? As we learned from Olivia's story, the stereotypes of eating disorders make it much harder to notice eating disorders when they don't look like the expected thing—*the stereotype of a frail, skeletal female concerned mainly with appearance.*

Much of the research you will find on "childhood obesity" causes, factors, and interventions remains quantitative—researchers look at numbers and weight loss as the key result. Qualitative data—the *needs, values, perceptions, and experiences* of the children involved—gets much less attention. Meaning that what you will find is: X change in weight occurred over X weeks in the group that did XYZ intervention. Then they'll compare weight change results in the weight-loss intervention group to the non-weight-loss intervention group and say, "See, this group lost weight, therefore this intervention is recommended." Sounds okay, right? Well, the truth is that this style of research is missing the fact that humans aren't machines. These studies do not consider how weight-loss interventions actually impact the whole person beyond their relationship to gravity. Another problem you'll see is very little or only short-term follow-up (usually less than two years). Most importantly, what is missed by this kind of research on children is the ways in which said interventions may actually *create* harm, internalized diet mentality, shame, body dissatisfaction, and a disconnection from trusting one's inner experience of hunger and satiety. We know that dieting has these results. Children (like all of us) are whole humans, not just bodies to be judged and manipulated. If we want our kids to believe that we truly believe they are lovable, worthy, amazing humans regardless of their body size, we must stop the intense scrutiny and focus on body size and BMI. Instead, we need to start trying to understand what we can be doing to help them feel confident and empowered in their bodies.

How often have you read a headline that says something to the effect of: *"America's Kids Are Obese and It's Getting Worse: Junk Food, Lack of Exercise to Blame for Childhood Obesity"*? (Remember that NBC News article we mentioned earlier? This was the actual title.) Do you immediately start worrying about children's bodies? Your child's body? Have you ever thought about what it must be like to be a "subject" in one of these studies? Being reduced to your body size for the sake of science? And, in the mind of a child in a weight-loss trial, even if you understand that all this is for science, you aren't developmentally advanced enough to realize that it's not because you did something wrong. You just know that the adults (who you're supposed to trust) are so fixated on your size, rate of weight gain, every morsel of food you put in your mouth, every serving of leafy greens you consume, and every step you take daily to reach their ten-thousand-step goal on the fitness tracker they have attached to your arm twenty-four hours a day. The researchers—who are willing to feed you less than you actually need for growth and development, ignore what the likely long-term impact of that restriction is on your body, and never stop to understand your experience, or consider that there could *be nothing wrong with your body at all*—are doing this to you. How does this feel for a ten-year-old, twelve-year-old, or sixteen-year-old who is trying to find their way in a world that is actively trying very hard to figure out how to get rid of bodies just like theirs?

There are clinical studies taking place right now on kids and teens, using intentionally low-calorie diets and fasting—enacting restriction and harm—and despite petitions, letters, and public calls to halt these studies, they persist. Money and funding can control more than we realize, and money that comes from the diet and weight-loss industry is extra deadly.

Diet culture and diet mentality align with the Western sociocultural belief that thinner is better. This hurts *everyone*. One of the most harmful results of weight stigma is that bigger people often experience shame in their body throughout the course of their life, and smaller people often live in constant fear of gaining weight. Even when it's not explicit, these messages and fears still exist. You don't have to be on a diet to be unknowingly up to your ears in diet culture. You have to choose to opt out, and you can't do that unless you're aware of the ways in which it causes harm, trauma, and oppression to you and everybody else.

Not everyone has the ability to simply opt out. In fact, the closer your body is to the social ideal of "healthy," the more privilege you have, and the more choice and freedom you have to walk away from dieting. This is known as thin privilege. Thin privilege provides those who have bodies that are within what society considers a "normal" or "acceptable" size range with the freedom to not have to be constantly trying to lose weight, dieting or starving for approval or for ethical and fair medical care, or be continuously oppressed, bullied, and ostracized.[37] *Thin privilege doesn't mean that you have never experienced body dissatisfaction, fear of weight gain, health problems, or weight stigma. It's simply the experience of living in a world that was made for your body to fit into.*

It's important for you to be aware that your child—no matter their gender, weight, able-bodiedness, or if they are neurotypical—lives in a world that emphasizes worth, productivity, and value based on appearance. This elevation of appearance standards as something we all should be striving to achieve is making people more vulnerable to disordered eating, more likely to diet and weight cycle their way through life, and much more vulnerable to anxiety, body dissatisfaction, binge eating, loss of self-compassion, lowered self-esteem, and depression. In fact, the cultural belief that thinness is a major requirement for attractiveness is one of the primary reasons why even highly educated psychologists and medical professionals—who are absolutely capable of interpreting the same research we are sharing with you in this book—have a hard time letting go of the belief that healthy weight control and permanent weight loss is possible, when there isn't one credible long-term study showing it is.[38]

THE DIETING MIND

You don't need to define yourself as a dieter or be "dieting" to be tied up in diet mentality. We are defining dieting as any manipulation, elimination, or restriction of a food, food groups, or calories for the intent of weight loss or the prevention of weight gain, or for the purpose of "wellness." (There are valid medical concerns that require restriction of certain foods or eating in a certain way. These are often referred to as diets but aren't the type of diet we are referring to here. Dieting isn't the same as avoiding peanut butter if you have a nut allergy, or avoiding gluten if you have celiac disease.) Dieting is tied to weight bias and appearance, and isn't just about health. If it were just about health, we would not prescribe calorie restriction to someone with diabetes, knowing that the calorie restriction itself is likely to cause muscle loss, episodes of overeating, and increases in shame and guilt. Not to mention increased urges to binge eat, none of which are helpful for improving diabetes management. On the contrary, Intuitive Eating has been shown to improve health across many measures.

Dieting is a risk factor for negative psychological and behavioral health outcomes. It comes with a number of proven, predictable outcomes that are the same for most people regardless of body size. The extra harm that we can inadvertently cause kids with early exposure to dieting is *because they are sponges*. Up until about seven years old, kids are unconsciously absorbing everything they hear you say and see you do. The way they hear and see you treat your body, talk about your body, and talk about food greatly influences the patterns and core beliefs they will hold about their own body image and self-worth.

It's probably becoming pretty clear that dieting—or diet mentality—is a strong predictor of future disordered eating. But if it's still a little hazy, here are some of the evidence-based outcomes of dieting:

- Predicts weight cycling—gaining and losing weight repeatedly over time.[39]
- Increases "all-or-nothing" thinking about food.[40]
- Doesn't result in lasting weight loss for nine out of ten people. No study has shown that weight loss is sustainable in the long term; although some people do experience sustained weight loss, they are outliers.
- Worsens health and metabolism, which has a negative impact on bone development for young people, hormone disruption, and slowed digestion.[41]

In 2016, the American Academy of Pediatrics (AAP) recommended not talking about weight with young people, including kids and teens. That seems reasonable after everything you have just read. The AAP is using the same research we are, and they are making a recommendation to reduce the risk to a vulnerable population. They are doing this despite the diet culture we are constantly steeped in. In these recommendations, five family-based behaviors were identified as highly associated with eating disorders and weight fluctuations such as gaining and losing weight outside of a child's natural growth curve—also described as weight cycling. Of these behaviors, three are high risk and two are protective.

THE FIVE BEHAVIORS INCLUDED IN
THE AAP RECOMMENDATIONS[42]

Avoid these three behaviors in the home, as they are likely to increase risk of developing an eating disorder and weight cycling:

1. Dieting—defined as caloric restriction with the goal of weight loss.
2. Weight talk—defined as comments made by family members about their own weight or comments made to the child by parents to encourage weight loss.
3. Teasing about one's weight.

Emphasize these two protective behaviors against eating disorders and weight cycling:

4. Eating family meals together.
5. Cultivating positive body image.

We truly appreciate and want to highlight these recommendations from the AAP, but we are frustrated and repeatedly heartbroken at how frequently we sit down with yet another young person who was told by their pediatrician to lose weight. This criticism coming directly from a trusted source isn't a benign recommendation and isn't likely to lead to improved health, well-being, or a positive relationship with food and body.

It's quite possible that you don't talk about weight in your house at all—yours, your kids' weight, or anyone else's weight. If that is you, awesome! Keep that up.

Parents have a responsibility to provide their kids with foods that will help them thrive, and a routine helps make this possible. Parents also have the responsibility to help kids learn that their bodies are very wise, and equipped to help them know what, when, and how much to eat. This is a gift you will give your child that will benefit them throughout their entire life. It's also very understandable that some parents see teaching weight control as a gift, as they are "sparing their child" from the potential stigma, trauma, and harm that happens in our culture to people with bodies that are larger than the societal ideal. What we want you to know is that your intent to spare your child harm is loving, but the impact can be detrimental. If you experienced bullying or shame around your body size as a child, you may be doing this because you don't want your child to experience the same thing. We know you want the best for your kids. Your child can live a vibrant, meaningful life in their natural body size—it isn't your job to try to control it.

In order to identify what could be happening at home that is potentially problematic, here are some examples and behaviors that model diet mentality to kids even if you don't call it dieting and even if it's not openly talked about:

- Eating light meals or diet foods to save calories, while other family members eat higher-calorie foods.
- Having diet beverages or coffee in place of a meal or snack.
- Talking about other people's weight or bodies in a negative way.
- Hiding treats and fun foods from your kids, or sneaking them.
- Sighing with disappointment or disgust when you see your reflection or refusing pictures.
- Tracking calories burned, steps taken, or needing to burn calories to earn your food.

OUR CULTURE REWARDS THINNESS, BUT AT A COST

What is thin privilege? Thin privilege, or having a body that more closely aligns with the societal ideals of size, is something that most of us can identify, even if it feels difficult to name. It comes with a lot of advantages—privileges. The desire we have to manage body size in order to prevent bullying or to help our kids be happier and more successful is about wanting them to have thin privilege. These privileges for kids are probably familiar to you because they are pretty identical to the way thin privilege socially empowers adults: thinner kids are more likely to be accepted in certain social circles, more likely to be picked to play a game, have an easier time buying clothes, are viewed as productive by peers and teachers, and are less likely to be bullied for appearance. Further down the line as adults, thinner people are able to fit in public spaces comfortably, are not shamed by healthcare providers for not managing their weight, are more likely to go to college and have a higher-paying job, and so on.

Being thin, conventionally attractive, and white are three things that provide an enormous amount of social power and safety to people, and yet by far the majority of people do not meet these standards.

As much as people want to think that diet culture is about improving health, it's just not. Diet culture exists to sell you things: diet books, diet foods, pills, supplements, weight-loss plans, bariatric surgery, clothing, beauty products; we could go on and on. It is directly connected to the predictable outcome that the more you diet, the more you'll keep coming back, because *diets don't work*. Weight Watchers (now WW) would never have been as profitable if it "worked" in the long term. In our opinion, Weight Watchers' definition of "work" is more along the lines of "our plan will successfully lead you to believe you cannot trust your hunger and you cannot be trusted to eat freely without counting your points. You need to keep returning to the program to keep yourself in check, particularly when your natural body response to calorie deprivation will be to think about food more intensely, feel hungrier, and break your diet as often as possible." That doesn't sound like the outcome everyone is hoping for when they are starting a diet.

IT'S SO HARD TO SAY GOODBYE— BUT WHEN YOU'RE READY, YOU CAN DO IT

It's hard, *so hard*, to simply let go of diet mentality—don't expect yourself to do so right away. Remember, diet culture surrounds us. You've been conditioned to it likely since the day you were born.

Take some time and really let the above information settle. If it's the first time you're broaching some of this with yourself, go easy. There's no race to undo your diet mindset, and the more acceptance and self-compassion you have, the better.

Letting go of the idea that you need to control your child's weight and their eating, however, is worth the effort. When we perpetuate the idea and teach our kids that weight equals health, we are worsening their chances for long-term health and well-being, as well as interrupting their ability to eat intuitively. The focus on health has become so skewed to be about weight that we've lost sight of all the factors that contribute to health and well-being. Moreover, if you can model body respect, self-care, emotional attunement, and permission to eat, you can be a powerful force for supporting your child to develop a healthy relationship with food and body.

Get curious. Let's stop and ask a few questions:

If your child lives in a thin or "average"-size body, do you want them growing up to believe that if their body should change at some point and become larger than average they should drop everything and start focusing on weight loss or else they aren't as healthy, valuable, worthy, attractive, lovable, or respectable? Dropping a truth here: your child is very likely to experience weight-gain spurts and body changes throughout their whole life. If your answer is *My kid probably won't ever become bigger than average*, you may be quite wrong—and even if they never live in a larger body, don't we want to raise kids to respect others and body diversity? At the very least, is that a gamble that you're willing to take? We also acknowledge that kids of all sizes and weights struggle with body image, weight concerns, and appearance. That's what makes the 3 Keys important for *all* kids, not just higher-weight kids. We can help lessen the value of appearance overall, and focus on who they are, their gifts and imperfections, to support their confidence.

If your child lives in a larger-than-average body, do you want them to miss out on developing their natural talents or experiencing joy in their body because of its size? Would you want your child to believe that there is something wrong with their body and therefore they aren't allowed to eat as much as they're hungry for, enjoy the range of foods that their peers enjoy, or feel ashamed about how they look or what they want to eat?

Is controlling your child's food (and weight) worth the risk of diminishing or destroying your child's confidence and self-love for their natural body? Or worth the risk of developing an eating disorder?

We imagine that your instinctual responses to these questions are: *Of course not!* When confronted with the real costs and risks attached to believing all that diet culture teaches us, parents tend to realize we want to stand up to it, teach our kids resilience, body respect, and body kindness. The status quo can look less appealing when we are shown the real impacts that can alter a child's experiences for life.

These lessons apply to everyone. The cultural conditioning that begins so early means all of our kids are at risk for the negative effects of diet culture. Our kids need our protection and guidance. That's why it's so important to close the awareness gap between what parents currently are told about feeding kids and what they need to know to help promote physical and mental well-being in their growing child. Learning about and implementing Intuitive Eating in your life closes this gap and can protect your child in a world where we all have to work very hard to not fall prey to diet mentality.

When it comes to eating disorders, as with mental health in general, you cannot see the full picture by someone's outward appearance. Eating disorders, which occur along a spectrum of severity and symptoms, happen to people—including kids, teens, and adults—of all sizes. We hope knowing more about the prevalence and signs of disordered eating helps parents see how eating disorders can look a thousand different ways, can change and morph over time, and **aren't just a problem when your child is underweight.** Eating disorders are deadly, associated with a nearly twelvefold increase in risk for suicide,[43] and increase the potential for substance use and self-harm disorders. Eating disorders are very good at robbing someone of their joy, personality, authenticity, creativity, intimacy, and desire to live a full life. The more we can be aware of what eating disorders are, the more we can intervene early and protect our children from being robbed of their true selves and life potential.

Although there is a strong genetic component to one's risk for developing an eating disorder, dieting and diet mentality, weight stigma, and the way food and bodies are talked about—what is modeled to kids—has a substantial and lasting impact on them, even if they never develop an eating disorder. **Modeling is one of the primary and most effective ways of teaching kids their food values and about body appreciation.**

The spectrum of eating disorders is broad. On one end it starts with casual dieting, to occasional binge eating or restricting, all the way to a clinical eating disorder.

The belief that working on losing weight—or controlling one's weight—is good for your health is so normalized in our culture that it may even be surprising for you to learn that dieting alone is a major risk factor for developing an eating disorder. You might be thinking, *I diet and I don't have an eating disorder.* That may be true; not everyone who goes on a diet or who tries many different diets in their life will develop an eating disorder, but there's no escaping the truth that dieting has negative psychological and physical effects.

Dieting comes with a cost. Even if dieting is cloaked in *I'm just trying to be healthy, eat clean, or live a healthy lifestyle*, it has many sneaky ways of outwardly not looking like a diet. In fact, so many of the adults and adolescents that come to see us for help with their eating—whether they have general health or weight concerns, want to work on Intuitive Eating, or have disordered eating—are recurring dieters. Many of our clients have never been diagnosed with an eating disorder, but that doesn't mean they aren't suffering. Almost every person we see with an eating disorder has dieted at some point in their life.

So, ultimately, why should we be so concerned with dieting, diet talk, and focus on weight around our kids? **Dieting at its worst can be the first behavior in the development of an eating disorder, and at its best is simply not likely to work** for nine out of ten people who attempt it. Would you want a doctor to prescribe you a medication that has a 90 percent failure rate and comes with a host of serious risks? We wouldn't either.

If parents knew the short- and long-term effects dieting has on kids, we don't think they would continue to do it themselves, or even think of it for their kids. Or at least not nearly to the extent that many parents are currently actively dieting and conditioned by diet culture.

Over the last few decades, research has consistently demonstrated that young children are aware of their parents' dieting behavior as well as the societal thin ideal for females and the muscular ideal for males. By the age of four, they can begin to understand that if you talk about eating certain foods as "healthy" it is connected to the goal of "thinner." So it's not just dieting for weight loss that can have risks; it's the extent to which our culture has become overly obsessed with "healthy eating," which has become synonymous for many people with "weight management." "Healthy eating" and "weight management" aren't the same thing. How so? Well, our bodies are designed to manage our weight without us consciously having to intervene or count calories, through a complex system of hunger and satiety hormones, neurochemicals, and metabolic processes. Trying to control your weight or lose weight is more likely to result in weight gain. Yes, weight can shift either up or down as a result of moving away from disordered eating, eating for reasons other than hunger, or stopping the diet-binge cycle, but this is different from directly dieting with the intention of weight loss.

That being said, healthful, nutritious eating is something that should be accessible and an option for anyone who wants it no matter their size—unattached to the outcome of weight loss. Sadly, the reality is that healthful eating and weight management have become synonymous because of a diet culture that views only thinner bodies as healthy bodies. Big-name diet companies are changing their names to get away from weight loss as the primary goal, but are still about restricting calories to inadequate amounts. The "health goals" that other companies or plans promise are thinly veiled weight-loss goals. The "healthy," "happy," "better you" messages are almost always related to weight loss. "Diet" has become a four-letter word, and even the diet companies are trying to distance themselves from it. But if it looks like a duck and quacks like a duck, well . . .

That duck is still a diet.

Although eating disorders aren't the focus of this book, and this isn't a treatment approach for eating disorders, the huge awareness gap about eating disorders is real for many parents. Knowing the signs and symptoms of eating disorders and the risks we undertake when we engage in a diet are necessary. Understanding more about eating disorders helps the message that Intuitive Eating is *protective against eating disorders* click into place. **If you can reduce your child's risk for developing disordered eating and negative body image, you're going to also have a huge impact on their physical health, growth and development, social anxiety, confidence, risk for depressive symptoms, and general well-being.** The "why" of raising Intuitive Eaters for you is important and can help you fight the status quo when it's all around you. We can't give you your "why." But we can give you the chance to make an informed choice.

SUMMARIZE AND REFLECT

You've now read about the status quo and the ways control, restraint, rewarding, and dieting are harmful. These are the evidence-based reasons why we need to say no to the status quo. Control, which includes pressuring, restricting food, and rewarding or punishing with food, and dieting (both cultural and parental dieting behaviors) are common, encouraged, and even considered normal in our current social climate and in what parents are often instructed to do. Intuitive Eating is the next best step when we are ready to ditch diet mentality in our homes. We want our family members, every single one of them from all backgrounds and cultures, to grow up to become adults who are making a difference in the world. To raise these difference-makers, who are confident, capable, and compassionate, we need them to love their bodies and themselves. **We all need to be more powerful than diet culture.**

We want to leave you some things to think about. Ask yourself these questions and reflect on your answers and how you feel. Many of the chapters have these reflective questions to help you integrate this information for yourself and your family. They are *big* questions. There are no right or wrong answers.

- *Are you firm and rigid with your child's eating? How about your own eating?*
- *How often do you treat (reward) your child with food for good behavior?*
- *Do you threaten no dessert (negative pressure) if a meal isn't eaten to your approval?*

How are you feeling? Are any of the things mentioned above standing out as things you say or do? Are you scared you've permanently altered your child's relationship with food to a state of unrepair? If so, that might sting; but let's try to move forward. Notice what you're learning, and then act based on what you now know. This is where that compassion gets to come back. We know you've only been doing what you have thought of as harmless and healthy, even proactive. You're not alone, and if damage has been done, guess what—Intuitive Eating can help you repair it. You're not a bad parent. It's just a great time to recognize how your child may be interpreting some of what they observe you doing.

Personal Reflection Questions

- *In what ways have you been held back by the thin ideal, or by dieting?*
- *How does it feel for you to imagine your child believing that they too have to achieve thinness or a certain body type in order to be happy?*
- *What if your child's body isn't genetically designed for the body you think they should have? Do they deserve happiness in their natural body?*

If you're questioning what you're reading . . .

It would not be surprising if the thought you continue to have is *But I want my kids to be happy—and how can you be happy if you're fat?*

Deep down, we all know that happiness isn't about being a certain size or looking a certain way. Feeling well, being strong, having energy, and inherently knowing that you're treating your body kindly are all things we understand to contribute to happiness. Those things aren't directly tied to a body size. You and your child's happiness depend on life experiences, quality of relationships, fulfilling one's desires, reaching accomplishments, having a sense of purpose, and so much more. There are many people who have "normal" BMIs and aren't happy or healthy, and there are thin people who are depressed or ill and higher-weight people who are living their best life.

Happiness isn't something that gets assigned to a person when they are a certain size. There is a very strong belief that thinness will bring a person happiness, but this thinking is flawed. We don't want to ignore the truth, that those who are thinner face less oppression, less marginalization—but that doesn't equal happiness.

THE PATH FORWARD

Diet culture and its influence are daunting to think about. It might feel impossible to overcome. Or it might feel like the only alternative to rules and restrictions is chaos and carelessness with food. Luckily, there is another way. A way that isn't actually chaos, even if it can feel scary and exceptionally difficult at times. Learning how to raise an Intuitive Eater offers that alternative. We can help lead you in the right direction. The choices are still yours to make. And the wisdom is still yours to gain. Yours and your child's.

Intuitive Eating isn't our concept. It's not a new idea or one that is exclusive to this book. You may even have decided to read this book because you know exactly what Intuitive Eating is. Intuitive Eating has been around for decades; it was pioneered by two registered dietitians who noticed that their clients' attempts at dieting—even the gentlest lifestyle changes among them—continued to lead to failure, shame, embarrassment, guilt, and more dieting. And often, more weight gain. *Intuitive Eating* was recently published in its fourth edition and has been released in more than twelve languages in many countries. In fact, both of us are certified Intuitive Eating counselors and have studied directly with those original pioneers, Elyse Resch and Evelyn Tribole. Intuitive Eating has been studied, researched, and published about more than 130 times. This research continues to show us that not only can Intuitive Eating be healthy and safe, it can be incredibly protective against eating disorders and disordered eating—and many other health conditions that we often associate with poor nutrition or high BMI. **Intuitive Eating can be healing.**

Even in mainstream nutrition advice, we've heard more and more about how diets don't work. However, because diet culture has such a deep stranglehold on our ability to coexist with food and to have a pleasant relationship with our bodies, we often don't see the research that shows just how bad dieting can be or how helpful Intuitive Eating can be.

THE HAZZARD STUDY

The Hazzard study has some of the most profound results showing the protective benefits of Intuitive Eating. This study alone is worth its weight in gold, and we could've written a book with just this as the evidence.[1]

The study examined a large community sample of adolescents over a span of eight years, from 2010 to 2018. The researchers analyzed data from 1,491 students over twenty public middle and high schools in and around the Minneapolis–St. Paul metropolitan area. The data included eating behaviors, physical activity, weight status, and also analyzed factors related to socioeconomic status (something many studies overlook). The researchers also included a diverse mix of races, genders, and ethnic backgrounds. The results they measured were relevant to Intuitive Eating in three important areas—Intuitive Eating measures, psychological health outcomes (like depression symptoms, self-esteem, and body dissatisfaction), and disordered eating behaviors.

The data they gathered and how they conducted the study are important, but the results are even more important. They learned that teens reporting higher Intuitive Eating scores to begin with, *and/or* those who showed improvement in Intuitive Eating scores over the eight-year span of the study were associated with lower odds of having high depressive symptoms, low self-esteem, and high body dissatisfaction. The kids who were Intuitive Eaters and those who improved their IE scores over the period of the study were less likely to engage in unhealthy weight-control behaviors, extreme weight-control behaviors, and binge eating. Basically, the kids who either started out as Intuitive Eaters or learned more Intuitive

Eating habits over the course of the study were less depressed, had higher self-esteem, and were happier with their body image *and* were less likely to use extreme behaviors to manage their weight and were less likely to binge eat.

The strongest protective association was for binge eating. Improving their IE score just 1 point from baseline over the period of the study was associated with *71 percent lower odds of binge eating at follow-up*. That even a small increase in IE behaviors led to such a significant decrease in binge eating should be huge news! Binge eating is something that we often fear as an outcome of letting go of dieting, but studies such as this one show that it's the opposite—a side effect of dieting.

Most weight-loss or diet studies take place over the course of two years and tend to be pretty small samples—so the length and diversity included in this study makes it particularly powerful.

THE STUDY FROM LIPSON AND SONNEVILLE

Lipson and Sonneville's study was published in 2017 and conducted on nearly 10,000 college students across twelve campuses. They found high (what we believe to be alarmingly high) rates of disordered eating among this age group: 49 percent of students identifying as female and 30 percent of students identifying as male (within the previous four weeks) reported binge eating and compensatory behaviors such as vomiting (30 percent female, 29 percent male). By the time kids who are raised in a society that places BMI as a primary indicator of health reach college, they have a very high chance of developing disordered eating.

The study found that students on the higher end of the weight spectrum are more likely than lower-weight students to have symptoms of disordered eating, including binge eating and dangerous weight-control behaviors. This was not found exclusively among female-identifying students; researchers found no difference between genders when it came to compensatory behaviors—including vomiting as a means of controlling weight, abusing laxatives or diuretics (aka water pills), taking diet pills, and using exercise to "burn off calories" in a driven or compulsive way. They also found that the risks for disordered eating are also present for students across racial and ethnic identities. Higher weight was shown as the most consistent predictor of eating disorder symptoms, underscoring the importance of not treating "obesity" as a problem of overeating and physical inactivity, and that being "underweight" isn't the most prevalent indicator of an eating disorder.[2] The misperception that we should "treat" people with higher weights for "obesity" distracts us from the very real risk of those same people developing life-threatening eating disorders. This is weight stigma.

Our kids are facing more pressure than ever to achieve ideal body and appearance standards, and this cannot be separated from the pressures that have been placed on parents to manage or control their child's weight. *If we can start to create a lifestyle and mindset that can reduce the risk of disordered behavior as much as Intuitive Eating can, most parents would jump right in.* Dieting, including in childhood and adolescence, doesn't predict weight loss—but it does predict disordered eating. Dieting behavior can so closely mirror disordered behavior that it can be hard to tell the difference.

Even though there is a chapter in *Intuitive Eating* by Resch and Tribole about raising Intuitive Eaters, it's only one piece of what we are discussing here. We need so much more than a chapter to really develop the skills we need as parents to continue this work for our families. As you learned, part of Intuitive Eating is to use the logical and reasonable part of our human brain (our thought process), *to use our thinking skills*, to decide what to eat and when to eat based on what is available. Kids really need their caregiver to do that thinking part of the process for them, to set them up to be able to rely on their natural hunger and fullness sensations to eat the amount they need of what is provided. Parents have responsibilities as caregivers to feed little people. So, we knew we needed an entire book and an entirely different framework dedicated to the struggles, confusion, myths, stereotypes, and problems parents face when it comes to feeding children. Many of us parents come to raising our kids and feeding our kids with something called *generational dieting*. Generational dieting is the idea that we have been impacted by the way our parents, our grandparents, and so on have been impacted by dieting and food issues.

> The 3 Keys model and *How to Raise an Intuitive Eater* were created to help you understand two things: (1) what your child needs from you to remain or return to being an Intuitive Eater, and (2) how you can overcome the confusion and diet culture messages you may have internalized throughout your life that impact the way you feed yourself (what you model) and the way you make feeding decisions as a parent.

This model is intentionally a guide for you, not a set of rules. You can take in the guidance, and then you make your own decisions about what works best for your family. But we can help you see what the status quo is and teach you how to remove yourself from that way of thinking. We can help to break the pattern of generational dieting. The 3 Keys, which we mentioned in chapter 1, are an adaptation of Intuitive Eating combined with evidence-based recommendations specifically for feeding kids to promote a healthy relationship with food and body in the long term. So many parents love the concept of helping their child have a healthy relationship with food and body *and* are very confused, frustrated, and even scared when it comes to knowing how to feed their kids. This pattern of confusion you may have about your child's eating results from a conflict between what you know in your heart, that a healthy relationship with food and body is really important, and what you hear all around you: *Prevent childhood obesity, Avoid processed food,* and *Make sure your kids eat their vegetables or there'll be no dessert!* It's normal—but incredibly confusing—to hear these mixed signals.

It's not enough just to not diet, or to not talk about your weight in front of your child; you have to intentionally be pro–Intuitive Eating for yourself and for your children.

INTUITIVE EATING BENEFITS FAR OUTWEIGH THE ILLUSION OF WHAT DIETING CAN GIVE US

What we now know, after decades of reliable science, is that people don't fail at diets—diets fail us. The chances of a diet working—defined as resulting in weight loss that is sustainable for the long term—are quite slim. About 0.02 percent—which statistically speaking is a success rate similar to the chances of someone "studying Powerball winners to see how to become a multi-millionaire and then, armed with that information, quitting your job to play Powerball full time and winning the lottery."[3] In fact, there is very poor-quality scientific evidence that any intervention for intentional weight loss has been proven effective for longer than two to five years.[4]

Intuitive Eating was born out of the need for people to find a way to move forward with life unburdened by the constant drive to diet and lose weight. Tribole and Resch wanted their clients to have a dedicated way of relearning how to eat with peace and permission, and to ultimately rediscover the joy and pleasure of eating while enhancing their well-being and health.

Here is an overview of the ten principles of Intuitive Eating. This list might be worth highlighting, saving, or even copying and sticking on the fridge. It can be helpful to have reminders within arm's reach. Without further ado:

1. Reject the diet mentality.

Throw out the diet books and magazine articles that offer you the false hope of losing weight quickly, easily, and permanently. Get angry at diet culture that promotes weight loss and the lies that have led you to feel as if you were a failure every time a new diet stopped working and you gained back all of the weight. If you allow even one small hope to linger that a new and better diet or food plan might be lurking around the corner, it will prevent you from being free to rediscover Intuitive Eating.

2. Honor your hunger.

Keep your body biologically fed with adequate energy and carbohydrates. Otherwise you can trigger a primal drive to overeat. Once you reach the moment of excessive hunger, all intentions of moderate, conscious eating are fleeting and irrelevant. Learning to honor this first biological signal sets the stage for rebuilding trust in yourself and in food.

3. Make peace with food.

Call a truce; stop the food fight! Give yourself unconditional permission to eat. If you tell yourself that you can't or shouldn't have a particular food, it can lead to intense feelings of deprivation that build into uncontrollable cravings and, often, bingeing. When you finally "give in" to your forbidden foods, eating will be experienced with such intensity it usually results in Last Supper overeating and overwhelming guilt.

4. Challenge the food police.

Scream a loud *no* to thoughts in your head that declare you're "good" for eating minimal calories or "bad" because you ate a piece of chocolate cake. The food police monitor the unreasonable rules that diet culture has created. The police station is housed deep in your psyche, and its loudspeaker shouts negative barbs, hopeless phrases, and guilt-provoking indictments. Chasing the food police away is a critical step in returning to Intuitive Eating.

5. Discover the satisfaction factor.

The Japanese have the wisdom to keep pleasure as one of their goals of healthy living. In our compulsion to comply with diet culture, we often overlook one of the most basic gifts of existence—the pleasure and satisfaction that can be found in the eating experience. When you eat what you really want, in an environment that is inviting, the pleasure you derive will be a powerful force in helping you feel satisfied and content.

6. Feel your fullness.

In order to honor your fullness, you need to trust that you will give yourself the foods that you desire. Listen for the body signals that tell you that you're no longer hungry. Observe the signs that show that you're comfortably full. Pause in the middle of eating and ask yourself how the food tastes, and what your current hunger level is.

7. Cope with your emotions with kindness.

First, recognize that food restriction, both physically and mentally, can, in and of itself, trigger loss of control, which can feel like emotional eating. Find kind ways to comfort, nurture, distract, and resolve your issues. Anxiety, loneliness, boredom, and anger are emotions we all experience throughout life. Each has its own trigger, and each has its own appeasement. Food won't fix any of these feelings. It may comfort for the short term, distract from the pain, or even numb you. But food won't solve the problem. If anything, eating for an emotional hunger may only make you feel worse in the long run. You'll ultimately have to deal with the source of the emotion.

8. Respect your body.

Accept your genetic blueprint. Just as a person with a shoe size of eight would not expect to realistically squeeze into a size six, it's equally futile (and uncomfortable) to have a similar expectation about body size. But mostly, respect your body so you can feel better about who you are. It's hard to reject the diet mentality if you're unrealistic and overly critical of your body size or shape. All bodies deserve dignity.

9. Movement—feel the difference.

Forget militant exercise. Just get active and feel the difference. Shift your focus to how it feels to move your body, rather than the calorie-burning effect of exercise. If you focus on how you feel from working out, such as energized, it can make the difference between rolling out of bed for a brisk morning walk or hitting the snooze alarm.

10. Honor your health—gentle nutrition.

Make food choices that honor your health and taste buds while making you feel good. Remember that you don't have to eat perfectly to be healthy. You will not suddenly get a nutrient deficiency or become unhealthy, from one snack, one meal, or one day of eating. It's what you eat consistently over time that matters. Progress, not perfection, is what counts.

(From *Intuitive Eating*, 4th edition, 2020)[5]

Intuitive Eating will not look the same for everyone; in fact, it isn't at all about food recommendations for each individual. Remember, the goal of Intuitive Eating is about establishing and supporting a healthy relationship with food and body, no matter what a person needs to eat, chooses to eat, or wants to eat.

We've taken these ten principles of Intuitive Eating, as well as its goal of equality and body acceptance, and have added a focus on embodiment, along with mixing in well-researched concepts around the child's mind and parenting.

ALL KIDS AREN'T BUILT THE SAME

Some children have needs that aren't addressed by Intuitive Eating. This is expected, as we acknowledge the vast diversity among us. There isn't one approach to feeding kids that will meet every family's needs. Although we'd love to be able to provide a catch-all how-to guide for every parent's feeding questions, we can't, and we don't pretend to be the experts on every child. For some children, it may seem challenging or impossible to let hunger signals guide their eating. Here, Intuitive Eating principles will still be useful in some ways, such as in reducing the influence of "good" and "bad" thinking with foods, allowing all well-tolerated foods as part of the feeding routine, and focusing on eating foods that are enjoyable and that promote energy, growth, and development. Still, being an Intuitive Eater will not look the same for everyone, and there's nothing wrong with that. Some kids need to rely on external cues like the clock to know when to eat. In fact, most kids are distracted easily by the world around them and are often unaware of early hunger signs, just as some adults who have been dieting for a lifetime can be unattuned to their hunger cues. Part of the 3 Keys is that the caregiver implements a feeding routine and a schedule to set the child up for eating consistently and adequately throughout the day. **Kids need the safety and structure established by their caregiver. Intuitive Eating for kids doesn't mean meals and snacks are dictated by the child's hunger alone.**

WHAT IS A POSITIVE RELATIONSHIP
WITH FOOD AND BODY?

The truth is, everyone's definition of this will be different. How do we put words to something so personal, abstract, and complex? Practically every person you meet will have a different definition. (It's important to note that we will sometimes use the word "healthy" instead of "positive" when we talk about this relationship. But healthy isn't a word that everyone identifies with as their goal, and the same goes for the word positive. As you read this you'll see both words used interchangeably.)

We've already mentioned "positive relationship with food and body" a couple times by now, so let's talk more about what that can be. What if the basics start with changing the way we associate with our body? Instead of something to overcome, to improve upon, and to exist in spite of, what if our body is something that we can learn to be grateful for, something that deserves innate respect just because it exists, and is a worthy part of us all the time? What if food were no longer something we are only supposed to derive energy from? What if we did get to find pleasure and joy in food, while getting enough of it *all of the time*? Those questions might seem impossible, or distant. They might not be present for you now, but what if they could be? What if that's the relationship with food and body that your child gets to develop for themselves?

BENEFITS OF RESPECTING YOUR BODY
OVER TRYING TO CHANGE IT

If you're feeling unsure as to the benefits of pursuing this state of mind and body, let's talk about some of them. We feel these are truly benefits parents will get behind, and yet you may not have ever realized the connection that exists with food, body, eating, and empowerment and resilience.

When a person cares about their own body, and respects their body, they are more likely to be assertive and resilient in the face of difficulty, including gender-, ethnicity-, sexuality-, and race-based discrimination. They are less likely to believe they are bad or unlovable based on appearance, and more likely to have healthy and empowering relationships not just with their own internal self, but with others. There are also physical benefits to having a positive relationship with your body, including the freedom to move and be physically active in ways that are enjoyable (for reasons that don't include changing your body). You can develop a deeper sense of body respect, which in turn leads to being more likely to assert agency and protection against unwanted sexual attention or any physical violation such as sexual coercion or rape (we acknowledge that these are not within anyone's full control), or saying no to drugs, alcohol, and other substances under peer pressure. You're also better able to engage in self-care that stems from fulfilling needs and desires, like being in tune with what your body needs in terms of rest, comfort, healthcare, and movement. When we are less tied up in body dissatisfaction and comparison, we are so much more capable of tuning in to the needs and desires our body has around food. And finally, when we have a positive relationship with our own body, we are less likely to engage in a lifetime of yo-yo dieting—which isn't good for our health.[6]

Can you imagine how different your life would be had you been raised and supported to believe that you deserve to love yourself unconditionally? This all-important concept is known as *radical self-love* and is fundamental in forming a trusting relationship with our own bodies, and therefore food. This might feel like an extreme concept, and might not always feel possible. Radical self-love is about the respect that your body is always worthy of, and the food and kindness your body is always worthy of—regardless of its state. Radical self-love, a term coined by Sonya Renee Taylor, author of *The Body Is Not an Apology*,[7] is the most powerful instrument we have to break down diet culture's power over us. Taylor—who is a renowned poet, activist, artist, and thought leader—brings to light through her writing and activism that only through stripping away the pressure to conform and self-silence (what diet culture tells us to do) can we engage with our full potential, power, and liberation to help ourselves and others. Consider what it would mean for your child's future self to help empower them with the superpower of radical self-love. Radical self-love might be a future state that you move toward as you and your family establish positive relationships with your food and your bodies.

Helping you and your family move toward a more embodied, positive way of living (including how you relate with food) is one of the primary goals of this book. Embodiment is another concept that isn't new; it was fostered by Dr. Niva Piran. It's a framework that encourages us to look beyond perfectionism, and to being our authentic selves—regardless of the societal expectations that have been placed on us. Through working toward embodiment, we develop the opportunity to develop all those benefits we listed a couple paragraphs back.

There is no perfect relationship with food and body. As humans, we are living imperfect and uncertain lives; therefore, something so key to our human experiences as our relationship with food simply can't be perfect either. Part of being human is learning to accept difficult or painful experiences and to live a life that includes various pleasant and unpleasant things. When it comes to feeding our kids, part of the pressure put on us as parents is to "perfectly" feed them. We are told to do this in order to ensure they are healthy now and in the future. This is the part of the illusion that our diet-centric culture has created. But perfectionism is unnecessary; in fact, it's hurting us! Perfectionism doesn't let us be human.

The Intuitive Food and Body Relationship Model provides a way to explain how the elements of food and body interact, creating our relationship with our body. Each piece is one aspect of the whole relationship, and they all interact together (along with aspects of life that aren't included—like spiritual practice) to bring us closer to or farther away from an embodied relationship with food and body. This model may be just a starting point for you, and it can be an incredible tool for the work ahead.

A RELATIONSHIP WITH FOOD AND BODY ISN'T ONE AND DONE—IT EBBS, FLOWS, AND FLEXES

Because these pieces are all intertwined, when one element changes, the others may flex. As a result, our relationship to food and body might feel more positive or more negative on any given day. It can be easy to feel like we are supposed to be positive or we've failed, but this is called all-or-nothing thinking, and it's a mindset that needs to be challenged. It's a form of perfectionism. The relationship with food and body isn't something that is described as "good" or "bad," and it certainly can't be perfect. Rather, your relationship with your body fluctuates across a spectrum, landing in various places depending on what is happening, the state of your body, and so on. It can move to a more positive place or a more negative place depending on the elements of the Intuitive Food and Body Relationship Model. It's likely to be forever evolving as we learn new ways of being in the world, and as our bodies change in different phases of life. Many people can relate to having a "bad body image day" or a period of time when it feels exceedingly hard to have compassion or appreciation for your body. For many people, these difficult feelings may describe most days for as long as they can remember. This is a common experience, something that makes us human in a society that is constantly telling us we're not good enough (thanks, capitalism, white supremacy, and patriarchy!). By practicing acknowledgment of the different interactions and how they are impacting you on a day-to-day basis, you can provide yourself with the support you really need to get through those times.

> Having a positive relationship with food and body doesn't mean you always feel amazing. It means you have access to some guiding behaviors, practices, and beliefs that minimize harm, reduce the time you spend feeling negatively toward or in your body, and optimize the way you take care of yourself to live a life that is more liberated and creates an overall greater sense of well-being.

THE INTUITIVE FOOD AND BODY RELATIONSHIP MODEL

Relationships with food and body are complex. Each positive element plays a role in your relationship with your body and has an opposing element. More experiences with the positive elements will result in a more positive relationship overall, while experiencing or practicing more opposing elements will feel less positive and result in reduced overall well-being.

> Notice how the more privileges a person has, the fewer barriers they are likely to face that will get in the way of experiencing the positive elements.

> Elements of an intuitive relationship with food and body:
> - **Comfort:** opposed by stress
> - **Permission:** opposed by restraint
> - **Trust:** opposed by mistrust
> - **Flexibility:** opposed by rigidity
> - **Satisfaction:** opposed by deprivation
> - **Connection:** opposed by disconnection

One important thing to note (and we will note it again and again) is that a positive or healthy relationship with food and body isn't just the absence of a negative or disordered relationship; that is just a neutral relationship. We need to go above and beyond for our kids to foster a positive relationship because they are living in a world that is constantly working to disconnect them from their body and profits off devaluing it. A positive relationship with food and body also doesn't

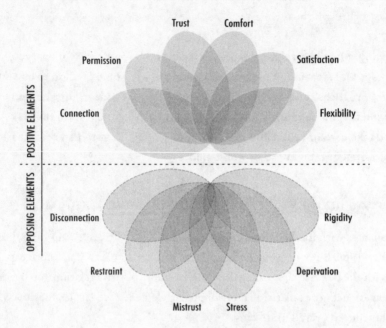

Trust   Comfort

Permission   Satisfaction

POSITIVE ELEMENTS

Connection   Flexibility

OPPOSING ELEMENTS

Disconnection   Rigidity

Restraint   Deprivation

Mistrust   Stress

have anything to do with what your body looks like, its ability to perform work, function, or its size or shape.

Positive embodiment isn't something that everyone will consciously desire to have or will be capable of achieving. This can be caused by many things, including—not least among them—trauma. Additionally, not everyone will attain a sense of comfort in their body—they may never feel safe as a result of their lived experience, even after dismantling diet mentality and weight stigma. Trusting one's body is also not going to be equally accessible for everyone. We recommend you don't view these positive elements as individual choices, but rather points for understanding how you or your child may be experiencing their body. Just because we know that lowering our stress will likely result in increased comfort, it doesn't mean that it will be simple—or even possible—to do.

MODIFYING THE FRAMEWORK SO IT FITS FOR YOU

It's important to make this information relevant to you as an individual. A person who has experienced trauma, which manifests in the body physically (as trauma so often does), may not want to include comfort, or trust, or connection in the definition of their relationship with their body. It's possible for some—through the process of healing, gaining trusted support from others, and with time—to be able to access more or all of the elements, should they wish to do so. No person is by any means expected to define their relationship with their own body in this way. We encourage you to use this framework as a stepping-stone to what works for you.

Interestingly, so much of what we think of when we typically talk about health is an outward image of what a body looks like or how well it works. (*I can run a mile!* Or: *I lost 5 percent of my body weight! I fit into my high school jeans!*) Neither the way you look nor your body's ability to function define your health, nor are they necessary to build a healthy relationship with food and body. A person doesn't need to change their body size, achieve a certain function, or lose weight in order to tune in to these elements.

The 6 elements of the Intuitive Food and Body Relationship Model

- **Comfort:** This is the sense of comfort you feel in your current body. It's not about always feeling "comfortable" the way we might expect, but rather it's about being able to identify that your body isn't "bad" for feeling discomfort. Knowing that despite physical discomfort, your body still offers you comfort in the way that it's *home*—a place that deserves care, respect, pleasure, and compassion. **Your body deserves to seek and receive comfort, comforting care, and this never ends.** Comfort incorporates the belief that you deserve to take care of yourself, more than the actual comfort you attain. *Often, people who experience negativity about their body don't identify as feeling worthy of comfort or rest or that they deserve to feel comfortable.* Much of this stems from a lifetime of being told that their body isn't good enough. When you hear this over time, you internalize this oppressive messaging, and believe it.

- **Comfort's opposite, stress:** Stress is a response that manifests in many different ways, but it can come from facing stigma and oppression through those harmful messages. Stress can be emotional, psychological, and physical. It's due to constantly feeling like you have to "fix" your unworthy body. Stress can also be a direct result of the attempts you make to change your body, such as the stress of dieting, restricting, overexercising, and so on. It can also be experienced due to circumstances outside your control. Things that can contribute to stress can be marginalization, abuse, violence, and many other things. On the other hand, believing that you—in your current body, no matter what—*do* deserve to seek comfort, pleasure, joy, and peace in your body is a measure of your relationship with yourself. For many people, additional healing is needed to bring them back to believing the truth they were born knowing: that they're deserving and worthy of feeling and seeking comfort, if they want it.

■ **Permission:** Having unconditional permission to eat is a main pillar of Intuitive Eating. Permission is about allowing yourself (or your child) to have food for all the different reasons you may need or want it. Including: permission to eat because you're hungry, because you want something, or for pleasure or comfort. Permission is the truth that you're allowed to eat what you want and need, to experience pleasure with food, and you inherently are worthy of eating all foods. Permission is a launchpad for being able to eat with awareness and in a way that feels good for your body. Permission extends beyond food and eating, too, to include permission to rest, to say no and have healthy boundaries, and to take care of your needs.

■ **Permission's opposite, restraint:** Restraint is the opposite of permission and it's a reason why diets fail. Restraint sets up the mind to want to overcompensate for what is being missed. Restraint theory tells us that the foods a person limits or is deprived of are likely to be the foods they will eat more of at a later time—be it when the diet ends, when they are emotionally vulnerable, very hungry, or any other reason. Just like permission, restraint can be applied to other needs beyond food and hunger: we have needs for human connection, choice, time to process or be alone, recharge and rest, to name a few.

■ **Trust:** The element of trust is how well you *trust the signals* from your body and how much *your body trusts* that its needs will be met by you. Specifically, your hunger, fullness, and satiety cues. There are other ways to experience trust with your body as well—do you trust what a full bladder feels like and head to find the nearest restroom? Do you trust that feeling you get when your head becomes foggy and your eyelids heavy, as signs that you need to get some sleep? Trust is how strongly you believe that your physical sensations are signs of your body's true needs and that when your body communicates something to you about what it needs, you're allowed to act on it. When you have a strong sense of trust, you believe your body will send a signal and that your mind (your conscious self) will respond to that need the best you can. Trust goes both ways—you trust your body to tell you when you're hungry, and with Intuitive Eating your body then trusts that it will get the food it needs within a reasonable time frame.

- **Trust's opposite, mistrust:** Loss of trust, or mistrust, occurs (for example) when dieting or during times when food is scarce. You stop giving your body the food it needs and then your body responds by enacting changes in hormones and neurochemicals that create urges to overeat or binge, compensating for the lack of food. This is the beginning of a cycle of mistrust and disordered eating. Trust goes both ways, from your body to your mind, and from your conscious mind to your body. Trust for a person is developed long before we make choices about food; it begins the day we are born when our cry for food is responded to quickly and we gain trust that our caregiver will meet our needs. This kind of trust can be broken at any point in your life, but the good news is, after it's broken, it can also be repaired—which is a lot of the work you may find yourself doing with your child using the 3 Keys.

- **Flexibility:** This element is specifically speaking to both body image flexibility and flexibility with food and eating, and we often find that once people see the value in flexibility in these areas, they are able to apply that same flexibility to other areas of their life. As Dr. Niva Piran writes in *The Handbook of Positive Body Image and Embodiment*, "Body image flexibility is rooted in psychological flexibility, a model of psychological health and well-being that emphasizes awareness and openness toward ongoing experiences to allow for action toward chosen values, even in times of great discomfort or distress."[8] What this essentially means is that the more mental flexibility you have, the more you can stay focused on what matters most to you without making choices or engaging in behaviors that ultimately take you away from the things you truly value.

- **Flexibility's opposite, rigidity:** Rigidity is the inability to adapt and adjust your actions or behaviors, even when it means sacrificing something. Eating disorder behaviors are a clear example of rigidity. Not being able to flex and adapt to your child's day or eating schedule because your plan went awry is an example of rigidity. Examples of rigidity are endless, but it might look like having a rule that your kids can't eat after a certain time in the evening, or not allowing a food with a certain number of calories or grams of sugar, or that certain foods are absolutely off-limits based on diet culture beliefs. Rigidity, sometimes a symptom of perfectionism, is when you feel you must follow food rules that lead you to eat less than you need or restrict, or miss out on valuable experiences like a celebration with family or friends because you won't be able to adhere to disordered rules.

- **Satisfaction:** Described by Resch and Tribole as "the hook" of Intuitive Eating, satisfaction is the element of your relationship with food and your body that gives space for pleasure, enjoyment, and fulfillment. Specifically, when it comes to eating, satisfaction is a place you end up when you intuitively feel you're getting enough to eat, and the food you eat is meeting your needs for taste, texture, flavor, aroma, temperature, and so on. What you need to feel satiated and satisfied will vary day to day and moment to moment (hence the need for flexibility!), and your body cues and internal wisdom let you know when you're getting closer to satisfaction. The more you're able to feel satisfied, the less need you have to continue searching for what will meet your needs. On a deeper emotional level, satisfaction also applies to your needs beyond food—we seek satisfaction in relationships, in our careers, in our life purpose, and in many other areas.

- **Satisfaction's opposite, deprivation:** Deprivation is what we experience when our needs aren't met. Deprivation is a feeling of being unable to achieve satisfaction. In a dieting mindset, deprivation is intentional, often with the purpose to lose weight. When kids experience deprivation, it's an expression of their needs not being met—sometimes by a caregiver. That unmet need contributes to an experience of feeling like they aren't worthy of having needs or that no one will hear their needs. Deprivation felt by a child can be a lifelong journey to heal from, where the grown person needs to experience a reparenting, either by someone else in their life, or by themselves.

- **Body connection:** Body connection is (for the most part) being willing to stay connected to your body—connected to hunger and fullness signals, and to thoughts, experiences, desires, and needs. This involves a level of mindfulness and awareness that is organically enhanced through the practice of Intuitive Eating. Connection becomes possible with the inclusion of trust, comfort, and permission. You need to be comfortable enough to hear your signals; then your trust will allow you to believe and form the connection to your body. This happens when you give yourself permission to slow down, be mindful, and experience your feelings and sensations. Body connection does require some level of mindfulness—which is something you can begin practicing at any time, just by pausing, tuning in, and noticing how you feel. Once you have some practice under your belt, this gets easier and more intuitive. Kids are generally much more likely to naturally have body connection because they haven't been conditioned for decades to disconnect like adults have.

- **Body connection's opposite, disconnection:** Because connection comes when trust, comfort, and permission are accessible, disconnection can occur whenever one of those elements isn't present. Disconnection may also be completely out of your control; perhaps it resulted from trauma (physical or psychological). In fact, you might be sitting in disconnection right now. That isn't uncommon. So much of the world—from diet culture to work-life balance to chronic stress and trauma—disconnects us from our body. Remember that this relationship isn't all or nothing: connection and disconnection will ebb and flow.

PUTTING THE PIECES TOGETHER

Now that you have learned about embodiment, a positive relationship with food and body, and had a crash course on Intuitive Eating, we can talk about why you're here and what the path away from the status quo can be. How do we put all of these elements together and help our children grow up with them? This very question is why we developed the 3 Keys for parents and caregivers—to help guide our future generation toward a more positive experience with food and body.

We know you really want to learn all about the 3 Keys now, but first we need to talk about someone else: *you*. You play an integral role in helping your child form their future with food and body. You're influential and powerful as both a role model and a supporter. First, we will focus on you and help set you up for success on the path to raising an Intuitive Eater. We are rooting for you and ask that you give yourself just a little more time to set the stage. The next part will strengthen your capacity to invest your energy into Intuitive Eating for the long term, which for many kids is what they really need from their parents and caregivers. We know you can do this.

SUMMARIZE AND REFLECT

Over the last three chapters, we've challenged the beliefs of our culture. The way diet culture impacts everything from our wallet, to our food choices, to our very own feelings of self-worth. We've talked about the harm dieting can do to us and our kids, as well as the protective effects of Intuitive Eating. Now, take a deep breath and some time to reflect on these questions:

- *What is your definition of a positive relationship with food and body?*
- *Does embodiment and the 6 elements feel like a space you would like to move toward? Why or why not?*
- *Try to tune in with your body for one minute. See if you can sit with the physical sensations you're having right now. Can you name one sensation you're feeling? Hunger? A need to pee? Thirst? Tiredness? What do you learn by intentionally pausing and checking in with your body?*

We're sure you're anxious to start helping your child on their journey, and because we need to talk about the important role you and your relationship with food plays first, here are some tips that you can implement *now*.

TIPS TO GET STARTED WITH
INTUITIVE EATING AT HOME

Consider the next five points as the CliffsNotes to this book. These are things you can start doing *today*, while in the process of learning more about how to move your family toward IE:

1. Try to stop talking about weight (*yours, your child's, anyone's!*). Remove the scale or at the very least hide it. If your child asks where it went, you'll see that they were noticing more than you might have realized. Tell them, *I'm learning that getting on the scale isn't something I need to do to be well or to take care of myself. I thought it was*

helping me, but it turns out it's not! So, our family is saying goodbye to the scale!

2. When you talk about food, recognize when you might be unintentionally or automatically bribing, coercing, or pressuring your child to eat (this might be a habit you need to start breaking). Don't beat yourself up if you catch yourself doing this. You'll learn a lot more about this as we go, but for now try to just know your job is to provide food regularly at consistent times throughout the day, offer a variety of foods based on what is available to you throughout the week, and only go so far as to think about gentle nutrition: a balance of carbohydrates, protein, fats, fruits, vegetables, and sweet foods at meals. You don't have to be perfect.

3. If you aren't already, eat with some awareness. Get curious about your own sensations of hunger, fullness, and satiety. You don't need to measure, portion out foods, count calories or points or macros. We know this may be drastically different from what you're used to doing, and we know that a big change can be anxiety-provoking, or even unearth some more serious disordered eating patterns. If you need help with this, we encourage you to reach out to a supportive friend, or if it's accessible to you, an Intuitive Eating–trained therapist or dietitian for more personal support. This isn't easy, and you're not alone. The point of tuning in to your eating isn't to make you eat less (a common misconception and a common way diet culture has co-opted Intuitive Eating). The point is to get in touch with satisfaction and your body signals. You don't have to do this tuned-in eating thing "perfectly" and savor every bite—keep it natural, and do what feels right for you.

4. Use positive talk about bodies and food: *I love that my arms and hands are part of my body so I can hug you and play with you!* Or: *I'm so looking forward to this delicious cornbread.* It will take time for you to recognize your automatic negative body and food talk and then decide to replace it with positive talk. Be compassionate with yourself; take it one moment at a time. If you make a mistake, you can repair it with an honest statement about how you didn't mean what you just said, and you're trying to not talk about food and bodies in a negative way anymore. Our bodies are precious and inherently good!

5. Change your mind (and your talk) about "good" and "bad" foods. Kids aren't motivated to eat any particular way by fear of health problems down the line. What teaching kids about "bad" and "unhealthy" foods does do quite effectively is scare them. Kids are very concrete thinkers. They aren't able to discern what you mean if a food is called a "bad" food, or if you say you're *so bad for eating X food*. For some kids, this can easily be the mindset that pushes them directly into a restrictive eating disorder, and for others it can create an internal dialogue of judgment and guilt. Over time, as they hear less fear-inducing language with food, their thoughts will begin to mirror your new, positive associations. This reduces the shame they feel when they want to eat something that was previously "bad" or "unhealthy," and the less shame, the better.

PART II

THERE'S NO SUCH THING AS A PERFECT PARENT

GETTING TO KNOW YOUR OWN INNER CHILD

It's time to talk about you. You're such an important part of your child's life and development that we can't help you help your child without focusing on you first. One of the most important phrases to hold from now on is *There is no such thing as a perfect parent*. Parenting is hard. We will mess up. We already have. Our parents weren't always right and probably did things that negatively impact us today, even when they had the best of intentions. Impact is always more important than intent.

Both of us have been through the process of healing from disordered eating and have spent a good amount of time working through the process of healing our inner child. Reflecting on your childhood and examining how your experiences with food and body influenced you might be a neutral, if not pleasant, experience. However, for anyone who has experienced trauma, abuse, neglect, body shaming, or food scarcity, this can be far more challenging. Again, we are going to encourage self-compassion, patience, and grace, as well as professional support, if you can get it. At the outset this chapter might feel unnecessary if you don't identify as having had any food or body struggles in your life, but we encourage you to read through it anyway; you just never know what could be hiding in a memory, or where diet mentality may hang out in your everyday experiences that you haven't previously recognized as anything to be aware of.

What is the inner child? Well, it's the part of you that holds the lessons you learned, the traumas that you may have experienced, as well as the joy and excitement you may have felt. Those experiences are still impacting you, even if subconsciously. Healing this inner child allows us to heal any negative experiences and to know what it's like to experience the parenting we needed. This can be incredibly difficult work, depending on how much trauma and re-parenting we need to do, and that's okay.

The point of unpacking how you were raised to relate to food and your body, and to other peoples' bodies, is never about placing blame on the person or people who raised you. The purpose is to come to a place of understanding what happened and how it impacted you, so that you can learn from it. Then you can learn what is keeping you from having a positive relationship with food and body and from being an Intuitive Eater. If you don't feel like an "Intuitive Eater" at this point in your life, there may have been moments in your past when that voice was present. How well you remember it—or even feel able to identify as an Intuitive Eater—is likely related to how early in your life you were taught to mistrust that voice. Are you able to identify when Intuitive Eating was interrupted for you? There is a great deal of healing in this. Even if you find yourself experiencing emotions like anger toward your parents, this is a common stop on the journey that is this work. That anger or grief—and any other feelings you may experience—are valid. Maybe this began with your parents or caregivers, maybe it began with their parents, or a peer group at school, your college dorm mates, or maybe it began with another influential person or force in your life. Regardless of the reason or source, it deserves that care. Time and again, the interruption in a person's positive relationship with food and their body is caused by *generational dieting*.

Generational dieting is the compounded effect of our parents dieting, and their parents, and their parents. It's something that our children will feel too. When we say "dieting," we know that not every family was "on diets" the way you might think of them. Generational dieting includes family patterns of upholding the ideal that a thinner body is better than a fat body, and that you should eat to control your weight rather than to honor your hunger. Generational dieting shows up in endless ways, unless we break the cycle. The reasons your parents had certain food beliefs and behaviors may be much clearer when we are able to dial in to the generational dieting. As an example, if your parents were very diet-minded, weight focused, or controlling about food, it's highly likely they too lived through an experience as a young child that caused them to disconnect from their internal Intuitive Eating ability or to value appearance so strongly. We aim to understand and look at the way you were raised, while also leaving space to be compassionate for what your parents or caregiver may have gone through as well.

UNCOVERING WHAT HAS INFLUENCED YOU

It's important to ask questions to remember how we were taught to relate to food and our body. How was your body talked about as you were growing up? How was food talked about? How was your eating or your siblings' eating talked about? Did your parents grow up with having enough food on the table for every meal? What could have been some reasons behind being encouraged to eat more than you wanted when you were young? When did your body become something more than a body—something that needed to conform to external beauty or health standards?

Now for some good and bad news: you alone are never going to be the problem or the solution to your child's relationship with their body. You can set them up to believe and trust that they are unconditionally loved, and their worthiness doesn't depend on their appearance or abilities. But the fact is we live in a culture that teaches us all that we should feel shame and loathing about our bodies if we don't meet the status quo and should always be trying to better ourselves. That is how diet culture works. If the companies who profit off people believing they need to look different, be better, be thinner, have lighter skin, straighter hair, bigger muscles, smoother skin, less fat (you get the idea) didn't exist people would feel differently about bodies. There is more to the story: our body-image suffering doesn't just come from companies trying to profit off us, although that is a huge factor. There is an entire history linking fatphobia to racism and white supremacy centering and idealizing whiteness, thinness, and, of course, money. These things, whiteness, thinness—along with being male and having money—give you relative power in our culture. You aren't to blame for how your child and eventually your adult child feels about their body, and you aren't the only influence. You aren't going to be able to control their social surroundings, positive or negative lived experiences, whether or not they develop an eating disorder, or many other factors that influence embodiment. The best we can do as parents is set them up to have a strong and healthy relationship with their body regardless of what the world throws at them. You don't need to blame your parents, and you certainly don't need to blame yourself. Instead of blaming, think about understanding, uncovering, and moving through your past for a better future for both you and your child.

LEANING ON SELF-COMPASSION

We've mentioned self-compassion a couple times, and we'd like to talk more about what that means. Self-compassion is so important for moving through this work and parenting in general.

Self-compassion involves:

- Treating yourself kindly.
- Knowing you aren't alone in your thoughts and experiences—many others are having the same experiences.
- Having mindful awareness of your thoughts and sensations—noticing your thoughts as they arise, and knowing they are just thoughts—and practicing noticing without being judgmental.[1]

We want to help you feel empowered to have a positive influence on your child, without feeling like you have to do everything "perfectly." You do not have to be a perfect parent, or perfect at Intuitive Eating, to have a significant positive influence.

A LOOK AT PARENTING TODAY

At the moment we are writing this, we are eleven months into the global pandemic of COVID-19. The world as we knew it a year ago when we began writing this book, five years ago, and a decade ago seems to be vanishing into thin air. Globally, communities are going through serious and necessary growing pains of historical social uprising for the Black Lives Matter movement and political unrest, and the future for everyone seems to be impossible to get a grasp on.

Underneath the massive social, economic, and political issues we're facing, many parents are overworked, financially stressed, emotionally taxed, and struggling with their own relationships with food and body. All of this is happening while everyone is just wanting to do what is best for their kids. No matter what is going on in the world around you or when you're reading this, you want what is best for them.

You, your child, and your family can heal and find a more peaceful way to relate with food. There will be ups and downs, but one thing to keep reminding yourself of is: **You do not have to do this perfectly.** Write this on a sticky note—tape it to your bathroom mirror so you see it every morning—let go of perfectionism and embrace your humanity, flaws, habits, history, triggers—this is your story. We all have a story with food and body, and yours is your truth.

It's not your job to fix everything for your child. Once we settle into our role of helping them down the path of the healthiest relationship with food and body that we can, we can then let go of unrealistic perfectionist expectations. The following are lessons that you will read more about throughout the rest of the book.

Your role is:

- **Get to know your inner child**: Understand and unpack your own history with food and your relationship with your body.
- **Put on your own oxygen mask first**: Take care of yourself when and where you're able to so that you're able to do the emotional and mental work of helping your child. Taking care of yourself includes: eating and sleeping enough, getting emotional support, going to the doctor or healer, taking medications as prescribed, and healing from disordered eating, among many other things. You aren't expected to be perfect; do what you can.
- **Feed your child**: Provide enough food at consistent and reliable times. Offer a mix of familiar and preferred foods, along with new foods. Reliable and predictable meal and snack times create a sense of safety and prevents your child from having a fear of deprivation or famine. Kids need the structure you create for them. You, for the most part, decide what is served while taking your child's tastes and preferences into account. The decision about what is served is gradually shared as your child develops more independence. Having space between meals and snacks offers the opportunity for them to show up to the next eating opportunity comfortably hungry.

- **Let them experiment and learn from what their body tells them:** Your child has a natural curiosity to try food, experiment, taste, and come to their own conclusions about what they like and don't like and how much they need to eat. You can consider this an essential part of the process for them. Let your child explore with fullness—they may have times when they eat more of something than they were hungry for and feel the discomfort of being too full. For children, Intuitive Eating is an embodied experience; it doesn't happen through logic, or by reasoning as a cognitive process. Charts and scales with cute pictures that try to teach fullness and hunger to kids can't create the same impact on the inner Intuitive Eating process that this embodied experience does. We don't have to "get" them to eat a certain way; rather, we create an environment that supports them by allowing them to have their own experiences.

- **Model Intuitive Eating and decide to stop dieting:** Use your Intuitive Eating voice. This may be a gradual letting-go process for you, and that's okay.

- **Get the grown-ups on the same page:** Communicate and align caregivers to send a consistent message to your child: their body is worthy as it is today and they deserve to get enough to eat, to eat food they like, and to not feel bad about what they want to eat. Grown-ups provide the food and what is offered, while kids decide how much to eat of what is offered.

- **Create a respectful home environment free of shame and weight talk and one that promotes body respect:** This builds your child's inner voice and establishes resilience for when they are outside the home and away from you.

- **Really show up for your child:** Help your child feel fully seen by you. Tune in emotionally to them. This helps their unconditional worthiness develop as a core belief.

- **Take the pressure off what your kids eat:** Use an "add-in, pressure-off" approach to help encourage nutritious eating. This means: think about what foods you want to add in to your family's routine of meals and snacks, instead of a "take away" or a restrictive approach that is based in diet mentality and will have the opposite effect from what you intend.

- **Be kind to yourself:** Use self-compassion, curiosity, and the 3 Keys model to start the journey along an Intuitive Eating path for you and your family.

Your role isn't:

- To control how much or what your child chooses from what is available.
- To create rules around food instead of boundaries.
- To foster a fear of getting fat or fear of health problems related to eating, or project your own fear or to "manage" anyone's body size.
- To motivate your child's eating behavior with fear, shame, guilt, or pressure.
- To bribe or coerce your child into eating "healthy" foods.

Now that we've covered the general role of a parent or caregiver in raising an Intuitive Eater, we are going to take a little trip down memory lane.

WE WANT TO PROTECT OUR KIDS

Each one of us has an inner child. Many parents express the desire to "save their child" from experiencing what they went through, like bullying, shame, or negative body image. The experiences we've all had with diet culture and that pressure to be in a certain body have given us reasons to want to protect our kids. Unfortunately, this desire to protect them through weight control actually reinforces body shame and leads straight into a diet cycle. That desire to protect our kids from the same negative experiences we had or saw is our inner child coming to the surface. We also want to help our kids step out of the same body-shame cycle that we may have known. In order to do that, we need to help that part of ourselves heal.

VICTORIA, AVERY, AND SUGAR

Victoria is a mother of a six-year-old girl named Avery. She came to me (Sumner) worried about how much Avery appeared to love eating sweet foods. Victoria described some of the things that worried her, as she had been reading articles about sugar addiction and eating disorders. Often, her daughter would wake up and ask to have chocolate for breakfast, or an entire extra dish of syrup with her waffle to eat on its own, and she said she would almost always choose to eat desserts like cookies or candy over other foods when given a choice. As I was moving through our assessment, I took care to not jump to conclusions quickly, but rather wanted to be sure I was really getting the full picture of what was going on with Avery. Through the assessment, I learned that Avery had no growth concerns, no nutrition deficiencies, no trouble sleeping, and no lack of energy. In fact, Avery was incredibly energetic, and for the most part really "normal"— which meant she was playing well with friends, having typical meltdowns, doing well in school, and asserting the usual signs of autonomy and independence that six-year-olds do. When I asked some more questions, I found out that Avery was also eating foods other than sugary ones— although she did have limited food preferences and was not a very adventurous eater. The list of preferred foods was: Rice Krispies, berries, pasta and rice, French fries, chicken and salmon, spaghetti, carrots, milk and yogurt, sunflower seed butter, breads and muffins, apples, chips, popcorn, and crackers.

As we worked together over the next few sessions, it became apparent that what was bothering Victoria most had nothing to do with Avery— it was her own inner shame about being a bad parent and her unspoken fear about her daughter's eating. Victoria shared her experiences of being yelled at by her mother for wanting a second serving of dessert or asking for sweets. She remembers her mom and grandmother constantly bashing their own bodies and her mother using words like "disgusting" and "baby belly" (long after she had babies) to describe her body. Victoria recalls the scale in the bathroom being very important to both of her parents. She had tears in her eyes as she remembered that her mother would never swim with her during the summer or at the beach because she didn't want anyone to see her in a swimsuit. Remembering how she was taught to feel around food and the way she was shown to feel about her body was painful, and these memories were showing up unconsciously for Victoria every time Avery wanted sugary or sweet foods. The anxiety, fear, and shame that was showing up was impacting the way she was interacting with her daughter. She also recognized an inner voice that was constantly in her head and told her she was a failure as a mother if her daughter didn't eat healthy enough. Through our work together, Victoria was able to recognize and start re-parenting her inner child. When Victoria was able to see that Avery was actually just fine, eating enough variety, and exhibiting very typical eating for her age, she was able to relax and feel better about allowing her daughter to eat sweet foods. Over time, Victoria was able to trust that if she continued to offer balanced meals and snacks and not shame Avery, her eating would stay balanced and peaceful. Along the way, Victoria came to see what a gift it would be to not put her daughter through the same gamut of guilt and shame that she went through with food growing up.

PSYCHOLOGY THAT'S NOT FROM PSYCHOLOGISTS

We are dietitians. We don't psychoanalyze or treat clients around their mental health and traumas. What we *do* do for our clients is best explained by Elyse Resch: "We can help them understand why they have the feelings they have about food and body, and the significance of their eating disordered voice." We help parents to understand how and why their inner child shows up when it does and impacts not only their relationship with food but their child's relationship too.

When we have a negative relationship with food, we often feel unable to trust our body because we are taught that our appetites and cravings aren't what's best for us. Diets are the only way to go when you don't trust your body and your hunger. Trust is a critical element to establishing body connection (remember the Intuitive Food and Body Relationship Model?). Without it, we can't believe that we can be okay in our body. According to Erik Erikson, the very first psychosocial developmental stage humans go through is *Trust vs. Mistrust*.[2] During the first eighteen months of life, a brand-new human is very uncertain about the world and they look to their caregiver to provide a sense of safety, comfort, and security. Developing a sense of trust is one of the most important goals at this stage of life. What is the first thing newborns do when they're born? They seek to nurse—they are hungry! They can sleep and go to the bathroom on their own, but in order to eat, an infant is 100 percent dependent on their caregiver. When babies aren't able to fully develop a sense of trust in their caregiver at this stage, it can result in a state of fear and anxiety that the world is unpredictable and not a safe place.

Developing trust in this stage isn't specifically about whether they had breast or bottle; this is about a caregiver consistently and reliably meeting the needs of the baby with food and comfort. With this information, it's easy to see that eating is our most primitive need, and if it's not met, this can begin the development of a sense of mistrust and disconnection from Intuitive Eating. If an infant receives inconsistent responses to their cry for hunger—or, in more traumatic situations, they are neglected—they are likely to mistrust their hunger signals, and mistrust that their needs in life will be met.

According to Erikson, when our needs are met in each stage of development, a person will acquire a virtue that is an essential part of healthy cognitive development. In the stage of *Trust vs. Mistrust,* the virtue acquired is hope. Hope is how a person responds in a time of crisis—do they trust that there is a real possibility that someone will be there to support them in a time of need? Without hope, we will seek to get our needs met in other ways as a substitute for reliable people. Food can become that reliable sense of comfort in times of crisis.

WE CAN HEAL FROM OUR UNMET NEEDS

Where development at any stage isn't fulfilled, any unmet needs can be met successfully later in life. For many people, this is what is happening as they decide to heal their relationship with food and body. They are successfully resolving their needs that were not met in childhood and learning to acknowledge their needs compassionately, be it a need for food or other emotional needs. When we are given a chance to re-parent our inner child, we have a shot to re-experience that stage of development and create the safety we needed (and still need), and we can pass that healing on to our children.

The next stage we encounter in Erikson's theory is *Autonomy vs. Shame and Doubt,* and this happens between one and three years old. If you've already had a kid pass through this phase, or currently have one in it, you know the autonomy those littles are learning to assert. It can be an ego struggle! Two-year-olds can be very determined to do things all on their own, including making decisions about what they eat and what goes on their plate.

The drive to assert our autonomy and set boundaries is something we naturally develop as toddlers and never really lose. When children aren't adequately supported by their caregivers, they can fail to develop a strong internal will, which is the result of successfully gaining autonomy. Without a strong internal will, they may struggle with establishing healthy boundaries and will rely on being told what to do instead of listening to their own intuition. This probably sounds familiar. Dieting is a really powerful example of relying on external instructions for how to eat and not listening to your inner voice to lead you. One way we help kids to assert their autonomy with the 3 Keys is by setting compassionate boundaries (for example, saying *Not right now* to a requested snack thirty minutes before dinner that may spoil their appetite) so that at mealtime they are comfortably hungry, internally motivated to eat what they choose from what's available, and use their autonomy to direct what and how much they eat.

DEPRIVATION AND MASLOW'S HIERARCHY OF NEEDS

We want what we can't have. Maslow's Hierarchy of Needs is another important psychological theory behind Intuitive Eating and raising Intuitive Eaters. According to this theory, we need to have certain needs met first in order to achieve higher-level needs, ultimately leading to self-actualization. Before we can focus on one need, we need to meet the needs that are required for life and safety. If we don't have a basic need met, it's unrealistic to think we would want or would be able to pursue a need on a higher level. We naturally strive to get our needs met, and if we are deprived of something, there is a consequence; with food it's often a behavior that emerges with the intent to fulfill our need. Binge eating is a behavior that emerges when a person isn't getting enough to eat. When we feel a sense of deprivation, we feel a biological need to meet that need and find food. Our most basic needs for survival include food, water, warmth, and rest. If we aren't fed enough, hydrated adequately, sheltered, and getting some sleep it will be very difficult to make any of the next-level needs a priority. Having the goal of getting a

Maslow's Hierarchy of Needs

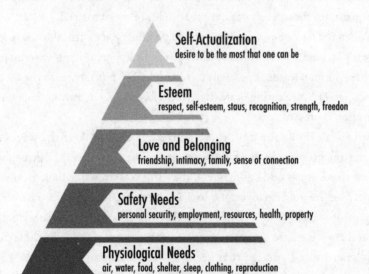

Self-Actualization
desire to be the most that one can be

Esteem
respect, self-esteem, staus, recognition, strength, freedon

Love and Belonging
friendship, intimacy, family, sense of connection

Safety Needs
personal security, employment, resources, health, property

Physiological Needs
air, water, food, shelter, sleep, clothing, reproduction

promotion as a priority when we don't have housing or food doesn't make a lot of sense. Just in the way that making happiness and self-fulfillment a goal when we aren't eating enough is fighting against our own biological sense. People in a state of food deprivation, be it from dieting or from an eating disorder, begin to distance from social interaction and become hyper-focused on food. What this looks like in a dieter's mind is that a significant portion of their waking thoughts become centered on food and body, such as reading cookbooks, fantasizing about the next meal, making exercise plans, obsessive calorie counting, obsessing about food in general, or binge eating. Hyper-vigilance and overthinking about food are actually symptoms of an eating disorder. When you're not eating enough due to food insecurity, restriction, and/or dieting, your brain becomes fixated on food and thinking about food, and you experience increasing cravings for higher-calorie and sweet foods to get your body the energy it needs. This is because our body doesn't experience intentional restriction much differently than it experiences genuine food insecurity. As soon as deprivation builds up (which can take anywhere from a few hours to many days or months), it's very natural—and helpful for survival—that we have a tough time sticking to any diet.

YOUR EXPERIENCE OF DEPRIVATION

If you have been on and off diets your whole life, it might be relieving to hear that it was the dieting itself that was leading your brain to want to eat past fullness or to eat certain foods to compensate and protect you. Your brain and body are trying to maintain those levels of safety that they are wired to need.

When the lack of money forces you to go hungry, it's natural to crave a binge or to eat past comfortable fullness when given the opportunity in order to protect your basic human needs. You aren't a "failed dieter," but rather it's the diets that are set up to fail you: eating more than feels okay and food cravings happen when deprivation is present.

When we think about all those truths and then look at the way we have been putting pressure on our kids to eat less, or eat right, or eat healthier, we can see how those are at odds. Of course, they will feel the same biological need to be *safe*. We are told that weight loss is achieved through a negative energy balance—if we use more calories daily than we take in, we'll lose weight—but only in theory. Because humans aren't so straightforward, we have these psychological systems and our ego that keeps us from being so robotic. We have responses to this deprivation. The most likely biological response to being in negative energy balance—even for kids, who have increased calorie needs for growth and development beyond weight maintenance needs—is to increase the drive for more food, to sneak food, to hide food or to binge in secret for the body to get its needs met.

The narrative that diet culture has perpetrated is that those biological needs are just our base impulses that we need to overcome, and it's all about willpower. This narrative saturates everything from the media to the doctor's office. So, even though we know that this backlash happens when we restrict—that it's just activating our survival impulses—we will likely still hear recommendations to limit food or change our child's weight. Your child's body is *smart* and will fight for its safety. In homes where there isn't enough food all the time, we know there is a significantly higher risk of developing an eating disorder as a result of unreliable food availability. This is another space where healthcare providers (even dietitians) are often undereducated: how the body and brain will seek out food when it's safe to have and available because your body is putting its survival and safety above all else. Biological drives are hard to ignore—and they shouldn't be ignored. Even though there is air pollution, we would never advocate for you to hold your breath, even if the air isn't entirely safe, because the biological need to breathe is the most important. This is left out in conversations about eating disorder treatment; we try to fix the individual and don't acknowledge the way other societal influences have contributed.

Many things can contribute to our child's (and our own) ability to feel trust and safety in their body. Remembering that we need to acknowledge everything from sleep, to physical safety, to affection, to food in order to work toward their happiness is important. Because they (and we) will never move into a place of food and body peace without first meeting that basic need to be fed.

IF YOU HAVE AN UNTREATED EATING DISORDER

Perhaps at this point, after reflecting on your own history and your food and body story, you're noticing disordered eating or eating disorder behaviors of your own. Eating disorders are common, not your fault, and treatable. If you're suffering on any level from disordered eating, we encourage you to seek support and ideally, if you decide to work with a trained health professional, find one who works from a weight-inclusive, Intuitive Eating–informed approach. One of the best books available to learn about medical complications from eating disorders that isn't weight-biased is *Sick Enough: A Guide to the Medical Complications of*

Eating Disorders, by Dr. Jennifer Gaudiani.[3] In her book, Dr. Gaudiani explains that you don't have to meet certain criteria, be "underweight," or experience any of the other stereotypical representations of what most people assume mean you're sick enough to get help. You deserve to get help as soon as you're ready, or even if you don't feel ready but know there's a problem, and in fact you're allowed to make your own recovery the priority before you move any further along in this book if you need to.

OUR INNER CHILD IS OFTEN STILL THE VOICE WE HEAR

The goal of resolving your own past isn't to make the voice of your inner child go away—it's to understand your story, resolve the pain, respond to your trauma responses with compassion and non-judgment, and to see how that voice shows up for you now, as a parent. By understanding your history and moving forward with the intention of taking care of yourself and meeting your needs in ways that may not have happened in the past, you can help yourself and your child.

So often as adults we ignore our needs—we have been taught to be tough, just keep going, and make other things the priority rather than ourselves. Sometimes, of course, we can't stop and soothe ourselves, but often we can do *something* to help. Helping and soothing our wounds regarding food, deprivation, body shame, and neglect are important places for healing if we want to be able to help our kids with these same concerns.

REFLECTING AND SUMMARIZING

Take a few minutes and reflect. You may not know exactly how your caregivers were supporting you as a baby and a toddler, but you can start to piece together your experiences and their impact. Often, the ways caregivers were responding to your needs very early on are similar to how your needs may have been met—or not met—as an older child, and you may be able to form some general understanding of it.

Here are a few questions for you to reflect on:

- *Did you experience food insecurity, was your access to enough satisfying food restricted, or were you introduced to dieting at a young age?*

- *Are you hopeful in times of distress that you will find the support you need to survive and thrive?*
- *Do you listen to and trust your inner voice, set boundaries, and feel that you strive to get your needs met?*

Perhaps your parents did everything they could to keep you fed, but there were times when there just wasn't enough food. Perhaps you often had all you needed, but the few times you experienced deprivation created a strong protective response that became a lingering worry that there wouldn't always be enough. Maybe your parents withheld food to discipline you or teach lessons, or they struggled with their own trauma. It's possible that a parent who struggled with an untreated mental illness, PTSD, or depression was not able to nurture you or meet your emotional or physical needs, and this caused you to experience deprivation or neglect. Maybe your parent(s) initiated you into dieting at a young age, and the trauma and shame of that experience created a lasting sense of perceived deprivation (*the thoughts that you can't or should not have what you need to feel satisfied, even if there is enough food available*) and that sense of perceived deprivation is still with you today.

In their book *The Power of Showing Up: How Parental Presence Shapes Who Our Kids Become and How Their Brains Get Wired*, world-renowned doctor Daniel Siegel and Tina Payne Bryson, a PhD social worker and psychologist, write: "When you develop what we call a 'coherent narrative' about your own past, you can be much more intentional and consistent as a parent, and much more effective in the ways you show up for your kids."[4]

UNDERSTAND YOUR FEEDING LEGACY

Feeding Legacy Tool

[Copyright © Jo Cormack, 2018]

Johanna Cormack, therapist, writer, feeding consultant, and mom to three kids, developed the Feeding Legacy Tool. This is a set of questions for you (and your partner if there is another co-caregiver doing this work). Jo describes your feeding legacy as "the sum of influences over how we feel about food and feeding."

Going through the questions will help you gain a better understanding of your feeding legacy, which will in turn help you with your child feeding experiences and raising an Intuitive Eater.

1. What is your happiest memory about food, from your childhood?

2. What is your worst memory about food, from your childhood?

3. What were the family rules about food and mealtimes when you were growing up?

4. How are they different (your answer to question 3) from the rules in your family now that you're a parent?

5. Pick three words to describe mealtimes when you were younger.

6. Which aspects of your upbringing (in relation to food) would you like your child to experience?

7. Which aspects of your upbringing (in relation to food) would you not want your child to experience?

8. Describe your grandparents' attitude to eating and their relationship with food. You may need to ask other family members for information about this.

9. Describe your parents' main beliefs and feelings about food.

10. Where do you think these beliefs came from?

11. Can you see any traces of your answers to questions 8 and 9 in your own beliefs, feelings, behaviors, and thoughts about food and eating?

EMBRACING YOUR ROLE AS AN IMPERFECT PARENT

How do we move from re-parenting our own inner child to helping our children through the formative years of creating a healthy relationship with food and body? As a parent, your role in your child's life is to meet the emotional and physical needs of your child. What this role entails changes throughout their life. The needs of a young baby are far different from those of a second-grader—and even more different from those of a high schooler. In the same way, the support you provide while raising an Intuitive Eater evolves throughout their life. However, there are two constants that we can always provide: the boundaries we create to provide support and the way we model a positive relationship with food and body.

One of the most important lessons to learn in raising an Intuitive Eater is acknowledging and accepting that you will never be a perfect parent. That is a big statement and might feel scary to read. Maybe it feels like a no-brainer. There is no hope that any of us will do it all perfectly. Not with feeding them, disciplining them, protecting them, or role modeling for them. Being alive means being in a world that exists with uncertainty. This can be a very uncomfortable truth. Parenting is real, intense, and full of screwing up before we figure it out. We do it because we love our kids and are just trying to do the best we can for them.

YOU WILL MAKE MISTAKES. YOU'RE ALLOWED TO BE IMPERFECT. THIS WILL MAKE YOU A BETTER PARENT.

Imperfection is part of being a parent and is vital to role modeling for our kids. If you're imperfect, it means you will make mistakes—you will have to repair, you will have to be wrong, you will have to grow. For children to see that imperfection is normal and accepted sets them up to trust themselves in all of their own humanity.

Role modeling provides us the opportunity to not only teach our children something, but to show them what it's like to practice it. You won't be perfect—that is part of the modeling we provide for our kids too. In fact, role modeling is key to the ways we can help our kids in their relationship with food and body; it's far more powerful than conversations, rules, or foods we let them eat. It shows that not only do we want them to believe this, we believe it and we live it.

WEIGHT TALK AT HOME

Let's look back at your childhood: Do you remember weight talk in your house? Even if you weren't encouraged to diet or weight wasn't mentioned, you probably heard the grown-ups talking about their bodies, the diets they went on, or the ways they "needed" to change. Those conversations, those incidences of negative self-talk you likely heard, started to develop your sense of how you should think or feel about food and body. These influences can be so deep and subtle that we might not even recognize how much they impact us today. If you can't remember any of those incidences, it's possible your parents modeled really positive relationships with food and body.

How big is the impact weight talk has on kids? Well, luckily, we have data. One study looked at over 350 adolescents and the way parents or family members talked in the home. Fifty-eight percent of the participants reported that weight teasing was happening at home and their parents often commented on their own weight or the daughter's weight; 45 percent reported that their mothers encouraged them to diet. The researchers concluded: "Parent weight talk, particularly by mothers, was associated with many disordered eating behaviors. Mother dieting was associated with girls' unhealthy and extreme weight control behaviors. In no instances were family weight talk and dieting variables associated with better outcomes in the girls."[1] They found that not only was negative talk and dieting that was directed toward the child resulting in increased disordered eating, but just the mere fact that there was weight talk in the home led to increased risk of extreme behaviors. There is *no* level of weight talk at home that brings positive outcomes toward embodiment. Even if you have fears about weight in your family, you cannot shame someone into better health. In fact, weight shaming or talking about a fear of weight gain is very likely to create disordered eating or an eating disorder, and also more likely to lead to weight gain over time.

Another study looked at five-year-old girls and their mothers and found that the young girls' ideas about dieting were influenced by their mothers' weight-control strategies, ideas, and beliefs. Out of 197 girls in the study, more than 90 percent of the mothers reported recent dieting and up to 65 percent of the five-year-olds already had ideas about dieting. Most of the dieting moms reported risky behaviors such as purging, smoking to suppress appetite, and fasting as part of their diet strategies.[2] We know how easy it is for our kids to hear us talking about or doing things that we don't want them to see. But see it, they do. My (Amee) six-year-old regularly brings up conversations that she wasn't part of or even in the room when they happened. Kids are more aware than we know.

BEGINNING TO CHANGE WHAT WE MODEL

How do we start to change the way we role model, especially if we've not been entirely aware of what we were already modeling? We've come up with nine behaviors that you can start to model for your kids. Something to notice here is that none of these explicitly tell you what or how to eat—that's not the behavior to model. It's the practices around food and body that we can model; what and how you eat is up to you. One of the ways diet culture encourages body distrust is by creating outside rules for eating. We aren't going to follow the same system. Because we trust your body, even if you don't just yet. The beauty of starting to change the way we model is that we can start even when we don't fully believe that we can trust our body. The feeling that you need to be told what to eat will fade as you build back trust with your body.

The nine behaviors that are crucial to practice modeling for your kids are:

1. Body appreciation and positive self-talk
2. Well-being over weight

3. Experiencing pleasure and satisfaction
4. Mindfulness
5. Self-care
6. Autonomy
7. Body appreciation through movement
8. Eating a variety of foods
9. Emotional attunement

BODY APPRECIATION AND POSITIVE SELF-TALK

We are conditioned, especially those socialized as female, to criticize our appearance. It's almost a stereotype that when women get together they will, at some point, complain about their bodies or appearance. It may seem like it's not a big deal—it's common. But the mere fact that it seems so normal is a clue to how conditioned we are to it. In fact, next time you're in public and around groups of people, listen to the conversations you hear. You may be shocked by how often you'll hear conversations about bodies or diets.

If you reflect on your own childhood, do you remember the way your mother or mother figure talked about her own body? Or even the way your father or father figure talked about his body? How do those memories make you feel today? When we are little, we don't see our parents as anything but perfect. To hear that kind of self-negativity coming from someone who we see as near-perfect can nearly tear out our heart. My daughter (Sumner) often comments on my body with the curiosity and low filter that most kids have. Although it was hard at first as she became more aware of other people's bodies, including mine, I decided to try my best to never be apologetic about my body. When she says, "Mama, your belly is squishy!" I say, "Yes, it is. I love my belly!" When she says, "Mama, your bottom is big," I say, "It's big and fabulous!" And we do the shake-your-booty dance together. Did it feel natural or even honest to do that at first? No way—I live in the same messed-up culture you do. But over time, I've seen that she has body appreciation for not only my unique body, but also hers. I can only hope this will help build resilience for her as she grows. I know I can't control everything that influences her, but I can do my part to model appreciation for my body. This helps encourage body satisfaction, and higher body satisfaction at any size is protective against disordered eating, specifically binge eating.[3]

Choosing well-being over weight is an active choice with steps you can take. Some things are very simple: removing the scale at home, declining weigh-ins at the doctor's office (if that feels helpful to you), and asking your pediatrician (*privately, not in front of kids*) not to discuss weight in front of your child. You have the option to decline weigh-ins at the doctor's office unless it is medically necessary, and while it can be important to have your child's weight recorded, there is very little good that comes from discussing it in front of your child. There is no age that is too young to start having this conversation with your pediatrician.

You can begin to stop all body bashing toward yourself and others—this includes negative talk about wrinkles, belly size, cellulite, weight, arm fat, and all the other things that we hear all around us. Talking positively or neutrally about bodies is important, as is talking about bodies in positive and respectful ways openly. This can help in making bodies less mysterious for kids. Don't engage in unkind "fat talk" with friends, and if you hear kids or adults body bashing anyone, try to make the brave move to interrupt it. Make the effort to verbalize and model being able to see your body in the mirror without a grimace, accepting that all bodies are different. Go out of your way to show bodies of different sizes and shapes and comment on how each one is unique in its own special way. Recognizing how it harms your child when they observe you talking negatively to yourself can be a wake-up call. However, that doesn't mean it's easy to stop, especially if it was modeled to you from a young age. Your child is listening, even when you think they can't hear you or don't understand. What you say is likely to be what they will say to themselves.

How do you talk about other people's bodies? Friends, family, strangers? Shut down negative body talk about anybody when it comes up. Stand up for people in public who are being body shamed. Remember that having thin privilege makes it easier to stand up to those negative voices than it is for those in larger bodies. We are raised to believe that fatness is something to be shamed. Use your thin privilege, if you have it, and set an example for your child about the importance of putting a stop to weight discrimination and bullying.

Research has shown that the desire for thinness—which isn't related to biological urges but stems from the societal preferences toward thinness and the way that beauty is presented to us—emerges around age six and that a child's body dissatisfaction is influenced by their perception of their mother's attitude toward her own body. If we, as parents, as mothers, have the chance to put a stopper in the obsession with thinness and appearance that we all recognize and so often wish we could break out of, what would stop us from changing our behavior?

EXPERIENCING PLEASURE AND SATISFACTION

Be vocal about enjoying food, pleasure, rest, the sun on your skin, or the cool fresh air in the morning. The more your kids can hear that you have permission to experience joy and pleasure in various ways, the more they will internalize that message and believe they deserve to experience pleasure too. I (Sumner) have a funny habit of making "*mmmm*" noises out loud when I'm eating things that I really enjoy. My husband knows he's really done well with dinner when the noises start! Over the years of becoming an Intuitive Eater, the now-automatic mindfulness with which I enjoy food has caused this reaction to really come out. It's a bit of a joke in our house, but I believe the way I outwardly express enjoyment and pleasure with food is rubbing off on everyone.

You can express pleasure without guilt—you deserve it, and by showing that you allow yourself pleasure, your kids will know they can experience pleasure without guilt too! It's common in our diet-filled culture that pleasure is something we are supposed to deny. Or a sign that we like things like food too much. But the truth is, finding pleasure in things is a biological drive.

We all have individual pleasures. I (Amee) have worked with clients who are distressed that their child isn't interested in the type of activities they believe are "healthy." Some kids are more interested in reading a book or playing with blocks than they are in riding bikes and going on adventures, and that is okay! I will never have an interest in running like my partner does; to me it's boring. And he will never be as interested in reading as I am. No matter what influences us, the things we find pleasure in will be our own. We, as parents, can encourage that. Food is pleasurable, and seeking different tastes and textures and ways to enjoy food is part of the experience.

MINDFULNESS

Mindfulness isn't necessarily a behavior or mindset that others around us can see. But the extreme awareness that kids have comes into play here. They might not notice every incidence of mindfulness, but the more we practice it ourselves, in many different areas of our life, the more it will be apparent to those spongelike minds. The goal with this behavior to model is, of course, to make mindfulness a normal part of life for our kids.

Mindfulness isn't what you might think: sitting on a cushion on the floor in an empty room cross-legged while meditating. You certainly can do that as part of a mindfulness practice, but it's much more than that. Mindfulness, sadly, has been hijacked by diet culture (and so has Intuitive Eating). We have had many conversations with clients who had previous negative experiences around mindfulness work that looked very much to be not another diet approach but turned out to be centered around the goal of eating less and losing weight. When they didn't sustain weight loss through a mindfulness practice (because the mindfulness practice was actually a diet, not a mindfulness practice), they felt more failure, shame, and hopelessness.

We describe mindfulness as a level of awareness. Mindfulness allows you to have more choices by being present with your thoughts. Thoughts such as: *What do I really want? How much am I hungry for? I can trust my body.* Instead of eating something just because it's there, you can check in with yourself if you want it, or about how you'll feel physically after eating it. Mindfulness allows you to hear the diet rules in your head, and instead make a choice based around permission, pleasure, energy, and appetite. You can eat intuitively when you have some space and the opportunity to be present with your thoughts, body signals, and with your decisions. There isn't one goal of mindfulness with eating, such as to eat less or to lose weight because you're satisfied with less food. **The larger goal is to empower you to turn away from rules, to a practice of eating in the way that works best for you in the given moment.** Living in a very busy culture that pushes productivity, scheduling, performance, earning money, and perfectionism takes away from being mindful. Even as an Intuitive Eater you may not always slow down and savor your food—*life happens!* Sometimes we have to eat on the run, or fit in a snack or lunch while on a short break. There are all kinds of reasons why you won't be able to (and why you don't need to) believe the story that every time you eat you have to savor every bite or you're doing something wrong. You can choose how to practice more mindfulness. The keys are choice and freedom, two things you'll hear about throughout the book.

HOW TO GET STARTED BEING MORE MINDFUL

When beginning to live with more mindfulness, many people want to start simply to be more aware in the present moment. You can practice mindfulness in your car while driving, while cooking, while cleaning a closet, while working—pretty much any time. Envision a gentle back and forth between checking in with your body and thoughts, and doing another task. In the shower, for example, you can intentionally experience the drift back and forth from feeling each sensation of the hot water, the steam, the sounds, the temperature on your skin, to getting a bit lost in your thoughts about the day ahead, then back to the sensations of being in the shower and what's happening in the moment. This is all natural; the back and forth is the process. It can be incredibly straightforward and simple, or complex and meditative, but it's like a superpower for people who tend to move through their life fairly unaware of what's happening in the present, or unaware of how their body and their emotions are responding to events. **Mindfulness is like your secret code to changing behavior. We can't make different decisions about how to eat, how to talk to yourself, how to respond, and so on if we aren't aware of what we're doing or thinking in the first place.** It's how we can hear and understand our body's signals, so true Intuitive Eating is practically impossible without it. The more we practice this, the more aware of our interoceptive (internal) signals and emotional states we can be and the more we can share these strengths with our kids.

> **Note:** Those who find mindfulness very difficult or inaccessible, or for trauma survivors who feel unsafe in a state of mindfulness, can still practice many facets of Intuitive Eating without a focus on mindfulness—such as choosing foods you enjoy, ditching the diet mentality, honoring hunger and fullness, and having unconditional permission to eat.

There are so many ways to start to incorporate mindfulness into our day-to-day life, so here are a few ideas for how to start to work it in:

- Use a guided meditation app to help with exploring meditation or relaxing.
- Stop and notice if you're clenching your jaw or drawing your shoulders up to your ears.
- Check in with your body and emotions and see what it is you need right now (a cup of water, to use the restroom, to ask for some help, to take a deep breath?).
- When eating a favorite food, like a piece of chocolate, eat it slowly and truly let the flavor wash over you. Let those "mmmm"s come out.

Remember, there are countless ways to practice mindfulness, and approaching it with an open mind is the first step.

SELF-CARE

Self-care is an umbrella term for describing the things we can do to take care of ourselves. Self-care can be everything from the mundane—like taking a shower, taking your medications, and feeding yourself—to the more luxurious—going on a date, taking time for a walk or a bike ride, or buying yourself something special. In times when you're more vulnerable, such as being really tired, stressed, hungry, unsafe, feeling depressed, and so on, your self-care might fall by the wayside. When we haven't spent our lives believing that we are worthy of being a priority in our own lives, it can be easy to slip into taking care of everything and everyone else first.

Perhaps you're someone who saw their parents always put everyone else first, or perhaps your identity—such as the color of your skin, your immigration status, your ability to work, your gender identity or sexual orientation, or your religion—is more marginalized in the culture you live in. You may feel you're often busy surviving, making ends meet, and caring for others, which results in self-care being commonly sacrificed for those other important priorities. Self-care often is only fully realistic for the most privileged. Showing your child that even boring self-care can be difficult but still worth prioritizing is important. Parenting is one of the greatest life challenges—you need to take care of yourself through the moments when you've been sleep deprived, lived through something scary like a family injury or illness, or the everyday occurrences like balancing parenting and working, being walked in on in the bathroom, bitten, screamed at, or tugged on to play while you're trying to do the laundry. Some of self-care comes from learning about boundaries and establishing them in our own lives. In other ways, it's more straightforward: fifteen minutes of peace and quiet, scheduling some "me time" on a weekend, taking a walk and moving your body, saying no to another request from your volunteer committee, or simply giving yourself permission to talk and vent to someone you trust. People who face discrimination need even more; they need those with privilege to stand up and take the lead, to speak up, to face the oppressor. Our self-care demands that we have others in the community (in our household, spiritual community, in our friend circle, and so on) who will help us get our needs met.[4] This isn't an individual responsibility. If you're unable to access self-care, *you will not be failing at raising an Intuitive Eater.* Maybe just noting that self-care is important will allow you the space to prioritize yourself, even just once in a while. You're the only one who can identify what self-care—and how your child will see you model it—will look like for you.

Au•ton•o•my

1: the quality or state of being self-governing

especially: the right of self-government

2: self-directing freedom and especially moral independence[5]

Ditching dieting and eating intuitively is one of the many ways you can model autonomy for your child. Dieting and moralizing food—such as counting points, calories, or macros—isn't autonomy. When you diet, your eating is being directed by an external expectation: these are the diet's rules. Feeling that there is something wrong with your body or weight when someone else or society has told you there is is another example of how we lose autonomy. *These are ways that you're giving away your autonomy to diet culture.* Sadly, many people may feel obligated to do what their doctor says because it's the only way to receive the medical care they need (we call this *unethical weight-centric medical care*). Not everyone is safe to exercise their autonomy in a culture that is oppressive, racist, and fatphobic. It speaks to how much work we all have to do to change the structures and systems in place that keep forcing people to give up their body autonomy—this is why body liberation is political. If you're able to, shift some of the ways you have lost your autonomy, get it back, and model it. Communicate that *you* decide what you're hungry for, what you want, and what you need. Autonomy can be saying no to someone who is pushing food on you when you don't want it. It can be asking for food even when no one else is eating if you're hungry. It can be demanding that you receive the same ethical healthcare that thin people receive. For more support on this and many other topics, check out the resource list at the end of the book!

BODY APPRECIATION THROUGH MOVEMENT

There is so much to love and appreciate about movement, although at times movement might feel like a chore. For some people, movement is a way to make themselves more mobile or able, to improve strength, or to support mental and physical health—all things that are benefits of movement but not tied to size. Everyone has an individual relationship to movement because everyone has a unique body. The emphasis on appreciating your body via movement means focusing on your internal desires versus what you "should be doing." In the same way we naturally rebel against food rules, we will rebel against required movement. Appreciative movement can and will look different for every person. Movement does impact health and provide some physical benefits, but not nearly as much as diet culture tells us it does.[6] All movement "counts" toward the beneficial amount; it doesn't have to only be heart-rate-elevating, sweat-inducing exercise. Moving with appreciation means you honor your autonomy (you have choice), recognize what your body is asking for and what feels good, and ultimately move your here-and-now body by doing what you *want* to do, not what you "have" to do. **Taking back your autonomy and choice over movement and relating to it with body appreciation is transformative.**

The messages from diet culture about exercise and movement have dictated the rules instead of us deciding what we want to engage in. This harms our relationship with our body because it interferes with our innate feedback: the noise in our head—the pressure—from diet culture distracts us from our natural desire for movement. When we move, we receive physical benefits in our body, as well as emotional and psychological benefits. Physical movement can boost your inner sense of happiness, hope, connection, and gratitude, across all stages of life. Kelly McGonigal, author of *The Joy of Movement*, found evidence that shows that movement actually can increase the joy you experience: "Over time, regular exercise remodels the reward system, leading to higher circulating levels of dopamine and more available dopamine receptors. In this way, exercise can both relieve depression and expand your capacity for joy."[7] And the compound experience of moving to music (dancing) with others leads to an extra release of endorphins (feel-good hormones)—which is why we highly support living room dance parties.

We want you to rethink your relationship to exercise. Are you moving out of a sense of obligation or guilt? Are you hoping to lose weight or change your appearance in some way? If we can shift the way we relate to and engage with movement through body appreciation, we can start to model what that positive relationship can look like. Moving to change your body size or shape is rooted in diet culture, punishing oneself, body dissatisfaction, and the thin ideal. The truth is that exercise isn't a guaranteed way to lose weight (nothing is), but there are true and meaningful health-promoting effects of movement when it comes from a place of being motivated by joy or by the intention of empowering yourself with strength, flexibility, or rehabilitation. The wonderful mental health benefits of physical activity aren't present if we are full of shame or guilt. You may even be in a place where movement sounds unappealing or untangling it from the web of diet culture feels too complicated right now, and that's okay. Movement can wait; modeling a healthy mindset around movement is more important. When you're ready, move in a way that feels right to you, that is a choice, and begin to cultivate a new relationship that stems from deserving to move your body in ways that honor your uniqueness and your interests. Take your time here.

EATING A VARIETY OF FOODS

There are many things that influence the types of food a child is willing to eat, and role modeling is just one. Some are related to privilege and are difficult to change, such as the social and environmental factors like availability of fresh foods, or the ability to purchase food. For the millions of kids who are facing hunger in America today, focusing efforts on community and municipal structural barriers to accessing a variety of foods will go much further in benefiting kids than talking about role modeling. If you can't bring home a variety of foods, or can't be home to cook a meal and eat with your children, then role modeling isn't what you necessarily need to be hearing about.

If access to food isn't a concern for your family, then eating a variety of foods can be an important behavior that parents can role model without creating rules and a power struggle. The goal most parents have is most often to encourage kids to actually like a variety of foods. Forcing or bribing kids to eat certain foods isn't effective in the long run, and it can actually have the opposite effect from what is intended. Role modeling is more effective, yet we still need to honor the truth that not every child will like all foods. A study investigating the relationship between kids and parents who role modeled fruit and vegetable consumption found: "Children who reported parental role modeling of vegetable consumption at snack and green salad at dinner were significantly more likely, than those who didn't, to meet the daily fruit and vegetable consumption recommendations."[8]

We aren't going to be advocating for any specific eating plan or encourage you to worry about getting your child to eat vegetables all the time. We are going to provide you with reasons for exposing and offering different foods and ways to try them. Keep in mind, one of the most important and influential aspects of modeling variety *is your attitude toward new foods, preparation styles, and flavors.* It could be that you yourself are selective with your preferences, but you make a point to model open-mindedness and interest in things like new cuisines, sauces, textures, or any new food or beverage. But we can't overstate the importance of modeling eating a variety of foods that you actually enjoy. Your child will observe you being open-minded, flexible, and curious about food in a positive way. If you're eating the same vegetables again and again and are barely tolerating them because you're "supposed" to eat them, that little spongelike brain will pick up on those nonverbal cues. A child doesn't have to eat the same foods every day or even the same quantities to get "enough" nutrition from their foods (vitamins, minerals, and so on). Simply having the goal of offering a variety from week to week is great. Diet culture almost always takes nutrition truth and spins it to make it feel urgent to "eat this, not that!," avoid something completely, or that a certain food will make your child act out in a tantrum. These claims are rarely—if ever—rooted in well-designed, ethical, unbiased science. We do not control our health with how we eat alone; it's just one of many determinants that impacts health and life span. By deciding to ditch diet culture, and instead just think about variety with food, you can take some of the stress off your shoulders, stay calmer with food decisions, and know that variety is wonderful and useful, and enough. (We'll get into more detail later about nutrition, as it's a complicated concept that deserves its own chapter.) As a role model, you don't even need to say anything about your eating or your child's eating, but you can turn to a "pressure-off" approach when it comes to eating fruits and vegetables. Repeated exposure (ten to twenty times of being offered a food is normal before some more selective eaters will be willing to even try) and you modeling eating the foods you hope your children will try are the goals of role modeling this behavior. Your child is ultimately in charge of their own likes and dislikes.

EMOTIONAL ATTUNEMENT

We left this one for last because it's a big one, and a tough one. Also, if you've had a rough relationship with food and body, you have likely experienced emotional disconnection as a way of surviving or coping. Emotional attunement can be described as being aware of what emotions you're experiencing and how they are showing up in your body in the present moment (sweaty palms, rising heart rate, knot in your stomach, headaches, and loss of appetite, for example). If this sounds similar to mindfulness and body connection, you're not wrong. They are very connected. They are all related to interoceptive awareness—which is how accurately you can sense the cues and sensations from your physical body. Broadly speaking, emotional attunement is your ability to identify your emotional state. With food and body and emotions all present, it's easy for these three to become one big chaotic cycle. If you're feeling stuck in that cycle of chaos right now, and identifying with emotional eating as a behavior that's not working well for you, here's our reminder for self-compassion. Pause and take a breath—*you don't have to be perfect at this.*

Emotional attunement is very interconnected with self-care and eating. For example: when you diet, you might notice that emotions pop up directly from the experience of dieting like anger that you can't eat something, hopelessness when the diet fails you, or anxiety about having to pick something from a menu. These are emotions that are cropping up simply from the experience of dieting. Additionally, as a living, breathing human being, you're always experiencing some emotion at all times—there is always something to notice if you're able to be present and attuned.

Modeling emotional attunement doesn't have one certain "look"; it's just you being your authentic self. The more attuned you are, the more you will model this. It might show up in the way of expressing your emotions more when you become more aware of them—*I'm having such a hard time trying to do three things at once* or *I'm really frustrated and I think I need to slow down and focus* could be examples of you expressing your emotions and modeling for your child what it looks like to notice and respond to what you're feeling. One of the ways I (Amee) have been practicing expressing emotions is by telling my daughter directly when I am feeling frustrated with her. And (as of the moment we are writing this) we have been in a global pandemic for months; both of us get frustrated with each other. Instead of letting it simmer, I look at her and say, "I'm feeling frustrated. I need to take a break so I can help you so we won't be upset with each other. Would you like a break too?" It doesn't always work. But we are trying and learning together.

Learning and modeling emotional attunement for your child isn't easy. Especially if these are newer practices for you. One of the 10 Principles of Intuitive Eating is "Honor your emotions with kindness." Each of these emotions, particularly the difficult or painful ones like sadness, anger, anxiety, loneliness, and boredom, trigger some kind of response. Being mindful of our own emotions—which comes with emotional attunement—and practicing self-care to tend to them when needed is how we can model this behavior to our kids. This is a huge topic and might be worthy of its own work. We encourage you to keep practicing, keep learning and noticing, and to seek professional therapeutic help, if needed (and I—Amee—believe most people could benefit from a regular therapist, if safe and accessible. There is no shame in that practice of self-care). Hold hope that as you practice these behaviors, you'll gain more clarity and a sense of direction.

SUMMARY AND REFLECTION

Being a role model for our kids is incredibly important. You probably already knew that, but maybe it was harder to notice how much *they* notice. They notice when we never get into the water at the beach or pool with them. They notice when we grimace over our vegetables. They notice when we put ourselves as absolute last and ignore our own needs. And telling them the ways in which we hope they live their life will never, ever compare to the ways in which they see us living our life.

This may seem like a lot of pressure, but the good news is we can be solid role models for our kids even while we're still learning. They will also have the benefit of watching us make mistakes and own up to them. To see us change and grow, and, hopefully, see us become more embodied adults who are working toward living their most authentic life.

Here are some questions to reflect on as you practice bringing these principles into your life:

- *How was weight and body size talked about in your home growing up? How do you talk about them now?*
- *How do you talk about food and exercise? How could you start to change the negative diet comments?*
- *What is your relationship to self-care now? How could you become more attuned?*
- *How often do you catch yourself in negative self-talk? Or diet talk?*
- *What fears do you have about letting go of expectations for your body? For your child's body?*
- *How do you know when you need some restorative self-care? What are some ways that you can practice self-care? Do you enjoy the foods that you choose to eat?*

THE DOUBLE-EDGED SWORD
OF PARENTAL CONTROL

From the beginning, raising an Intuitive Eater is about creating an environment where your child can feel comfortable and confident with eating, and where you support them with their inherent and natural ability to eat. We can't tell them what and how much to eat, restrict them from certain foods, and hope that simply teaching them what is "healthy" for them will allow them to fully develop a functional, natural way of eating as they become independent eaters. *This fails us almost every time.* (It's important to note that although uncommon, there are some people who seem to not be driven to eat by pleasure, and don't seem to react to the experience of restriction the same way most people do.) We need to create an environment for eating that facilitates their innate drive, models behaviors, and instills in children a sense of trust that we won't deprive them. **Their hunger isn't a bad thing, and they can trust their body.** How can anyone feel trust in their body and relaxed about eating if they aren't supported with practicing it?

We've already mentioned that attempts to control your child's food intake can—and often do—backfire. It's time to dig into this. We have been taught to think, either directly or indirectly, that the more negative control you exert over your child, the more they will comply with your wishes. In the short term, it may seem effective—but the reality is that it's a double-edged sword.

Have you ever had an experience where someone made you do something you didn't want to do? How did that make you feel? Did you want to just do the opposite, if only to assert your own voice? That is a natural human reaction to being controlled. Our environment, who we are with and what is happening around us, makes a difference in how we perceive our autonomy. Our job as parents is to create an environment around food and eating that is positive, with a sense of connection, so that our children feel free to assert their autonomy and have choice over how much they eat and what they eat of what is offered.[1] We all have a natural reaction to avoid being controlled. Psychological reactance theory (PRT) states that when something or someone threatens our freedom to choose how we feel, act, or relate to something, a natural reaction, opposite from the recommended action, feeling, or choice, is provoked, to restore the threatened lost freedom.[2] The human drive to establish and maintain our autonomy, something that starts to develop in toddlerhood and continues to grow all our lives, is designed to ensure our freedom. Freedom-threatening language (for example, "you must," "you have to," "or else") will elicit a stronger desire to disobey, while choice-enhancing language ("Which would you like, ___ or ___?" "You can have ___ now or save it for later; which do you choose?"), which is more implicit, reduces the threat or feeling of being controlled, resulting in utilizing what we know about the importance of autonomy to elicit self-directed behaviors. There is powerful research around reactance and PRT that looked at anti-tobacco advertising and adolescents. Take, for example, the truth® campaign, an anti-smoking campaign aimed at reducing smoking among teenagers. On the truth® campaign's web page, they state, "We've always been about exposing big tobacco's lies and manipulation. And while they keep adapting their tactics, we keep it real." Furthermore, the truth® campaign's messages consistently emphasize adolescents' autonomy in making their own informed decisions about tobacco use. "We're not here to criticize your choices, or tell you not to smoke. We're here to arm everyone—smokers and nonsmokers—with the tools to make change."[3] This has been cited as arguably one of the most successful public health campaigns in US history.[4,5]

The will to assert our autonomy is inherent in us as humans and is persistent. We all have experiences in life that thwart our autonomy when we have done something because we had to or would have faced punishment or backlash. Think about when a manager tells you how to do a project without letting you figure out how to do it on your own. Or how it feels when someone close to you, a family member, for example, is always telling you you're doing a task wrong, and you need to do it their way. Some autonomy-diminishing experiences are normal, and we can be resilient through them. But when we are raised or chronically stuck in an environment where we cannot assert our autonomy in an age-appropriate way, there are consequences. The risk of deep psychological impacts, particularly losing a sense of self-determination and the propagation of self-doubt resulting from the inability to establish autonomy, can be intense. Of course, there are times when parents need to be in control, for safety and because a child isn't developmentally capable of problem-solving or decision-making. We need to cut our young child's hot dog or grapes for them, because giving them a sharp knife would not be safe even though they are grasping for it, saying, "I do it! I do it!" Inappropriate parental control, however, diminishes child autonomy. They learn that their decisions aren't to be trusted. They learn that they can't be trusted or feel incompetent.

You're the person who is mostly responsible for keeping your kid alive, safe, sheltered, and protected. For helping them mature and grow emotionally and intellectually. Now, imagine you're able to put a big, protective embrace around all of the things you watch your child do in their life. You create safe boundaries so that they can explore the world, make mistakes, and become their own unique little person. As parents of school-age kids now, we (Amee and Sumner) have already witnessed the unbelievable transformation of baby to toddler to big kid, and are waiting with hope and uncertainty about the next phases to come of older childhood and adolescence. All parents, no matter your beliefs, your rules, your systems, or your upbringing, can relate to the truth that the ride of parenting is wild, uncertain, unpredictable, and at times very hard.

We use the word "boundaries" to describe necessary, positive parental control. The goal of creating boundaries is to help your child establish a healthy, autonomous self with food and body. *You can help them hear their inner Intuitive Eater. You create necessary boundaries, and allow them to do what they are capable of in their developmental stage so that they can grow into their confident, capable, adult self.*

Inappropriate parental control with food involves the two types of control in feeding practices we introduced in chapter 2: using restriction and/or pressure (rewarding, punishing, coercion).

RESTRICTION

Saying something like: *You can't have pizza because it's not good for you.* Or: *You can't have more than two slices of pizza until you eat your fruit salad.*

Other examples of restriction include: never allowing a certain type of food in the house even though you know your child likes it. Or never/rarely offering cookies when you know your child likes cookies. Or limiting snacks to only fruits and vegetables, when they may likely be hungry for something more substantial, with fat or protein, to hold them over until the next meal.

BOUNDARIES

Saying something like: *We're not having a snack right now, and dinner is coming soon, but we can have X food later when we sit down.* Or: *I'll add that to the dinner menu this week.* Or: *There are only two left, so you can have one, but we need to save the other for someone else.* Not allowing more than a certain serving size or portion because there's not enough for everyone to have more, or because it's a higher-value food and money is tight. *Boundaries aren't strict rules and don't look the same for all families. With the information you learn in the 3 Keys, you can trust yourself to make the right choice for you and your child in the moment. You can learn from what happens.*

SHAME AND ANXIETY AREN'T EFFECTIVE LONG-TERM MOTIVATORS

When it's time for potty training, despite there being various methods to this madness, you want your child to get it. You might even be eagerly anticipating no more diaper changing! You know that when the diapers come off—but before they know the true meaning of the potty—there *will* be accidents. You're probably very in tune with the fact that shaming your child and punishing them for an accident isn't going to help the process and would not be supportive of them feeling competent and relaxed about their ability to eventually "get it." We say "Oops!", clean it up, and head to the potty. Then when they wander there on their own for the first time and actually go in the right place, it's a party! Why does this work? *Because fear and shame and anxiety aren't effective motivators.*

There are many aspects of parenting for which we already know negative control and dominance will not help, and many parents who are tuned in to this choose to let their children learn from natural consequences. An example of parenting using natural consequences is instead of forcing your child to wear their coat, let them go outside and experience the cold, so that they come back asking to put it on when they're ready. Parents who use this approach in nearly every other aspect of parenting don't necessarily with food. This is the power of fatphobia. Parents may be too afraid of the possibility of weight gain to allow freedom and permission with food. Intuitive Eating challenges parents in this way, to move through their discomfort with even the possibility of weight gain, for the opportunity to wholly support their child to form a positive, respectful relationship with food and body. On the flip side—not necessarily from diet culture but from other beliefs that were passed down to you—parents may be pressuring a smaller-bodied child to eat more than they are hungry for or to finish their plate, unaware of how that pressure can further perpetuate food avoidance or anxiety. They may not realize this is likely to result in the opposite of what they want for their child and creates a rift in their inner Intuitive Eating process. As for our kids, we know they will make mistakes in all areas of life. We tell them to try again and learn from their experiences. Yet, when it comes to eating, our culture has adopted beliefs that go against this very mindset. By intervening and telling kids how much to eat, when to stop, dictating what they should eat before they can have something else, never letting them eat unconditionally because of our fear of them overdoing it, getting a tummy ache, or gaining "too much" weight, we aren't allowing them to utilize their natural abilities to eat and regulate their intake—and as a result they lose touch with the natural signals and abilities to regulate their food intake that they need to be competent and confident eaters for life. They aren't given the chance to test and develop a strong sense of autonomy around food. When parents intervene too much, the vital abilities children are born with start to fade. **If you don't use it, you lose it (though it can be found again with Intuitive Eating).** It's literally as if by asserting so much negative control over our child's eating, we are placing them in a diet mindset before they can even consent. When we place pressure (positive or negative) on a child to try to make them eat something, it can cause them to be even more averse. It just doesn't help for the long term.

Many parents turn away from the concept of Intuitive Eating, thinking it means a free-for-all where kids are directing all aspects of eating. Thinking about this isn't only hilarious, but really awful to imagine, especially for young kids! Older kids, however, will be able to take on more and more of their own decision-making, and we can allow that. But as for those smaller children, to let it be a free-for-all as a parent, I see peanut butter and jelly smeared across the furniture, and my son working his way through forty popsicles a day because he can't reach anything else and will need to satisfy his hunger. Young kids aren't ready to make all their decisions around food, and asking them to do so is placing a burden on them they can't handle. They need you to fulfill your role to set structure, safety, and adequacy in their eating routine (Key 2). They also need you to let them learn to trust their body and to explore eating and feeding in ways they can over- or undershoot the mark, and feel what it feels like to eat too much cake, or drink too much juice, or not eat enough and feel the discomfort of hunger between meals. (Just like they need to learn that it hurts to scrape their knees if they don't watch where they're going.) We know that kids benefit immensely from appropriate and positive control, healthy and necessary boundaries set by caregivers. They need to feel a sense that someone is in charge to keep them safe. However, we also understand how Intuitive Eating for kids can easily be misinterpreted by parents, given that *for adults* it looks very much like—and is—total freedom and permission.

HAVING A ROAD MAP, AND SOME STRUCTURE, SETS A STAGE FOR SELF-REGULATION

Even adults who are recovering from their relationship to food and body often need to start by creating some structure for their eating—a bit of a road map, including when to start eating, meal and snack times. Kids benefit from this same structure. Remember when we mentioned the need to sometimes revisit a stage of development and either receive some healthy re-parenting or learn to re-parent ourselves? This applies here too. If your own journey into Intuitive Eating is bringing up a fear of giving yourself unconditional permission to eat or a difficulty with eating enough food, re-parenting that part of yourself and providing a compassionate, loving structure (not the rigid, rules-based structure of dieting) for yourself might be a gentle step to take. Exploring how to set structure for your own eating if you're someone who wants to heal your relationship with food may begin with some curious contemplation. Ask yourself, *How would I feed my partner, my best friend, another parent? What would it look like to set up structure to feed someone else? Can I try to do that for myself?*

Eating is more than an action we want kids to do, it's an intricate and nuanced physiological process. For an example, we'll look at sleep: it's different from certain everyday behaviors we do and want our kids to do, such as brushing their teeth, putting dirty socks in the laundry, and cleaning up, in that it needs to be internally driven; it's a part of our biological makeup—sleep is, in fact, intuitive, even though we have some structure to it (wake-up times, naptimes, and bedtimes, with flexibility if we are more or less tired). We encourage you to think about the structure of daily eating in a similar way. Structure is important and helpful, but we have to remain open-minded and responsive to day-to-day fluctuations and circumstances.

By attempting to use negative control (*including restriction, reward, and punishment with food*) and pressuring kids to eat, we are creating a disconnect from their body cues. This comes at a huge cost—kids develop and grow up to think they can't control their eating (because they haven't been given a chance to!) and live in a somewhat constant state of shame and deprivation, or anxiety and avoidance. They focus on and want what they aren't given permission to have, and question their desires. We unintentionally create reactions that lead to eating more than they're hungry for, developing food anxiety, negative meal experiences, sneaking food, restricting food to control weight, hiding food, and feeling bad about their natural hunger. **We also can inadvertently cause harm to our relationship with them as humans.** Many adults are living this way and it's nearly impossible *not* to pass these behaviors and beliefs down to kids, given that role modeling is known to be one of the most significant sources of how kids adopt behaviors.

By raising your child to be an Intuitive Eater, you're facilitating self-regulation, the ability to know when to eat, how much, and how to stop when they've had enough so they may feel fully satisfied and can generally move on between meals and snacks without being preoccupied by food.

OVERCONTROL TAKES AWAY THE OPPORTUNITY TO BUILD SELF-REGULATION SKILLS

Contrary to many fears, and as we mentioned earlier, using an add-in, pressure-off approach with feeding kids doesn't strip a parent of all their control. We aren't suggesting that you should allow your four-year-old to start dragging the step stool over to the fridge to decide what's for breakfast every morning. Parents need to be in charge—we have decisions to make, budgets to work with, mouths to feed, and more. Positive parental control is part of establishing healthy boundaries and helping kids feel cared for and safe.

Parents can create an eating environment where they are fulfilling their role by providing consistent meals and snacks (while including a variety of foods and food groups) and allow the child to determine how much and what to eat from what is offered. This separation of roles between caregiver and child is commonly known in our field as the Satter Division of Responsibility in Feeding (sDOR).[6]

Autonomy support (*you making space for your child to be in control of how much and what they decide to put in their body without the external influences of praise or punishment*) also has another benefit—it will strengthen the feelings of closeness and trust, and the relationship you have with your child through feeding. When they were an infant, they trusted that you would feed them when they cried for food, and today, they still need to trust you in the very same way. They need to know that they can be finished when they've had enough, won't be blamed or shamed for their appetite or what food they want, and they can eat as much as they need to eat, unconditionally. If this trust has been broken after a pattern of attempts at overcontrol, it can feel overwhelming to think about how we can gain that trust back. You can probably identify a certain look on your child's face when they feel worried about how you'll respond to their request for another cookie: that is one example of a symptom of some broken trust. We know how hard that can feel to recognize it and to feel ready to take the steps to make the change. It's important to know that this can be repaired. It's never too late.

There is deep meaning in you promoting and valuing autonomy for your child. The decision to respect your child's eating style, preferences, hunger, and fullness signals communicates more to them than just *Mealtime will not be a battle for us anymore*, it communicates, *I hear you. You can trust your body. I understand. I trust your body. I respect your body. I respect you.* When you trust them, they will be able to learn to trust themselves.

You can be in charge as a parent, while not being controlling. *And this doesn't mean you lose control of feeding scenarios.* In the roles of child and parent, it's important for lots of reasons for parents to be in control—namely safety and meeting kids' needs, as they aren't developmentally capable of doing most things on their own until they grow into adolescents and adults. We can maintain control where it's needed, but can let go in areas where it doesn't help.

IF WE DON'T USE CONTROL TO SUPPORT OUR KIDS' EATING BEHAVIOR, WHAT *DO* WE USE?

The answer is something known as responsive feeding. A responsive feeding approach[7,8] is supported by research, and responsive feeding practices are considered to have a protective effect on maintaining a child's ability to self-regulate—that's the wisdom they were born with regarding knowing how much to eat, when to eat, and when to stop. Along with being a general approach to feeding for all children, responsive feeding is used in working with "picky eating" and in recommendations to prevent problematic or disordered eating. A systematic review summarized results from thirty-one studies. The most frequent finding, applied to ages ranging from infancy to elementary school, demonstrated that controlling feeding practices were counterproductive. Restrictive practices promoted more eating (associated with increased weight gain), and pressure to eat resulted in less eating (associated with decreased weight gain and low body weight).[9]

Every time your child hears you say *Just one* when they ask for another dinner roll, they are hearing you say, *I can't let you have as many as you want, because the amount you want is too much and that's not a decision you can make.* They feel both controlled and incompetent, and over time, they begin to believe this as truth. Then when their body wants more bread, or pasta or cookies, they have an internal conflict between what they want to eat to feel satisfied and what their internal narrative is telling them about being able to trust themselves. Over time, the use of even a simple overcontrolling statement like *Just one* has a profound impact on the child's self-regulation skills, even when you're not around. This kind of control can also impact their trust in feeling able to be open and honest with you regarding what they eat. Knowing that you said they could only have one roll and they had more can lead to them feeling like they have done a bad thing and may even fear telling you the truth. This is one way that sneaking and hiding food develops.

Wendy Grolnick talks about parental control in her book *The Psychology of Parental Control.*[10] She writes that the theorists who don't accept the positive effects of autonomy support and the negative effects of control are misinterpreting the meaning of autonomy to mean "independence" rather than "choicefulness." We want to be really clear, to avoid confusion, that autonomy doesn't mean you're giving your child the responsibility or independence to decide what is prepared or available to eat and when—that is part of your role. Supporting autonomy for your child isn't at odds with the feeding relationship that places you, the parent, in a decision-making role, and yet you don't need to be overcontrolling, to be in charge of what, when, and where your child is eating.

For many parents, one of the most misunderstood and uncomfortable things about the idea of raising an Intuitive Eater is the fear that not asserting control means their child directs all aspects of their eating, which could not be further from the truth. The practices of pressure, rewarding, and punishing kids around eating are socially ingrained. Most parents aren't trying to ruin their child's relationship with food; there has just been some really bad advice given over time rooted in diet culture and fatphobia and a hefty dose of very overzealous nutrition agendas put out in public health messages. **Kids need flexible structure, reliable feeding, and the chance to practice and trust their body cues and their emotional cues in a shame-free and judgment-free environment.**

INTUITIVE EATING TRUSTS THAT THERE IS AN INTERNAL MOTIVATION TO EAT

Giving kids more choice and reducing the pressure and control around eating and other developmental dimensions of their lives will strengthen their intrinsic motivation, self-esteem, will to learn and succeed, and natural desires to achieve healthy independence. Since the 1950s, researchers have been looking more closely at natural tendencies around intrinsic (otherwise known as internal) motivation and how it supports healthy development. It begins by recognizing that humans are born with an innate desire to explore, experience, grow, learn new skills, adapt, and master their worlds.[11]

The term "intrinsic motivation," which is the basis for self-determination theory (SDT), was coined by Harry Harlow. Self-determination theory is one of a few theories that are part of the responsive feeding umbrella approach. Having intrinsic motivation can be described as choosing to do something willingly, freely, and out of natural curiosity and enjoyment, rather than as a result of fear of punishment, reward, or pressure. What many feeding experts are currently investigating, and what we find so powerful in terms of feeding kids, is how intrinsic motivation isn't just related to psychological development, healthy exploration of the world, and building skills but is also very applicable to food and eating.

Self-determination theory outlines three psychological needs humans have in order to drive internal motivation: the need to feel autonomous, the need to feel competent, and the need to feel a relationship with others around us. The theory states that people are born with these psychological needs, and are most likely to have intrinsic motivation that directs them toward a meaningful and satisfying life when these three needs are met consistently.

Here is a brief but important lesson on SDT and the three human psychological needs that, when met, foster intrinsic motivation. This means that your child is born with internal motivation to eat adequately (when they drink milk) and from there we want to support our children to hold on to and strengthen that natural drive and curiosity to advance to eating a variety of foods as they mature. The number of different foods a person will eat naturally varies from person to person, and there is no "ideal." We support children in fulfilling their needs by avoiding the use of negative control, avoiding restricting their eating, by creating a positive feeding relationship, and building their competence. The three psychological needs of autonomy, competence, and relatedness can be described as a common thread that runs through all of us as humans. **Research and what we know about human psychological development tells us we can relax about food and that kids are wired to want to eat and to feed themselves well enough.** Many feeding difficulties may arise or are negatively reinforced as a result of the dynamics of the feeding relationship. As you read the descriptions of the needs below, you'll likely relate to how they feel relevant for you now, and also how they would have felt subconsciously vital for you as a younger version of yourself.

Autonomy: Humans need to feel that their actions originate from themselves. *We want to feel like we are doing what we want or choose to do, not what we are told to do.*

Competence: When we feel competent, capable, and effective, we are motivated to continue. *When we are asked or forced to do something we are unable to do, the experience of incompetence leads to feeling unmotivated to continue.*

Relatedness: Individuals need to experience love and interpersonal contact to develop optimally. *Even one safe, loving, warm relationship provides us with a sense of security and we can feel well-adjusted. This makes room for feeling curious, open, and trusting toward the unknown and the world around us.*

Autonomy, competence, and relatedness are all major players in the type of feeding relationship you'll have with your child. Foster these three needs, and you will be well on track to supporting the development and maintenance of a healthy relationship with food for your child.

YOU CAN BE IN CHARGE WITHOUT BEING CONTROLLING

Autonomy support is the degree to which parents create an environment that leads to fulfilling a child's need for autonomy—making some decisions of their own about food. **Autonomy support is one of the most important ways we allow our kids to maintain their natural ability to self-regulate, or if they have lost touch with that ability, regaining a sense of autonomy over their eating can help them recover it.**

Surveys done with parents describe one of the most common arguments *against autonomy support* to be the fear of lack of control at home. Although it's an understandable fear and it's easy to see how parents could be wary of, or even feel threatened by, the idea of giving kids autonomy and choice over their eating, we will emphasize again that *parents aren't losing control when they give kids more independence with their eating. They are letting go of the illusion, hope, or existing belief that they can control what their child eats and that it is helpful in the long term to do so.* When talking about barriers to supporting autonomy, there are many reasons why parents may not have the ability or the psychological bandwidth to offer autonomy support. We'll talk about those a bit later.

The main goal of mealtime is to have positive, social, or caring eating experiences to facilitate a peaceful eating experience and not one where kids may feel anxious, watched, monitored, or pressured. The goal isn't to "get kids to eat." Our own attitude and modeling to kids that we value positive mealtime experiences as parents can have a strong influence on creating a sense of **relatedness** at meals and snacks. If you struggle with letting go of the attention to what they are eating, try saying to yourself before meals, *I want to create a positive mealtime experience. I want my family to enjoy being at the table together first and foremost.*

It's easier to foster a positive and peaceful feeding experience when parents eat with their children if possible, no matter what that meal looks like. Things like fostering good, open conversation, showing an interest in how the other person at the table is doing, playing games that don't interrupt eating, and putting away screens and technology can all be ways to help create positive meal experiences. *What can you do that helps your child want to come to the table?* Help your child learn that all emotional experiences are okay to bring to the table and they are allowed to show up and be real. You're there to help support them, not to be the food police. *Connection is key.*

SOMETIMES PRIORITIZING AUTONOMY DOESN'T FEEL LIKE A CHOICE

In many cases, prioritizing autonomy and choice isn't an option. It also takes time to provide for and meet all the needs of a child, in particular the time it takes to shop, cook, and sit down for meals together—it isn't something all families even have the choice to do. Single parents are often dropping kids off at daycare or with another caregiver before sunrise, to work one or more jobs until midnight. Busy parents who work long hours, have multiple kids, or frequently travel for work aren't always, or even often, able to get dinner prepared at one time for the whole family. You may not be around when your child is eating their meals, and that's okay.

THE BEAUTY OF INTERNAL MOTIVATION

Remember that when the pressure and negative control are off, your child, like most humans, has an internal drive to eat in a way that will nourish them. We can trust that kids will be able to regulate their eating and eat adequately when the pressure is off and there is a structure of appetizing and familiar meals and snacks provided by a connected and tuned-in caregiver.

This isn't necessarily the case for children or people with eating disorders—anorexia nervosa, bulimia nervosa, binge eating disorder, other specified feeding and eating disorders (OSFED), and avoidant/restrictive food intake disorder (ARFID)—so this is a reminder that you do need to seek medical help from an eating disorder specialist to assess your child individually if you worry they may have an eating disorder or noticed they have stopped eating, have slowed or interrupted growth, or are losing weight.

Without measuring, calculating, and monitoring every bite of food your child eats—which in and of itself is unrealistic and likely to be inaccurate—aiming for some variety and trusting their internal drive to eat is the best bet for promoting balanced eating. Remind yourself that their internal drive to eat is what allowed them to cry for their very first meal. It's the default way of eating from birth, with an understanding that among individuals there will always be differences when it comes to preferences, likes, dislikes, and so on. Our ways of eating aren't exactly the same as everyone else's, and that's okay. A wide variety of foods that provide nourishment, energy, and pleasure may be ideal, but it certainly isn't going to be how every child eats. We can't force our kids to enjoy—or even eat—a wide variety of foods. But we can always keep offering new foods and modeling the enjoyment of them we hope they develop. With no pressure, the foods we are eating and enjoying can actually start to seem appealing and exciting.

NOVELTY

Just think, if you were to strip all diet thinking, nutrition rules, pressure, rewards, and punishments away from a young eater—how do you think they would eat? You might initially think, *Well, they would just choose juice and candy all day long every day!* Understandable that most parents immediately fear what their kids would choose to eat without pressure. In reality, when people have permission to eat all foods without judgment in an attuned way, we see the opposite of your worst fears—*but this unfolds over time as their relationship with food heals.* Excitement about having new permission and access to foods that were more off-limits is normal and expected. It can be quite difficult for parents to sit with the way the removal of restrictions around food are often followed by a period of overeating or, in some cases, bingeing. However, the more we continue to allow food with unconditional permission, the less of that brand-new appeal a food has. It's like a new toy right after a holiday: at first, it's super exciting and the child will carry it everywhere. But soon that excitement has worn off and they might even forget about that toy, but as soon as you try to give it away, they want it again. Both adults and kids will have a similar reaction to food in the process of Intuitive Eating. Similarly, the removal of pressure with a child who is more of an avoidant eater might lead to less variety and less food intake initially, but over time they will feel more comfortable to eat according to what they need and feel more relaxed and calmer around food, knowing there is no more pressure.

Children who have experienced food deprivation or semi-starvation may seem as though they are eating past comfortable fullness more often—this is a survival mechanism that their body has developed to keep them safe from the threat of famine. Overeating is much safer for our bodies than starving. Although some parents may understandably find this worrisome, a responsive feeding approach is the most compassionate, most healing path to helping a child who may be hoarding food, binge eating, or overeating. It may be a slow process, but it's far more likely to support long-term healing than an approach based on restriction, punishment, or overcontrol. Food is too much of a biological need to assume we can help or heal with rigidity, deprivation, or policing.

There is a period of time, typically about as long as the food was not freely available, before the food returns to an emotionally neutral place. The heightened interest we see kids (and adults) have in certain foods, let's say cake at a special occasion, is a predictable and natural response to the novelty of it. A child would likely not want to eat nothing but cake three meals a day, every day, for the long term. Also, even if they can't put words to it, or aren't really aware of it, eventually their body notices if it isn't getting certain nutritional needs met, or isn't achieving satisfaction from eating a variety of foods. Your child's appetite and cravings will change to support getting their nutritional and sensory (satisfaction) needs met.[12,13]

TWIZZLERS, CHOCOLATE MUFFINS, AND PEPPERONI STICKS

I (Sumner) enjoy eating Twizzlers, chocolate muffins, and beef jerky (pepperoni sticks, to be specific). Are you judging me yet? On any given day, I may really be craving eating those three foods and perhaps they are around. Let's say I'm on a road trip, forgot my cooler packed with lunch and snacks, and only have my Twizzlers, chocolate muffins, and pepperoni sticks from the gas station. (This is absolutely a selection of snacks I've had on a road trip, by the way.) I could eat those and enjoy and feel relatively satisfied and comfortable throughout the day, with no negative consequences. Eventually, however, if I were to experience multiple days of eating just Twizzlers, chocolate muffins, and pepperoni sticks, I would pretty quickly begin to start wanting other foods. I might also start to notice a cumulative negative impact of low energy, GI distress, fatigue, or just feeling blah. I might crave a juicy peach, a crunchy salad, a hot plate of Chinese food, or a tuna sandwich. My cravings would be changing as a result of a number of different things: (1) the wisdom of my body: I can feel that I'm not getting what I need; (2) a natural desire for a variety of tastes, textures, and temperatures within the diet; and (3) habituation theory: I would become bored eating the same thing over time and the novelty of my delicious Twizzlers, chocolate muffins, and pepperoni sticks wears off.

Children are equipped and designed (arguably even better than adults are because they haven't lived through years of environmental diet culture influencing their thoughts, eating choices, and inner critic) to eat a variety of foods. Also, notice how the three foods I ate on my road trip *do* provide a balance of macronutrients—carbohydrates from the Twizzlers and muffin, protein from the pepperoni, and fat from the muffin—yet, alas, macronutrient balance alone isn't enough to lead to satisfaction. *Satisfaction is the hook of Intuitive Eating.* This is the most common flaw in thinking we see from weight-loss experts and nutritionists: meal plans designed for weight loss are provided to people who have been sold the idea that they can simply cut calories, lose weight, and keep it off, with no acknowledgment of the importance of satisfaction.

FULLNESS VS. SATISFACTION

When you're craving something—like a slice of fresh-baked bread—and you attempt to replace it with a lower-calorie, more "diet-friendly" option, you aren't going to be satisfied unless that was in fact all you were hungry for. You might be full from food, but full isn't the same as satisfied. You can feel very full from a big bowl of steamed broccoli, but despite your fullness you may continue to seek something else to eat because you're not satisfied. Satisfaction isn't just about getting macronutrient needs met; it's much more complex. The internal system of satiety hormones, energy needs, and hunger signaling is profoundly accurate and the basis of why we need to lean into the idea of trusting one's body and appetite more than external rules of what is "healthy" and "unhealthy." **When we aren't satisfied, there will be some kind of consequence.** Usually, the outcome is overcompensating, "cheating on the diet," and for the vast majority of people, weight gain over time as the body strives to protect and defend itself from a state of caloric restriction. That weight gain is protective, based in survival and adaptation, and, for so many people who have dieted or lacked access to enough food, *life-saving.*

HOW WE THINK ABOUT FOOD MATTERS—A LOT!

We have talked a lot about what happens when we use pressure, coercion, restriction, or punishment to try to control our child's eating. It's interesting to add one more layer, though: *how our thoughts about food matter.* When a child has only had a forced-to-eat relationship with broccoli, they'll eventually develop some thoughts about broccoli that are not likely to be very positive. Other kinds of thoughts are also very powerful over our perceived experiences. One study investigated just how much mindset matters. Participants, on two occasions, were given a milkshake, and all shakes were the same 380 calories. Participants were told they were getting either a low-calorie "sensible" shake (140 calories) or an "indulgent" shake (620 calories). Researchers measured ghrelin in the participants' blood at three points—baseline, when they were anticipating the shake, and after drinking it. Ghrelin is a hunger hormone that is higher during hunger and typically decreases after eating, playing a role in appetite suppression telling the brain it's okay to stop eating. It's part of the communication system that signals to us we've had enough. What they found was astounding. When participants believed they had "indulged," they had a steeper decline in ghrelin levels, and when they believed they had been given the "sensible" lower-calorie shake, they produced a relatively flat ghrelin response.[14] In our work with clients, and in our own experiences from dieting, this makes a lot of sense. When people believe they haven't "overeaten," or believe "they've been good" because they ate the low-calorie ice cream instead of the full-fat version, they are more likely to keep eating, and this could have something to do with the possibility that our satiety hormones aren't just physiologically but psychologically induced.

NO CONTROL NEEDED

Both the psychological evidence of the approaches and theories we discussed earlier, responsive feeding, social determinants of health, psychological reactance theory, and the body of Intuitive Eating research, have formed a growing acceptance and understanding in the field about how to raise an Intuitive Eater. Without pressure—and with an adequate amount and variety of foods and a loving, connected feeding relationship—we can trust our children to know how much to eat. When we attempt to use pressure, rigidity, punishment, or shame, it backfires because our amazing little people are wired to assert their autonomy, trust their emotional signals, and heed the desires of their brilliant bodies.

WRAPPING UP PART 2

Pause here, and remember you're not alone. Diet culture is insidious, and many parents are stressed and confused about feeding their kids and want to do more to support a healthy relationship with food. You can do this imperfectly and still help your child. As parents, we are doing all of this with humility, imperfection, and self-compassion.

You're not required to be an Intuitive Eater—you're free to do whatever feels right for you.

It's possible to support your child with Intuitive Eating without being an experienced Intuitive Eater yourself. It takes time, sometimes years, for the change from dieter to natural Intuitive Eater to set in. The timeline will be different for everyone and there's no need to compare yourself to anyone else. Although it can take time, you can certainly experience benefits and freedom and peace very quickly once you start working on it, while also role modeling Intuitive Eating for your child before you feel like you've mastered it.

If you have no desire to be an Intuitive Eater yourself, aren't ready to give up dieting, or maybe don't identify with that label at all, you have every right to do what you want to do. Some of your behaviors of dieting, as mentioned earlier, will be visible and influence your child, but there is a lot you can do to reduce harm and express a more neutral attitude around your child just by changing how you talk about your eating and your body out loud. You should never feel guilty about how you decide to eat or take care of yourself, even if that includes dieting. Although we hope more people can move toward body appreciation, self-care through Intuitive Eating, and modeling that you value well-being over controlling your weight, we completely recognize that this doesn't feel like a choice for everyone.

Be aware of not turning Intuitive Eating into another diet or more rules. Nearly everyone who comes to find healing through Intuitive Eating has had prior experiences of dieting, food rules, and external direction telling them what, when, and how much to eat.

Stay true to your intentions and the reasons why you picked up this book in the first place. Be aware of how easy it could be to turn Intuitive Eating into another set of rules. Intuitive Eating isn't a "hunger and fullness" diet that means you can only eat when you're hungry enough and have to stop when you're full. Put conscious effort into tuning in to your body and trusting that your child can tune in to theirs, rather than getting fixated on how to do Intuitive Eating the "right way." If you ever start to feel anxious or unsure about what to do, take a few breaths, slow down, and ask yourself, *How am I feeling? What do I need in this moment?*

Think about the experience of eating from your child's point of view. How would it feel if someone told you, "You can have permission to eat whatever you want and need, *but* you must only eat when you're *actually* hungry and don't overeat!" You can probably recognize how this statement feels very controlling, and triggers a desire to rebel. That is exactly how both adults and children respond to any "rules" mode of eating, and it's true that even when practicing Intuitive Eating, if it's based on the goal of weight loss or "being good," there will be a reason to psychologically rebel and you'll feel like Intuitive Eating doesn't work.

Even a statement like *Are you really hungry for that? But you just ate!* can imply that your child isn't really allowed to eat unless they are "really hungry." Upon hearing this type of controlling statement, anyone may feel tempted to disconnect and be dishonest about how they feel in order to escape the feeling of overcontrol that comes from a rule about only being able to eat when hungry.

Here are some ways we have found people unintentionally turn Intuitive Eating into another diet (and diets are designed to fail and make you feel inadequate, so, don't believe these rules!):

RULE: You can only eat when you're hungry.

TRUTH: You have permission to eat whenever you want to! You can decide what will work best for you.

RULE: You have to stop eating at the "right" time to avoid feeling uncomfortable fullness.

TRUTH: You get to decide when you're satisfied and when the right time to stop is for you. You're allowed to stop eating something if it doesn't taste good anymore and you're allowed to keep eating past full if it's yummy and feels good for you to do so.

RULE: If you got uncomfortably hungry, you did something wrong.

TRUTH: There are lots of reasons why you may have been overly hungry when you ate—maybe you didn't have food with you, you were busy, distracted, more hungry than usual, and so on. It's a predictable and healthy body and brain response to want to eat fast, eat a lot, or eat sweet and dense foods when your brain is very hungry. If you want to, learn from what happened, and move on.

RULE: If you ate something that didn't make you feel well, you did something wrong.

TRUTH: No one can always predict how a food will make them feel. Don't judge yourself. Take note, take care of yourself, and move on.

RULE: If you are having chips, candy, ice cream, or another "junk" food, you have to pair it with a meal or more "healthy" snack.

TRUTH: Planning ahead can be great if you're a planner, but flexible, spontaneous eating is part of what is so great about having a peaceful relationship with food—enjoy what you want, when you want it.

RULE: Emotional eating isn't allowed in Intuitive Eating.

TRUTH: Emotional eating can be one way of soothing or coping in difficult times. With mindfulness and permission, you can decide how it looks for you to eat for emotional reasons, or to try to cope in another way. If you eat to cope, you aren't bad, you're just coping. All-or-nothing thinking around this can be very tricky and lead to feelings of guilt and shame for even having cravings, which ultimately adds another layer of emotional pain and suffering. This second layer of emotions is likely to end up in complete disconnection from your emotions and your body, often becoming the binge cycle for many people. So, go ahead, have the food if you want it. Think about really meeting all your needs, physiological for food, as well as any other psychological and emotional needs.

RULE: If you binged, you've done something wrong.

TRUTH: This happened for a reason. A binge itself isn't the problem; it's signaling that something else needed your attention or that your body needed to make up for missed food. Every binge has a message and a purpose even if it didn't feel good. What can you learn from what happened? What did you really need? What caused you to need to disconnect from your physical sensations or mindfulness?

RULE: You'll always want to eat the same thing in the same way as you ate it last time.

TRUTH: It's hard to predict what you will want to eat in advance. Sometimes the very same food you had at your favorite restaurant last time will not taste as great the second time you order it. Be flexible, be open, and remember that not every eating experience has to be a five-star experience. You won't always need the same amount of food for lunch, breakfast, or dinner—*try to eat for the present moment,* not for the past or the future.

PAUSE AND REFLECT

- *What fears do you have around Intuitive Eating for yourself and your child?*
- *Do you notice ways you may be overcontrolling with food? Do you notice a lack of structure or boundaries? What are the emotions and moods surrounding family mealtimes? How will these work in the short term? What about in the long term?*

- *As you start to be aware of potential stressful events that cause you to be rigid and strict with food, what would you list as a few scenarios that you can be mentally prepared for?*

ANNA'S STORY

Anna grew up in a house where thinness was equated with healthiness. There was (and is) a copious amount of health anxiety that drove disordered behaviors. This anxiety shaped the way that Anna and her siblings were raised around food. Even to this day, despite knowing the Intuitive Eating path that she is on now, Anna's mom will still comment on weight gain or loss, and has always been ecstatic when Anna lost weight—no matter how it happened.

Anna states that if you were to ask her mom about diet culture in their house growing up she would deny it. She firmly believed that the rules she imposed were all about nutrition and health. The amount of food wasn't restricted, but the types certainly were. Cookies and other yummy food weren't kept in the house because "no one could control themselves." Anna remembers going to her aunt and uncle's house, where all kinds of foods were available. She would eat so much there that they nicknamed her "Hoover."

Anna's parents didn't really officially diet until she was a teenager, when they joined Weight Watchers. They didn't push the diet on the kids, but they did all eat dinners that were made based on "points." When Anna got into high school, her mom encouraged her to join Weight Watchers as well. This was about as explicit as the messages got.

However, the implicit messages were all around. There were always comments about eating too much sugar, not eating enough vegetables, "being bad," or eating the wrong foods. And messages from her mom about how ashamed she was for eating foods she enjoyed eating. The message was there: you need to be healthy, and in order to be healthy, you must be skinny. It all came down to "health" and "nutrition." This implicit message also came from the way her mom treated her own body. She was always making negative comments about her size, wearing clothes that "flattered" or hid her body. This message was quite clear too: her body was never good enough. Even though no one said this directly to her,

Anna knew how it was supposed to be. You were an adult and you hated your body.

Anna believes her mom's health anxiety came from her own mother. Anna's mom didn't think of her own mother as the "epitome of health." She often drank alcohol and didn't put much structure into her children's food. Anna's mom would often make comments about how lucky they all were that she fed them vegetables because her own mom often didn't. She would talk about the unhealthy food she was served as a kid. Anna heard the message that her grandma didn't care about health enough to prepare healthy food.

Anna developed disordered eating for many years after this, with weight loss resulting in praise from her mom and weight gain resulting in censure. She reached a point where she decided to seek help and found an Intuitive Eating– and Health at Every Size–based dietitian to help her change her attitude toward food.

Anna now feels like she is doing all of the unpacking and emotional work that her mom hasn't done. She has a toddler now and she doesn't want to feed him according to her own anxiety. She started learning about feeding kids and raising them without issues around food and heard *Let them eat when they want and how they want* and thought, *Well, who's going to teach me how to do that?* This is all coupled with the differences in the way her husband was raised around food. He had very little structure and was rarely given vegetables or fruits. As an adult, he wishes it could have been different. This has put Anna and her family in a position to learn balance between negative control and providing structure and variety for kids. Anna has had plenty of concerns about her toddler's food (he loves carbs and rarely eats vegetables), but she has been able to reassure herself that it's normal. Anna is still working out how to cope with her internal fatphobia, especially the kind she feels that makes her want to protect her child from living in a fatphobic society and family. She doesn't want him to experience the marginalization that Anna, herself, has felt, but also doesn't want him to develop the same disordered eating that she did.

She wishes that she had known how little control you have over your child; it's actually something she still says to herself on a daily basis. Even though she wants to protect her child from as much adversity as she can, she knows that she "can't force him to like broccoli." Anna told us, "As a parent your product is your kid and you're being judged for everything your kid does." She knows that the internal fatphobia she holds allows space for fear about the judgment that would come if her son were fat later in life. And she believes her mom is ashamed that Anna is fat now. But she would "rather be fat and happy."

All the aspects of raising an Intuitive Eater feel so foreign when compared to the way she was raised, yet she knows that it's how she wants to raise her son. She knows she grew up with a lack of trust in her own body and she wants to change that for herself and help ensure her son never feels that way.

PART III

EMBRACING A NEW PATH: THE 3 KEYS

Now we've reached the point where we can dig into the heart and soul about the "how" of raising an Intuitive Eater. Each of the 3 Keys, all equally important, provides guidance around an area that plays into the big picture of how we support our kids and their innate Intuitive Eating wisdom. In the next few chapters, you'll have the chance to learn all about the specific ways to model behavior, the logistics of feeding kids, ways to support your child in processing and responding to their emotions with kindness, and how you can use your own voice to build compassionate self-talk that impacts the development of their own inner thoughts about food and body.

AUTOPILOT OR MANUAL: THE POWER OF INTENTIONALLY CREATING SPACE

Creating space for new behaviors is a way we can start to shift to making these intentional changes in our life. As you take in the 3 Keys, we'd like to introduce you to a helpful tool for implementing any new behaviors and processes you'll learn.

If there is one simple phrase to hold with you throughout the process of implementing these new behaviors as part of the 3 Keys (or *any* new behavior) it's this: *choose your response to what happens, instead of reacting out of habit.* This phrase, along with self-compassion, is one of the most important things to hold with you throughout the process of raising an Intuitive Eater and parenting.

Psychologists and researchers in the fields of parenting, mental health, behavior change, and related fields have been studying the impact that pausing before reacting has on our ability to change and grow, particularly in the area of behavior change for decades. With many behaviors, we are acting out of habit and conditioning. It's one of the ways the human brain is really good at learning and being effective. We have the ability to repeat behaviors until they become nearly automatic. This reaction-without-thought is commonly known as "autopilot."

There are plenty of ways that you go into autopilot every day. You wake up in the morning and you check the clock, brush your teeth, or make your coffee or tea. To drive somewhere, you get in the driver's seat, put on your seat belt, foot on the brake, and check your mirrors. When you first learned to type on a keyboard, you were very slow, and had to be careful and intentional—now, typing is automatic. Those are some obvious ways we go on autopilot and there are likely ways that autopilot kicks in around food, body, and even self-talk for you. How might you be acting on autopilot when it comes to feeding your kids?

What is your typical response when your child asks for a food that you might consider a "treat," like candy, cookies, or dessert? Is it *Sure, can I help get it for you?* Is it *No, you don't need that,* or something like *That's not healthy, choose something healthy?* Do you notice that you say something out of habit, without really considering the situation? Perhaps that is your response because it's what you were told when you asked for food as a child?

There may be many automatic reactions and behaviors that are related to food and body that you're already starting to notice. Something else you probably have noticed is that these automatic behaviors aren't going to change just because you're reading this book. *We need to evolve from "autopilot" to "manual pilot" in order for the changes you want to make to become habitual.* After a period of time of repeating new behaviors in "manual pilot," they may become easy enough that they are "autopilot" behaviors—just like checking your rearview mirror when driving. "Autopilot" doesn't mean bad—just habitual. No one wants to be constantly thinking about every decision you ever make. Learning the 3 Keys is one thing, but actually *implementing* them and making them your new approach for the long term is something else entirely. To reach your goal of raising an Intuitive Eater, it will take some time, practice, and mindfulness about the basic practice of creating space between what happens (like when your kid asks for something to eat or any other number of stimuli) and how you respond (your new behavior). This mindful change is what it takes to shift from "autopilot" to "manual pilot."

How do you take that intention and turn it into actually shifting gears? The way we act after a stimulus can happen in two different ways: we can **react** or we can **respond**.

React: stimulus (*something happens*)—**reaction** (*what you do out of habit*): In this mode, there is no space to think or even access the logic you might need to choose a "manual pilot" action. Reactions are automatic and habitual. This is autopilot behavior, and sometimes it's super useful! (Think about typing, driving, changing a diaper, or reading, just to name some examples.) Our brains are highly skilled at doing things in autopilot mode. Sometimes it's the reaction that we have had for so long when our child asks for an extra snack or a piece of candy.

Respond: stimulus (*something happens*)—**SPACE** (*the breath to choose your next action*)—**response** (*intentional choice*): In this mode, by working on mindfulness and intentionally taking a breath and making the choice, you can *choose how you want to respond*. This is manual pilot behavior: it's how we choose our response mindfully, instead of reacting. It can feel strange to intentionally make a choice that isn't what your "autopilot" is used to making, but we can start to have the responses we actually want. "Manual pilot" can feel challenging at first and it takes a lot of energy. However, the more you live mindfully in "manual pilot" mode, the less energy it takes, and you may realize it can provide a lot of benefits. Over time, we can shift from "manual pilot" into "autopilot" for the behaviors and changes we actually want in our lives—we are creating new "autopilot" behaviors. Most importantly, it's not an either/or scenario. "Autopilot" and mindfulness can coexist and are both important to this process.

Responding instead of reacting is a powerful and effective way to approach behavior change. Applying the technique of taking the *space* to make an intentional choice allows us, as parents, to change the way our kids perceive certain things. My (Amee) daughter will sometimes walk up to me and say, "I know you're going to say no, but . . ." and I know the end of that question is something I need to check with myself. Is that something that I want her to assume I'll say no to? Or is it something I want to keep neutral and not make off-limits? That's the beauty of responding instead of reacting. Her assumption that I will say no means that I have reacted that way in the past and maybe I will keep saying no. But maybe it's an "autopilot" reaction I've had in the past that I am ready to change. In the space between reacting and responding, I can decide based on my priorities, values, and goals. (We'll learn more about values later.)

Taking even just a couple seconds to breathe before deciding what you'll say or do next creates a mindful and intentional space. Even with a few seconds, you suddenly have time to assess the situation, look at your choices, and make a decision that is going to help you hold your intentions. This is one of the best ways we can effectively help ourselves create long-term behavior change, through committed action.[1] By consistently making new decisions that are more aligned with your goal, you're able to help your brain respond differently *automatically*. Greeting your challenges and decisions with the intention of creating space before you respond is a form of *mindfulness*. Intuitive Eating is a way of eating and living that relies on mindfulness. We have to be present in order to tune in to our bodies, to choose our responses to what we hear, and particularly to model behaviors we want to teach our children. Remembering to switch to "manual pilot" is an incredibly important practice to implement again and again while making the changes needed to raise an Intuitive Eater.

THE FOUNDATION OF THE 3 KEYS

The 3 Keys of raising an Intuitive Eater are a way to bring the principles of Intuitive Eating into parenting. As we explained in the introduction, Intuitive Eating is a dynamic interplay of emotions, instincts, and thoughts. These are the three significant areas of your child's experience that we focus on with the 3 Keys: their emotions, instincts, and thoughts. Raising an Intuitive Eater isn't as simple as giving guidelines for what and when to feed your child. There isn't a magic trick that will make your kid prefer spinach over chocolate. We also can't guide you by only addressing the emotional side of eating and feeding. We can't talk about any of these things without contributing some practical strategies, language, and responsive feeding techniques that can help you with the million different ways your child might eat, express needs, feel emotions, and respond to what they see on the plate in front of them. We need to see that the 3 Keys all work together, addressing emotions, instincts, and thoughts.

> Each of the keys can be viewed as an umbrella, and within each key you'll find a general overview, the science to support the information provided, practical strategies for how to do this at home, and stories about what this has actually looked like for real people.

3 Keys:
How to Raise an Intuitive Eater

1 Provide unconditional love and support for your child's body

2 Implement a flexible and reliable feeding routine

3 Develop and use your intuitive eating voice

KEY 1: PROVIDE UNCONDITIONAL LOVE AND SUPPORT FOR YOUR CHILD'S BODY

This key is first because we believe (according to the stages of cognitive development) that for a person to develop their own inner trust, body appreciation, self-care, and self-compassion, they need to have received it from a reliable caregiver and had their needs met from an early age. Otherwise, in order to heal their relationship with food, they will need to repair and revisit what was not established previously by a primary caregiver. This key is about more than just talking about food; it includes things that greatly impact eating: emotional agility and attunement, respecting body diversity, and promoting a connected relationship between parent and child. It may sound like plain common sense to many parents—of course you love your child unconditionally, and you want to help them learn to be resilient and flexible! But we want to dial in on how we may be *unintentionally* putting conditions on our love. We also have to acknowledge that not every parent has experienced unconditional love around their body; we weren't all modeled or taught to not abandon ourselves when things get hard. As parents, if we don't have these skills ourselves, it can be difficult to offer them to a child. Key 1 emphasizes how you can stay tuned in to your child's experiences, including the experiences around their body and eating to help them build a connected and compassionate view of their eating and their body, leading to them sensing your unconditional love and support for *their* whole self. This fosters the ability to maintain that same love for themselves.

KEY 2: IMPLEMENT A FLEXIBLE AND RELIABLE FEEDING ROUTINE

Incorporating nutrition science, a compassion-focused responsive feeding approach, Division of Responsibility, and flexibility, this key drives home the practical strategies that many parents are eager to hear about. Key 2 offers the how-to's of an *add-in, pressure-off approach*. The flexible feeding routine is a go-to starting point for many adults who enter into healing their own relationship with food, and it's equally vital for children to have a similar routine. Eating regularly, feeding your body with compassion and permission, while not implementing rigid diet-like rules, are foundational for *anyone* when it comes to Intuitive Eating. Many assumptions about Intuitive Eating for kids state that it sounds like "the absence of a plan" or "only feeding your child what sounds good to them in the moment." (*Yikes! These sound like nerve-wracking approaches to feeding kids.*) Key 2 debunks these inaccurate assumptions and provides clarity around what you can do. The feeding routine is important because it ensures adequate and reliable food that is hopefully tasty, familiar, and satisfying. It allows children to rely on and trust their hunger and satiety instincts, while suggesting that caregivers fulfill their role in providing the food.

KEY 3: DEVELOP AND USE YOUR INTUITIVE EATING VOICE

What children hear is what becomes their inner voice. Many adult clients have shared with us that their inner story—*the automatic thoughts they have about their body and eating*—sounds very similar to what they heard as a child from a caregiver or another influential adult. Sometimes these phrases were not directed at them at all, but they heard their parent saying something to themselves, which then developed into their inner dialogue and thought pattern. As parents, what we say, the language we use—whether it's directed at our own body, our child's body, or someone else's body—is incredibly influential. Key 3 explains the power of developing and using your Intuitive Eating voice, which, in turn, becomes your child's Intuitive Eating voice for life.

KEY 1

Provide Unconditional Love and Support for Your Child's Body

Unconditional love and support for your child's body provides them the opportunity to believe that no matter what their body looks like, you believe they are worthy and lovable.

You do unconditionally love your child, and . . . unconditional love and support *specifically for your child's body* may not be something you have ever thought about. Could it also be true that you aren't aware of how your own anxiety or dissatisfaction with your body, or your childhood body—or any number of the other million life circumstances related to your relationship with your body—creates unintentional messaging that may come across to your child that you may not have unconditional love for their current body?

We would have a small fortune if we had a dollar for every time an adult or teen client came in seeking support for disordered eating and body image distress and shared something along the lines of *I know my mom/dad/parents really genuinely love me, but . . .*

They never let me eat any of the "good" stuff that other parents let their
  kids eat.
They were always talking badly about their own bodies and weight, which
  made me feel really self-conscious about my own.
They were always warning me against gaining weight.
They frequently emphasized the consequences of not eating "healthy" enough.
They always said things that made me feel my appearance and my grades were
  more important than anything else.
They forced me to finish everything on my plate and in my cup.
They never talked to me directly about appreciating or respecting my body—
  not once.

The thing is, body shame isn't just a result of intentional judgment or criticism toward your child; it can develop from the beliefs and patterns that your
child experiences from you and others close to them about bodies, weight, eating,
health, and "right" and "wrong." You may never actually say anything, ever, directly to your child about their body not being good enough—they can absorb it
in nonverbal communication, observing how you treat yourself and others with
regard to their bodies and eating.

SELF-COMPASSION REMINDER: *Remembering that we are all imperfect
parents allows us to embrace the famous quote by Maya Angelou, "Do the best you
can until you know better. And when you know better, do better," and not get stuck
in our past mistakes, which most people simply do not even realize are mistakes.*

Providing unconditional love and support for your child's body means you're
doing a few important things to the extent you're able to. We use the acronym
REAL to teach the important pieces of this first key.

Reduce body shame.

Embrace their needs—
be present with your child and help them feel seen.

Accept their desires and appetite.

Love their body for the way it is today—
don't try to make it something it isn't.

Let's talk about shame. Shame shows up in many aspects of negative embodiment. Shame is like the mean yelling parent on the sidelines of your kid's basketball game—making a lot of noise but adding nothing productive. Shame interrupts the positive; it distracts us from meaning, from our purpose, and from our self-respect.

The thing is, you can't really provide unconditional love and support for your child's body if you also inadvertently or intentionally shame them for their cravings, hunger, size, or appearance. They can feel shame by the slightest action—a simple comment, a look of disappointment, or a "nice" suggestion to eat healthier. The feeling of shame can be imparted unintentionally, so even when we think we are being careful with our words, the message can still come across.

Unfortunately, there is no way to remove or erase shame from your child's lived experiences. Brené Brown, who has researched shame and written about it more than anyone we know, uncovered in her research that shame is universal; it's part of being human. It's the silence about and around shame that allows it to gain so much power over us. We have to talk about shame with our kids. As parents, we can play a role in reducing the body shame a child may feel by being open and straightforward about bodies, making space to share about bullying and teasing, and especially for questions kids have as they grow into new and different bodies through puberty and beyond.

Shame is more than just about weight or appearance. A child may experience shame from having a chronic disease such as diabetes, being neurodivergent, transgender, or nonbinary, or not feeling athletic enough, graceful enough, artistic enough, or smart enough. All of these experiences relate back to their body in some way, and feeling shame about these things will change a person's inner dialogue and the way they show up in the world. And when kids feel they aren't "good enough" in other ways, the pressure to "still look good" can markedly increase. Everyone experiences shame around their body in some way; there doesn't need to be anything unusual or particularly wrong for a person to experience shame.

When you're able to recognize the oppressive and shame-inducing structures that exist and work to reject them, you become aware and resilient. Your kids will see your unwillingness to accept these oppressions modeled to them and grow up with an understanding of how to build resilience against body shame and diet culture. The resilience you model for them will be an incredible tool helping them to know their worth as a human, despite living in a world that asks them to conform to limiting appearance standards and self-loathing.

NORMALIZING BODIES

All of our bodies do weird things that are actually only considered to be "weird" because they aren't normalized. The aspects of appearance that have truly been normalized in our culture are thinness, youth, whiteness, and attractiveness. But normalized doesn't mean that most people do or should experience these things. Skin isn't always smooth, hair is unruly, our fat jiggles and rolls. We have disabilities, cellulite, acne, stretch marks, and body hair. Bodies come in various shapes, textures, sizes, smells, and even make sounds that can trigger shame if we don't take steps to normalize them all.

One of the biggest problems we are seeing in regard to parenting and body shame in kids is that dieting and body shaming—as opposed to body appreciation—are what have been normalized. Studies estimate that half of girls and one-third of boys ages six to eight want to be thinner—the likelihood that your child of that age feels that way is shocking.[1] **We can see from observing the rates of disordered eating among young people that normalizing is in fact a very powerful influence—it's just that we have been unintentionally normalizing behaviors that are actually seriously harmful, not helpful. This normalization isn't something you did wrong; it's the way our culture has sought to suppress those who don't fit the mold.**

No one can argue when we say that most bodies simply don't look like what we see in advertisements, on social media, and on TV. Yet, if we aren't teaching our kids this, they will assume something is wrong with them when they look in the mirror and see a pimple, body hair, or weight gain. In her book *The Beauty Myth*, Naomi Wolf depicts and unpacks the complex history that generation after generation has upheld: that fat is unnatural, wrong, gross, and unhealthy. Western white culture still reproduces this today. According to Wolf, "Researchers found that parents in the United States urged boys to eat, regardless of their weight, while they did so with daughters only if they were relatively thin. In a sample of babies, 99% of the boys were breastfed, but only 66% of the girls, who were given 50 percent less time to feed." As quoted in *The Beauty Myth*, Susie Orbach wrote, "Thus, daughters are often fed less well, less attentively and less sensitively than they need."[2] Although for much of the last few centuries the beauty myth has been directed at women, it's just as oppressive toward males and people across the entire gender spectrum today. Males, in particular, are conditioned and taught not to show vulnerability, and especially not vulnerability around body image or self-esteem.

Your child is too special, too important, too much of a miracle to go through life not believing wholeheartedly that they are worthy and lovable for every single ounce of their body and being. You're the one who will prove that to them. You can help reduce their body shame—and we hope you will choose to try. We also want you to remember that you aren't responsible for eliminating their body shame, because so much more contributes to shame than just your actions and feelings.

DEMYSTIFYING OUR WEIRD BODIES

One of the things that makes kids so incredible is the ability to do things uninhibitedly, especially when it comes to what they say. Simply by being open and ready for the opportunities, you can help to demystify bodies for your child. An example is not automatically trying to shut your kids down for noticing things like cellulite, veins, wrinkles, loose skin, belly rolls, or body hair and asking you about them. If we shut down those conversations, we send the message very early on that those things aren't to be talked about and kids are left all alone to try and figure out if their body is "normal" or "good."

I (Amee) grew up with a mom who was disabled. She had polio when she was five and walked with crutches for the rest of her life. She would always notice when kids, with their lack of a filter, asked questions about her crutches or legs. She was never, ever ashamed of the questions that kids would ask—she felt shamed by the quick shutdowns and quiet shushes from parents while they avoided eye contact. We can't control the questions our kids ask or the things they see, but we can control our reactions to them.

Depending on the age of your child and their emotional maturity, try to make these conversations enjoyable and light. You don't need to sit them down (*although for some talks, yes—sit them down and get their full attention!*)—but rather think about making these conversations something that can happen on any day, at any time. That is an important part of the normalizing. Your child may say, *Mama, why do you have those weird lines on your skin?* (stretch marks), and you can say, *Oh, those lines? That's just how the universe (or God, or whatever feels right to you) made my body. I got these cool lines when I grew wider (or taller, or bigger, or had you in my belly!). Lots of people have them, and they don't bother me at all.*

The more you can practice this, the easier it will get. With your new mindfulness skills (remember: stimulus-space-response), notice the uncomfortable sensations that arise in you the first few (or twenty) times you engage and embrace these moments. That increased heart rate, tightness in your chest, or tingling skin are signs from your body that you're becoming activated—likely due to the discomfort of staying engaged in something new and uncomfortable. When you feel those sensations, instead of turning them off or shutting the conversation down, recognize that growth happens here. Then celebrate becoming braver and more confident in talking openly about bodies. The impact this can have on your kiddo as they develop and see their own body changing is profound.

Talking openly, especially if it was not modeled to you, is hard, but necessary. You want your kids to be getting their answers from you—someone they can trust, talk to, and from whom they can receive validation. In your child's mind, you're perfect, and if you, their perfect parent, still believe you're worthy and amazing even if you don't look like that impossible beauty standard, that begins to shift their perception of what beauty even looks like. *It probably looks more like you—more like them.*

YOU DON'T CONTROL ALL YOUR THOUGHTS— ONLY HOW YOU RESPOND TO THEM

Because of the cultural conditioning that you've been living in (especially if you were raised in a colonized, Western culture like the United States), you very likely have automatic thoughts about your child's body if they don't meet society's "ideal"—such as wishing they looked a certain way, wanting them to eat in a particular style to manage their weight, or wishing for them to be smart, driven, athletic, or talented. It's not your fault. These attributes earn people praise, opportunities, and power in a culture that rewards you for how you look or how productive you are. It's not that any of these things are bad—being a talented athlete, scientist, or artist can be wonderful—it's that we often don't stop to notice all the negative impacts we face as people living in a society that places so much value on appearance and productivity. Many young people feel pressure to look a certain way, earn top grades, and be high achievers. There is a cost that comes with all that pressure. Achieving a certain body appearance and health status goes along with this. When parents don't realize the toll this pressure is taking on their kids, they inadvertently add to the pressure. Support your kids, but see them for who they are, not who you wish they were.

All in all, demystifying bodies, normalizing real bodies (body parts, body functions, body curiosity), and choosing mindfully how you want to respond with your child all contribute to reducing shame for them. You can't save them from ever experiencing shame, or from body dissatisfaction (remember, these are universal experiences), but you can take steps to help them build resilience against it.

E: EMBRACE THEIR NEEDS

As their caregiver, it's your role to help get your child's needs met and to validate that their needs are important. Back to the stages of psychological development, when babies and very young children experience having their needs met (emotionally and physically), they successfully acquire the virtue of hope. They trust that when they are in need, someone will be there to help them fulfill their needs. As your child grows and matures, they eventually get to take over more and more of their own caretaking, and can meet their own needs in many ways. **When a trusted caregiver isn't around to fulfill a child's emotional or physical needs, this experience can begin a cycle of turning to food to cope and to soothe.** We need to fully tune in to our kids, try to meet their needs, and help them feel seen. This has nothing to do with managing body size, and everything to do with demonstrating our care and commitment as they are growing into their mature selves.

How does ensuring your child feels seen help with their relationship to food and their body? When we fail to see them, they could fail to fulfill their primal human need for belonging. As humans, we are built to be with others, to be in community, and to belong. From an evolutionary standpoint, many of the behaviors we inherently act on are designed to "keep us in the clan." Thousands of years ago, when every single person had a role to play in safety and survival, to be cast out from the clan meant certain death. Today, although we no longer live in clans and we have resources (and the internet) and beds to sleep in and grocery stores to shop at—we are still biologically wired to rely on a sense of emotional belonging.

In a busy world where we all are juggling life's demands, working, paying bills, managing kids, doctor visits, preparing food, laundry, caring for elderly parents, attending spiritual or religious gatherings, connecting with others, having a little downtime, sleep, and all the other things—parents often feel unable or unwilling to be fully present and tuned in to their child's needs. *You're doing the best you can,* and for many valid reasons, you may not have been tuned in to some (or maybe even a lot) of your child's emotional needs. Tuning in to your child's emotional needs is the emphasis in this key because it may be easier for a lot of us to meet our child's physical needs—food, shelter, safety, safe transportation—than to find the energy and the capacity to tune in to their emotional needs. Our kids will often do anything they can to avoid being a "burden" and may even seek to help us and take care of us when we are stretched too thin. This is why we have to do whatever we can to bring ourselves back—again and again—to the truth that our kids need us: they need us to tune in and really see them. When we fail to consistently tune in and come back to them, they can begin to lose trust that they are worthy of our love, time, and attention, and that narrative can begin to sneak in as their internal truth.

We aren't experts in parenting and we don't claim to have all the answers. We have, however, utilized the groundwork that has already been laid by actual experts. One of these critical pieces of groundwork we have to include in the 3 Keys to raising an Intuitive Eater was created by Dan Siegel and Tina Payne Bryson in their book *The Power of Showing Up*.[3] It's their model called the Triad of Connection.

THE TRIAD OF CONNECTION: HELP KIDS FEEL SEEN

Truly seeing our kids, as Siegel and Bryson write, is about three things:

1. Attuning to their internal mental state in a way that lets them know that we "get" them so they can "feel felt" and understood on a profound and meaningful level.
2. Coming to understand their inner life by using our imagination to make sense of what is actually going on inside their mind.
3. Responding in what's called a "contingent" way, where we respond to what we see in a timely and effective manner.

We can apply the Triad of Connection to how we respond and relate to our kids' styles and patterns of eating. In fact, when you truly tune in, you can see that when there has been a disruption in your child's Intuitive Eating, food and eating may be filling a need they have to soothe or distract or seek pleasure, or even serving as a form of nonverbal communication. Parents often understand the necessity of applying this kind of awareness to their kids' behavior everywhere else—but not to their eating behavior. Parents, thanks to diet culture, generally believe that eating is something that should be strictly unrelated to emotions and should be purely about nutrition or "health" rules. We know that most parents do not feel that the way they encourage their kids to eat is "diet minded"—the emphasis is on health. But often, health and "healthy eating" conversations have been overtaken by diet culture. The idea that eating should not be emotional is problematic—eating is often very much tied to emotions—and when you notice your child eating, then shame them for it and label it as "lazy, unnecessary, or wrong," you add another layer of shame on top of what may have been the reason for their emotional eating in the first place. This becomes complicated to unpack and even more complex for them to make sense of. Even many adults aren't able to easily make sense of their eating patterns in response to mood, emotions, and coping.

Your child's eating and your response to their eating becomes a bidirectional relationship. Your concern about their eating causes you to have a certain reaction, which continues to fuel the behavior you're worried about.

BRADEN'S STORY

Braden's story is a common one that we've heard many times in our work with families.

Eleven-year-old Braden is experiencing a difficult day at school and comes home feeling really bad. He doesn't feel seen or validated upon getting home from school—everyone is too busy or too preoccupied with other things to stop and care and listen to what his day was like. In response to feeling upset with no caring connection to help him process the disappointment, Braden turns to food to escape, relax, numb, soothe, or cover up the uncomfortable emotions. Soon after, a parent comes along and notices his eating; they assume this is simply a poor choice, and make a comment about his choice to eat "junk food."

A second layer of emotional suffering (shame about his eating) is added to Braden's first layer of suffering (a hard day at school), and he's now feeling guilty for eating in a way his parent was not approving of, and he may even be in trouble for it.

Braden might think, *I can't do anything right. I'm so bad for eating this way. Everyone hates me*, all while feeling alone, unseen, unworthy, and unlovable. It's very easy for Braden to ignore his emotional needs, and instead focus on his eating behavior, blaming himself, the food, and his body, instead of recognizing what really happened, which was: he was unconsciously attempting to soothe and comfort himself in the midst of difficult feelings.

Braden's parents weren't really seeing him—they assumed there was no underlying reason for his eating, and not only have they unintentionally made their child feel worse, they also have still not really seen the initial problem that was impacting him in the first place. This is a double layering of not tuning in, and adding shame on top.

Using the Triad of Connection, you can perceive, make sense of, and respond to what you see in your child's behavior. Don't react to eating behaviors; create some space when you notice your urge to react, and try to understand what could be going on that is leading your child to feel the need to use food to cope or soothe. If you notice they may be eating to soothe or eating for reasons other than hunger, direct your attention to finding out what they need, what the source of their discomfort is, and what you can do to support them, and resist any urge to talk about their eating during a vulnerable time. *The eating isn't a behavior to fix; it's actually a very understandable human response to an unmet need—we want to check in with our child and really see what it is they're trying to self-soothe for.* If they are open with you about their eating, telling you they're upset about it, be curious and non-judgmental. Most importantly, don't collude with diet mentality if they suggest to you they want to try to lose weight or eat healthier. Simply remind them they can eat however feels best for their body, in a way that is satisfying, enjoyable, and energizing. Check in with why they may be feeling compelled to diet or alter the way they are eating, as this can be a response to bullying, stress, or other negative situations too.

As often as you can, actively tune in to what your child is able to share from their day—really listen. Pay attention to nonverbal cues, their mood, and eye contact. As Siegel and Bryson write, "use your imagination," act like an investigator and try to make sense of what you see—*Does my child need anything from me right now? How can I show up for them at this moment?*

If you have a child who seems to have moved away from eating for hunger and you suspect they are using food to help calm, soothe, distract, or cope, do not make your attempt to connect with them be about the food or about any concern about their weight. The intention should be to show up for them, to listen to what they're going through, to understand and accept that food may in fact be what is helping them and to know that's okay.

If tuning in and really seeing your child isn't the way you have been able to interact with them, it's never too late to change that. *It may take time to right this ship, but you can do it.* Over time, they will begin to feel you are there for them, and their shame around eating will start to lessen.

If you notice any similarities between what was happening with Braden's family and your family:

1. Stop commenting on the food—try to avoid verbal or nonverbal body language communication about your concern around their eating or weight. It's vital to stop food shaming and food policing as much as you can, because this fuels the need for any person, especially a child or teen, to rebel and use food to send a message of asserting their autonomy. They will be naturally driven to do what they are being policed by you not to do.

2. Ask yourself to commit to tuning in—pay attention, and be there for them emotionally. Expect that it will take time for them to trust that things are shifting. *You do not have to be perfect at this.* For some kiddos, especially if this pattern of emotional unmet needs has been happening for many years, there may need to be space to work with a family therapist who can help you repair the emotional broken bridges. We encourage you to seek out support, and invest in doing that work if you can with a weight inclusive care–informed therapist who will not offer weight loss advice.

A: ACCEPT THEIR DESIRES

Remember when we talked about Victoria and Avery and sugar in chapter 4? Through her work with an Intuitive Eating counselor, Victoria acknowledged her inner story, that her own childhood shame of eating sugary foods and feeling bad for having wanted sweets was what was causing her to worry so much about her own young daughter's drive for sweets. Yes, it's true that Avery happened to be a child who was drawn to sweet foods, yet she also was eating enough of other things, had no health or growth concerns, and was doing just fine as a kid who enjoys sweets.

Desires and cravings are very primal. We actually don't know exactly what causes some kids to be highly driven toward sugary foods and others to have very little interest. What we do know is that diet culture has taught us a narrative of shame around this tendency, and parents often make sense of this by thinking they have somehow done something to cause their child to love—or be "addicted to"—sugar. (Remember that sugar, glucose, is what our brains and muscles use for energy—we need it, and it isn't "a waste of calories" to consume sugar. You'll have a chance to learn more about this later.) We also need other nutrients to thrive, and therefore we need some sugar and other foods and nutrients. Many parents develop this misunderstanding that they have somehow created their child's preferences for sweets, and that it's within their control to change them back to "healthy" preferences. This isn't true, and there's nothing wrong with kids who have a natural tendency to prefer and enjoy sweet foods. Negative parental control, restricting, or a strong emotional reaction to their child's desires is what is likely to cause an unhealthy relationship with certain foods, not the food itself. When your child learns they are "wrong" or "bad" for liking the foods they like, they will learn how to avoid your reaction and escape feelings of shame by learning to sneak food, hide food, and eat it when you can't see them. They will then likely develop a secondary level of emotional stress, which is feeling guilty for doing something you would not approve of, simply because sugar has been demonized. Reading this, we bet you can envision just how the process of developing disordered eating builds on itself: shame, guilt, desires, shame, guilt, desires . . . and the cycle goes on.

It will make most parents uncomfortable to relax about food, but you can do this. When your child exhibits a desire, lean into it with them. Ask them what they really want. Discuss when might be the next right time to have the food. Assure them that if they can't—or don't—have it now, they will have a chance another time. Allow foods—even sugary ones—to be available often. Can you enjoy it together, or add it to next week's menu? This may sound like a small act, but embracing and accepting your child's desire for pleasurable food (or something else they desire) is an act of seeing them, of stripping away the shame of food pleasure, and of allowing them to know they can have it if they want it and they don't need to feel bad about it.

L: LOVE THEIR BODY FOR THE WAY IT IS TODAY

The moment a child believes their body is no longer making you proud, or isn't acceptable to you, they will have also lost pride in their body. Your approval, affirmation, love, and support are the foundation for your child to have a loving relationship with their own body.

Most parents do not want their kids to feel like their worth is based on their body. However, we may also feel afraid for what will happen to them if they exist in a body that isn't deemed "good" or "healthy" enough. You can make sure your child knows that they will be worthy and loved by you no matter what their body looks like. By doing this, you provide them the chance to experience life on their own terms.

Examples of ways we accidentally place conditions on love through our attitudes on food and body:

- Overemphasizing physical traits, like mostly complimenting them on appearance or looks.
- Praising things that are out of their control, like appearance, quality of clothing/things.
- Punishing or shaming a child for something they ate out of fear it will cause weight gain or is "unhealthy" or "gluttonous."
- Spending more money/time on siblings who do sports than on those who enjoy nonphysical activities.
- Talking about how we, as adults, have to look a certain way or are only going to find success/attention/friendship/love if we are more attractive.
- Discussing other people's bodies in a derogatory way (For example, *Too bad she looks like . . .*).

When we place conditions on love, even accidentally, we make our kids feel as if they will be less worthy, less lovable, if they don't meet those conditions. Our society already places these conditions on us all—but we can either reinforce them or help our kids question the truth of these conditions.

MODELING KEY 1

Modeling Key 1 comes in the form of, you guessed it, expressing unconditional love and support for *your own* body. Does that make you want to run and hide? (You're not alone.) This is absolutely the opposite of how our culture indoctrinates us to feel toward our own bodies. We are told hundreds, if not thousands, of times a day that we're too unhealthy, we have too many wrinkles, and we ought to be constantly striving to improve our health, appearance, and productivity. Thank you, capitalism and the patriarchy. Actually—*no, thank you.* We've had quite enough of this and are completely ready to *stop passing this on* to the next generation. If we pass our dieting legacies on to the next generation, we continue to add fuel to the fire where our dreams (and soon after, our kids' dreams), desires, and voices go to disappear. It's possible to pursue wellness and health if you want to, without buying into the idea that you have to look a certain way or eat a certain way. Health isn't something you can see.

Expressing the same amount of kindness and compassion for your body as you want to for your child's body may, at times, feel like one of the hardest things for you to do, *especially if you were not modeled how to be kind or compassionate toward your body from a young age.*

Your child has loved your body since the moment they realized it was the one to hug them, rock them, feed them, and respond to their cries. They love you for all of you. They will question and feel confused when they see you not loving your body, or criticizing yourself, and then they will internalize that. *If my parent can't accept their body for how it is, that probably means I shouldn't accept mine. Especially if I am anything like my parent.*

PUT AN END TO YOUR NEGATIVE BODY TALK

You can decide that from now on you will not talk negatively or criticize your child's body, or your body. You're a human, of course, which means you will make a mistake or two. And when you do, guess what: you can repair.

REPAIR WHEN NEEDED

How can you model what it looks like to learn from mistakes, reduce shame, and stay open and honest? Here is an example of what you might say in front of your child if you happen to say or do something that you recognize after the fact is no longer in line with your new anti-diet beliefs.

> *"I think you heard me when I said _____. I didn't really mean that. I am so grateful for and proud of my body—it allows me to live here, to be your parent, and to be in my life. When I get tired, cranky, or stressed sometimes I say things I don't mean. I do not want to take my feelings out on my body. I'm sorry, body!"*

If a child believes they are doing something "bad" by eating something or wanting a second helping of ice cream, they often will think, *I'm bad,* because their behavior is viewed as "wrong." If they pick up on the fact that you judge bodies, you don't want your body to look big or fat, or that you don't like fat bodies, they will internalize that and adopt the same beliefs.

Key 1 helps you work toward the six elements of the Intuitive Food and Body

Relationship Model. With your unconditional love and support, your child will have more access to living with comfort in their body, feel they have permission to eat and satisfy their desires, trust that their needs will be met, both emotionally and physically, and not be faced with rigid rules around food and movement, allowing flexible beliefs and thinking to set in. All six of the elements of a positive relationship with food and body are addressed by providing unconditional love and support for your child's body, which is why it's the primary key to raising an Intuitive Eater.

SUMMARIZE AND REFLECT

Unconditionally loving your child's body may seem simple and obvious, but the truth is it can be so much more complicated than that. By providing unconditional love and support for your child—no matter their body size—you allow and encourage them to explore their own authentic existence in the world. You can provide them with a chance to be themselves, not what diet culture wants them to be.

Here are some questions to reflect on after everything you have read in the first key:

- *When do you notice yourself having "autopilot" reactions instead of "manual pilot" responses?*
- *How would changing those from reactions to responses change the way you interact with food and body? How about the way you interact with your child?*
- *What are some ways that you have been putting conditions on the love you give yourself? What about the love you give your child?*
- *Do you have fears about what might happen if you provide unconditional love to you and your child? What about hopes?*
- *In what ways can you discuss bodies and address shame more openly and encourage your child's natural curiosity?*

KEY 2

Implement a Flexible and Reliable Feeding Routine

As a caregiver, you can be in charge without being controlling. Kids benefit when you reliably and consistently provide food, while maintaining and modeling flexibility day-to-day. Routine, choice, and an add-in, pressure-off approach all foster Intuitive Eating.

WHY THE FEEDING ROUTINE IS SO IMPORTANT

The fundamental steps in ensuring that a child retains their innate ability around hunger and fullness are consistency and trust, in infancy and beyond. It's this internal wisdom that forms the basis of Intuitive Eating.[1]
—ELYSE RESCH

First, let's take a look at why the routine and the structure of feeding kids matters so much, and then we'll explore what we mean by flexibility and its importance. The feeding routine is what sets up your child for success to be able to self-regulate and hear their body cues more clearly. Even with adult clients, we will often start with implementing a flexible and reliable eating routine—this is an integral part of the Intuitive Eating process. When the body isn't fed consistently, it will adapt by shutting down some signals (regular hunger cues), and amplifying others (urges to binge) as a way of surviving despite inconsistent food availability.

A routine allows your child to build trust that enough food will be available, so they will be able to fulfill their job in self-care and eating, which is to rely on their intuitive wisdom—their body signals—to direct how much they eat. Without the routine—because kids are dependent on their caregivers to plan and prepare meals—they will be more likely to become disconnected from that innate wisdom.

AN EPIDEMIC OF HUNGER AND UNDERNUTRITION

In situations when a family doesn't always have enough money for satisfying or filling meals, the routine is disrupted. For any person, adult or child, facing food insecurity will naturally decrease the priority of Intuitive Eating, and bring their body to a place where the priority is seeking out any food, getting enough food, and even eating more food than feels comfortable when food is available due to the looming threat that there won't be enough later. Due to this shift in priorities—and due to the fact that millions of families in the United States and around the world face hunger and food insecurity every day—you can see the critical need for public policies and communities to be working on ways to get all kids fed, rather than focusing on "childhood obesity." Because of food insecurity and hunger, one of the adaptations by the body, as mentioned above, is binge eating disorder. Food insecurity is actually a predictive risk factor for the development of disordered eating and weight cycling. However, public health attention is always placed on weight, and not the true underlying health concern: an epidemic of hunger and undernutrition that disproportionately affects poorer groups.

Not only does the focus on body size and weight create shame, weight cycling, and disordered eating among kids, it unjustly keeps the focus on the wrong thing. A child who goes to bed hungry is still waking up to be taught in school that their parent is making the wrong choice by taking them to McDonald's for dinner (even if that's all they can afford or have time to eat) or that they should be eating more carrots and less potatoes. Public health efforts need to shift from fighting weight to fighting the systems that result in millions of children facing hunger and lack of equitable access to food every day.

- Means that the caregiver or parent provides food at regular and consistent times—about every two to three hours for younger children and two to four hours for school-age children, starting with breakfast soon after waking.
- Is individualized to each family based on your culture and your life.
- Is meant to support your child's need for consistency and trust—not to put pressure on you.
- Aims to offer nourishing and tasty foods, including a variety of grains/starches, protein, fats, fruits, and vegetables (remember that even sweet foods can be a regular part of meals and snacks).
- Understands that it's the child's job to decide what and how much they eat of what is served.
- Includes something that the child likes (*preferred foods*).
- Includes reasonable, realistic meals and snacks (*packaged food isn't "bad"*).
- Can be prepared by you or your child if they are developmentally capable of preparing food for themselves.
- Allows for food to be eaten in a flexible manner, such as *eating off the planned routine because someone offers something, because the child asks for it and you approve, because your child's needs are different that day (more movement or change in sleep), your schedule varies, and so on.*
- Isn't a rigid style of eating, but rather a guide of times to help you and other caregivers plan to meet the hunger needs of the child.

"Offering" means making food available for self-serving, or serving it without any verbal or nonverbal pressure. Some kids may have a habitual or conditioned response to say "no" to what you verbally offer. Instead of expecting them to say "yes" just because you're verbally offering, try serving a plate or dish of the food family style, where they are seeing and smelling the food up close, as part of the food experience, without feeling pressure to eat it. In general, family-style meals where people serve themselves (age appropriate) is a pressure-off way to offer food, while still making it available and allowing exposure. Remember that even watching your child for what they will eat is something many will be able to sense, and can feel like pressure or like they are being monitored. Try to keep conversation and attention away from what individuals are eating, and approach other subjects.

Observing young children's responses and interaction with the meal when serving family style is an eye-opening, enjoyable, and major difference maker for many families. Kids love and appreciate being able to do even the simplest thing for themselves—like serving their own noodles to their plate!

You've already seen this recommendation, and here is where it comes into play: *provide enough food at consistent and reliable times; offer a mix of familiar preferred foods and new foods.* Reliable and predictable meal- and snack times create a sense of safety and prevent your child from having a fear of deprivation or hunger. Parents ultimately decide what is served, and we encourage checking in with your kids about what sounds good to them. The sooner you involve them in the decisions, the sooner they can become familiar with the practice of checking in with their desires and appetites. As they become more independent with age, they will take on more responsibility for what they want to eat. Older children start to be able to come up with the ideas on their own, a skill we really want to support and reinforce as they develop more competence. Only you know the amount of independence that your child is ready for.

As we dive deeper into this concept, you may notice there is a lot to unpack, but, at the same time, it's simple. **Your most important job when it comes to food is to do your best to make food available at reliable times.**

This is the continuation of the trust that was established in infancy with feeding on demand at reliable times, and even though it's no longer formula or breast milk, and they can begin to talk and display food preferences, your child still is counting on that trust that food will be provided consistently. Young children don't have the level of consciousness to ask for food when they're hungry—they are easily distracted and in awe of the world around them and will likely not actually ask or show obvious signs of hunger until they are well past comfortable hunger. In most cases, the moment you realize your child is hungry and cranky for food, you need to act quickly because they are likely already experiencing a pretty high level of hunger.

Making a feeding routine a priority will help support your child to show up to meals and snack times hungry. This doesn't mean rigid meal and snack times—sometimes grazing between meals, even having milk or juice, can be important to allow because it's keeping food neutral and allowing them to honor their hunger. Sometimes, frequent grazing and asking for more snacks can be a sign that they need more to eat—or they need more satisfying and satiating foods at meals and snacks. When your child isn't allowed to eat when hungry, there will be consequences in their relationship with food and their body. This can be a reason why some kids start to sneak food. We want kids to feel like it's okay to ask for food and to eat food. When we flip the goal from fear of eating too much to ensuring they are getting enough, eating when hungry makes perfect sense. As parents, we are also allowed to say "not right now" or create a boundary around snacks. We encourage you to question the motives behind the "no." If it's because a meal is coming soon, communicate that and assure your child that they will be fed with yummy food soon and their hunger isn't wrong. The big picture of eating at consistent times throughout the day allows us to see how we can help to enable our kids to be satisfied from meals and snacks until their next chance to eat. Figuring out the times, types of food, and boundaries for kids eating between meals is something some families have to do. If a child is consistently showing up to the table at mealtimes not hungry, having a cup of milk an hour before the meal might be too close to that mealtime. In that case, move the milk to the previous snack or tell your child that they can have milk with dinner. There may also be other solutions that work better for your family. Your child's appetite will vary from day to day and the flexibility of the 3 Keys helps them get those needs met and eliminates deprivation.

You're more likely to reduce stress at a mealtime when you remember—and trust—that your child can self-regulate. If we allow self-regulation, kids will eat when they are hungry. Having a routine helps you and your child show up to the table with less stress. Without a feeling of hunger, being expected, forced, or pressured to eat goes against what their body is telling them, and can set the stage for disconnection and tuning out from their body's hunger and satiety signals. On the other hand, when a child is too hungry at mealtime, they might feel cranky or upset, get a headache, and not be as capable of sitting down respectfully to eat. We're confident that if you have toddlers or young kids you've already seen this happen. *It's hanger (hunger + anger) in full force!*

Now, can you hit the bullseye with this every time and ensure your child is always in the ideal place of hunger before meals? Nope! Do your best, and release the need to fully control this. They may be more or less hungry at certain meals. The add-in, pressure-off approach (*you'll learn about what this means next*) is meant to allow the child to adapt and eat according to how they are feeling in the moment. Intuitive Eating emphasizes eating for the present moment, not the past (what they ate earlier) and not the future (what they will eat later).

With a flexible feeding routine, there is no expectation for kids to always clean the plate, eat the same amount of food at dinner they ate the previous night, or even to eat all their vegetables. Encourage them to listen to their body, and support them when they do—this includes not having any rules about how they have to eat, not even a "no, thank you" bite (this is a common rule some families have about requiring at least one bite of each food served). **You can do this by modeling with your own eating: tasting your food, slowing down, eating what you like, and stopping when you've had enough, while also avoiding any verbal or nonverbal pressure on them to eat.** If mealtimes have been a battle in your house, one of the ways you can start to really turn this around is to relax about food. Serve what you serve, but put more attention on *how everyone is doing, not what everyone is eating*. If mealtimes have been contentious for your family, purposely taking all conflict away from the table will be an important step. We can aim to create positive mealtime experiences, every time, and emphasize the relationship with our child, and their relationship with their body, as the focus.

If your child shows up to the table ravenous, there is a natural tendency (*not at all due to a lack of control on their part*) to eat fast and eat a lot, because they are hungry after a missed snack or meal, are entering a growth spurt, have expended more energy, or possibly even for an unknown reason. If you start to notice that your child is often ravenous at mealtimes, the best approach to take is observing: maybe they are simply not getting enough to eat during the day, feel rushed, or have had the experience of losing their chance to eat if they don't do it quickly. No matter the cause or contributing factors, by stepping back and observing, we can practice resolving the issues and providing our child with the supportive eating environment they need.

THE ADD-IN, PRESSURE-OFF APPROACH

The add-in, pressure-off approach will help reduce stress you might be experiencing at the table.

Add-in

- Instead of focusing on what to "take away" from your child's eating routine, think about what to add in *without* pressure.
- Do intentionally try to offer a wide variety of foods; if your child is selective about what they eat, avoid wasting a lot of food by preparing a smaller amount to start.
- Continue to help them feel competent and trusting that there will always be a familiar food they like at the table (such as cheese, bread, tortilla, pasta), along with more variety.

- If you think your child isn't getting enough of a particular food group, try adding in more of what they *do like* from that group. For example, if your child only likes apple slices and you worry about their variety of fruit intake, serve more apple slices, often, and a small amount of various other fruits without pressure. Try serving other fruits family style, so they get exposure via their other senses without being asked to taste it. You want that desire to taste a new food to come from their *internal motivation.*

- Offer food groups in a variety of ways. Again using fruit as an example, if you only ever serve raw, plain fruit as a side, that can get repetitive and boring; try serving fruit with whipped cream, a dessert made with fruit, or fruit salad with yogurt to mix things up. There are many savory recipes that also include fruit—try to think outside the box. Dried fruit instead of fresh, smoothies with a meal, or mango or pineapple salsa on tacos, for example.

- Keep offering new foods, even when they've expressed dislike—you're offering *exposure without expectation,* and it can often take twenty or more exposures before a child chooses to eat a food for the first time. Just seeing the food served, having a role in preparing it, getting used to the look, the aroma, and the idea of it, all help make that food more approachable.

- Model eating a wide variety of foods (as much as is comfortable for you) to show that these foods are enjoyable and delicious. Not everyone has to or will want to eat a huge variety of food—it doesn't mean health will suffer.

- Do make sure to taste the food yourself to make sure it's appealing: *dried-out cut vegetables and mushy overripe or flavorless underripe produce can be a big turnoff.* If you wouldn't want to eat it yourself, don't expect your child to want to either.

- Season, season, season! Don't be shy about using oil, butter, and salt and seasonings, especially on vegetables, which can often taste bitter to kids as their taste buds are still developing. Add cheese, dips, dressings, and sauces too.

Pressure-off
- No coercing, pressuring, forcing, using bribes, rewards, or punishments to motivate your child to eat.

- You don't have to enforce a two-bite or "try one bite" rule.
- There are no rules about having to eat anything, other than coming to the table and joining the meal.
- Serve foods you and your family enjoy, without the expectation that everyone will like them or want to eat them.
- No requiring them to finish all their juice, milk, or vegetables (or any food).
- No comments meant to encourage eating, such as: *I can't believe you're not eating that, I made it just for you! Don't you want to try the green beans? You're only eating plain noodles? You're so hard to cook for. You asked for this so you have to eat it.*

In a pressure-off approach, focus on your role of providing the food at reliable times and let the child decide what and how much they want to eat.

Know that kids' tastes can change over time, so something they may really not like at one point could become one of their favorite foods when you continue to offer it in a positive, pressure-off way. For this reason, avoid saying repeatedly, *Micah really doesn't like cantaloupe, he tried it once and spit it out across the table!* Your child will hear this, and begin to believe they don't like cantaloupe, simply because that's what they've heard you say. Also avoid labeling your child as any kind of eater, such as a "picky eater," or "impossible to feed." They hear this and it becomes part of their inner narrative and belief system about their own eating style. They will also notice comments about your food preferences. Everyone is allowed to dislike foods, but avoid talking about how gross or disgusting you find a food—practice using language more like *That food isn't for me, but lots of people really enjoy it.*

Kids at all ages can evolve and eat more variety—but it doesn't involve making it "their responsibility," their weight, or how they look. Encouraging more variety without pressure does require you to fulfill your role, which is to be in charge of what's available, offer appealing foods, and model instead of pressure.

HOW MANY MEALS AND SNACKS—AND WHEN?

A general schedule of eating that will support most kids' growing bodies and high energy needs into early puberty (which can start around age nine) and beyond is three meals and two to three snacks a day—*or more.* Your family, or perhaps your culture, may have a variation of this schedule that works best for you, and we highly encourage you to retain cultural preferences and stay consistent with whatever is most comfortable for you and honors any traditions or customs, while keeping in mind that kids often need to eat every two to three hours on average.

Sample feeding routine: Younger child, school day
Breakfast—7 a.m.
Snack—9:30 a.m.
Lunch—11:30 a.m.
Snack—2:00–3:00 p.m.
Dinner—5 p.m.
Evening snack—6:30–7:30 p.m.

Another sample feeding routine
Breakfast—7–8 a.m.
Snack—9:30 a.m.
Snack—12:00 p.m.
Main meal—3:00 p.m.
Dinner—6–7 p.m.
Evening snack—8 p.m.

Sample feeding routine: Older child or teen
Breakfast: 9:00 a.m.
Lunch: 12:30 p.m.
Snack: 3:00 p.m.
Snack: 5:00 p.m.
Dinner: 7 p.m.
Snack: 9 p.m.

When more of the morning hours are spent sleeping (or your older child just doesn't want to eat breakfast early), they will be naturally hungry for more snacks later in the day. This helps them get all their energy needs met and keeps them satisfied at regular intervals throughout their awake hours, while it may look different from a traditional breakfast, snack, lunch, snack, dinner, snack routine. Some of our teen clients are eating their snacks at 10 p.m. and 12 a.m., and that is what works for them. It also may be different from how you would eat and that's okay. An older child or adolescent often has very different feeding needs than an adult. You may notice them eating two plates of dinner where you're full after one; the carbohydrate and energy needs of an adolescent can be the highest of any point in time in the life cycle. Infancy, adolescence, and pregnancy are generally the three phases when humans need the most calories per kilogram of body weight compared to any other times. You will notice this reflected in how often infants need to eat for their rapid growth, the increased appetite of your adolescent, and the shift in hunger and cravings that come with pregnancy. Despite these expected times of highest energy needs, appetite can change at any point, for anyone, which is all a part of the miraculous wisdom of the body to know when and how much food it needs, and to communicate those needs through neurochemical and hormonal hunger and satiety systems.

You get to decide what routine will work best for your family. The goal is to move toward having a routine (remember—this isn't rigid, it's a guide), to try and have at least one family meal together daily, if possible, and to be aware of not waiting until your child is overly hungry to start getting a meal or snack prepared. We know all families have various schedules, and you can come up with a meal and snack routine that best fits what you and your family are working around. This might take some trial and error to find the routine that is not only best for you and your child, but actually possible with your needs and responsibilities.

Take some time and write out what you think would be a reasonable routine for you and your child now. Think about what time your child wakes up, and what time you need to get to work and get them to daycare, school, or other commitments. Where is it possible to fit in a family meal together? What do you need to do to help provide snacks between meals?

FLEXIBILITY: WHAT IT MEANS, WHY IT MATTERS, AND HOW TO BE FLEXIBLE

Simply being a parent guarantees that you cannot predict your schedule or feeding routine on any given day. Planning ahead is great (and so nice when it works out!), but there is a real benefit to accepting that there will undoubtedly be interruptions in your plans. From what research shows us, it's the bigger patterns of behavior and the routine that matter, not being perfect or strict around a schedule. Don't get so focused on a plan or a routine that you lose the ability to be flexible. Show your kids that it's okay to change your mind or make a different choice when you need to.

PSYCHOLOGICAL FLEXIBILITY IS A FUNDAMENTAL ASPECT OF PSYCHOLOGICAL HEALTH

Flexibility means:

- You can identify the need to stray from the plan in the moment (this is an example of being present).
- You're mindful about what changes in the plan bring up for you. In a lot of unforeseen food situations, parents can be triggered by their own internal diet mentality or food police, and also be flooded with thoughts like *That's junk. My kid will be unhealthy if they eat that. I'm a bad parent if I let them eat that.* With mindfulness you're able to notice all the thoughts that come up before you decide how to respond.
- You can identify values to help guide you: the key in knowing how you want to act (the decision) is in identifying what is most important to you in the moment, and in the big picture. You can use your parenting values to ultimately help you come to the decision you think will work best in combination with what you know your child needs in their eating routine.

CONSIDER YOUR PARENTING VALUES

Your values can guide you in tough moments, or when your old, automatic reactions pop up. This is a vital part of the journey to raising an Intuitive Eater. Making moves that bring you and your family closer to the big-picture goal—that peaceful and positive relationship with food and body—becomes much easier when you have some clear guiding values to connect with in decision-making moments. Here are some examples of parenting values to get your mind opened up to thinking about your own:

Independence
Curiosity
Building trust
Spending quality time together
Making positive food memories
Tolerating disappointment
Having patience
Experiencing pleasure

Helping others
Being attuned
Fostering confidence
Modeling flexibility
Self-care

Reflection on values: What else would you add to this list? In your own words, how would you describe what's most important to you in how you parent around food? In what ways are you aligned with or different from other important caregivers for your child? Are your values similar or different from the values that diet culture places on you?

Psychological flexibility refers to the ability to recognize and adapt to situational demands, to remain aware and open to the present moment such that one can recognize and shift behavior strategies as required by situational demands, and to engage in actions that are congruent with one's deeply held values.[2]

This definition reinforces why flexibility is so important. Flexibility is what allows you to put your values over perfectionism. It helps you feel better about your actions and decisions, and helps you be clear on what kind of feeding relationship you want to create.

Imagine doing something fun with your family; for example, being at the zoo, a once-in-a-while, fun activity you do together. Your child asks for an elephant ear, despite having packed snacks available. It's understandable to think to yourself, *I went through all the trouble to pack food to help my child have a balanced snack, and now they just want an elephant ear.* See if you can slow down and consider this moment from your child's perspective. They see the elephant ear, and it looks so intriguing! It smells delicious, they rarely get the chance to have one, and it's a *fun food.* If the elephant ear is something you can afford, you could consider the value that this food may add to the experience of being at the zoo. You have the opportunity to model flexibility, spontaneity, and permission to eat all foods. Remember that those snacks you packed don't have to go to waste. One option is to say, *Sure, we can get an elephant ear, how fun! And we'll find a table so we can sit down and eat our snacks, before moving on to the next exhibit.* Or if you just had breakfast before going to the zoo you might say, *Sure, we'll get one a little bit later when it's snack time.*

If one of your parenting values is also to be consistent with your response to things like whining and complaining and your child is throwing a tantrum or crying for an elephant ear before you've even talked about it, then you may say, We've talked about whining. I know it's disappointing, but we aren't getting an elephant ear right now. Please think about how you ask for things and try a different way next time. *Notice that this response has nothing to do with the elephant ear being a "good" or "bad" food, isn't about nutrition or food rules, or rewarding or punishing behavior—it's simply about your boundaries and expectations for behavior. Establishing this as an expectation often and early can help to stop the whining and behavior you want to avoid.*

Being flexible gives you the opportunity to put values over perfectionism or planning when it works for you.

Flexibility uses tools derived from acceptance and commitment therapy (ACT). ACT is a form of mindfulness-based therapy that focuses on accepting and experiencing negative thoughts and feelings while living our best and most valued lives.

Tools of ACT we can use in decision-making:

- **Mindfulness:** What is happening in the present moment that requires you to shift away from the plan or routine?
- **Parenting values:** What matters to you most in this moment given the circumstances?
- **Self-compassion:** What would a self-compassionate decision be right now for you as a parent?
- **Taking action:** When you release the belief there is a "right" or "wrong" decision, what makes the most sense for you while also moving toward your big-picture goal?

Also important for relating your decision to a child:

- **Communicate clearly:** *Tonight I'm deciding that it's okay to have a show on while we have dinner, but this is a once-in-a-while thing just for fun! Is that clear?*
- **Follow through:** As much as you reasonably can, be consistent with your decisions and how you communicate. If you say TV during din-

ner is a once-in-a-while thing, but then have the TV on 50 percent of the time, that isn't a clear message to your child and they may understandably come to expect that dinner is often eaten in front of the TV.

If you find yourself wanting to say no to the elephant ear request strictly for nutrition rules, what would it be like if you backed off from those rules? Your child will not get a nutrient deficiency or develop a health concern from eating an elephant ear.

Flexibility is a critical part of the 3 Keys, because, well . . . *life happens!* As much as you may value having meals at the table, making home-cooked meals, or meal planning every weekend, that may not always be what is realistic, and it certainly isn't accessible for everyone most of the time. You also might encounter days or weeks when you simply cannot stick to a plan and you need to fall back on flexibility. Everyone can benefit from flexibility, especially our kids. They need to know that there are times when they can eat not strictly for hunger, but for pleasure, enjoyment, and tradition. They will notice whether you're rigid or calm about when the dinner plan falls through, or they forgot their lunch and need to buy it. Flexibility applies not just to the timing of when your child eats, but also, and importantly, to what they eat. Are you demonstrating to them that they have unconditional permission to eat?

FLEXIBILITY IS WHERE PERMISSION TO EAT MEETS HEALTHY BOUNDARIES

This can understandably be confusing—how can you give a child permission to eat, while also being responsible for the feeding routine? Tuning in to your child and what is going on for them is going to be really helpful in helping you make your decisions.

When a toddler wakes up in the morning, and fifteen minutes later starts asking for fruit snacks, does that mean you have to give them fruit snacks for breakfast? No. When you tune in to your two-year-old's mind, you realize that what they are probably trying to communicate is *I'm hungry and I need some food,* but they are only two, so they're unable to say, *Can you make me a breakfast that will help me feel satisfied until snack time?* They are inserting a food they know how to ask for, and telling you they're ready to eat. You can say, *I see you're hungry, I'm going to get breakfast for you. Can you come to the table?* Then you can bring them the meal you decide you're serving, and they can decide how much of it they'll eat.

If they keep returning back to the fruit snacks, you can either add some fruit snacks to the breakfast and make no big deal about it, or say, *We're not having fruit snacks right now, but we'll have them later.*

DON'T GET CORNERED INTO "RIGHT" OR "WRONG" THINKING

It's important to have both flexibility and a routine, although that sounds contradictory. Having both will help with this process in two ways: (1) you minimize the consequences that happen when kids skip snacks or meals, and (2) you can feel fine about the fact that what happens between meals and snacks is likely to be unpredictable.

Your neighbor might appear on your doorstep with fresh muffins, or you may have cookies left over from a party the day before and you want one after breakfast. The flexibility aspect of Key 2 is *as important* as the routine aspect. If you just have the routine without the flexibility, you might feel cornered into right-and-wrong, all-or-nothing decisions. Focusing only on the routine doesn't include listening to your body or your internal desires: *Do you want the muffin that your neighbor just brought over? How will it work for you, or feel for you, to eat it at that particular time?* Only following a routine and not being open to flexibility is actually disempowering and isn't supportive of true Intuitive Eating.

At the same time, if you don't have any routine, it will be more difficult to meet the needs of your children. Having no routine, for most families, also makes feeding kids feel more stressful. The routine is the guide, the flexibility is what helps you make this sustainable, positive, and intuitive.

Routine and flexibility are equally important. Without a routine, you live in randomness—this doesn't support children with the consistency and boundaries they need to feel safe, and model for them how to create routines for themselves later on in life. Flexibility doesn't exist without routine. A routine without flexibility can create challenges, reactions, rigidity, and anxiety when the routine falls apart. Without flexibility, we miss many important learning opportunities, such as important chances to model for kids how we trust ourselves, our bodies, and their bodies.

Does this look the same for younger kids and older kids? Generally, younger children, especially those around the ages of one to six, really need the structure of the routine. As we mentioned, they aren't likely to be tuned in to their early signs of hunger, and by the time they say, *I'm hungry*, they will need something very quickly. It's even more important to be mindful of your child's developmental level rather than their age: Do they seem to express and understand when they feel early hunger? Are they motivated to and capable of preparing their meal or a snack on their own? If so, you may be able to check in with them more—*Are you starting to get hungry for lunch?*—but for the most part, younger kids really rely on their caregiver to establish the feeding routine and times while older kids are going to naturally be more aware of their hunger and can communicate clearly or get their own food. We encourage parents to stay involved and engaged in their preteen's and teen's eating patterns, but you'll need to let go of being completely in control over their routine.

What do I do when my child asks for snacks right before dinner? One outcome of the feeding routine is that your child will be ready to eat right around the same time every day. This is helpful, but also can cause a lot of hunger to build up if, for example, dinner is running behind. Don't hesitate to put out a plate of something for them to snack on (consider it part of their dinner) as you finish preparing the meal. This is a great time to put a variety of colorful, appealing, and new or exposure foods out for your kids to have to prevent pre-meal meltdowns caused by being overly hungry. Or if you're doing takeout or fast food for dinner, and there is driving time in the car when someone may be getting really hungry, keep some snacks on hand to help prevent them from getting *overly* hungry. Being too hungry before a meal can set off a biological drive to eat fast and to eat more, simply as a result of being so hungry, which, although it happens to everyone from time to time, may leave you feeling sick and can spur a drive to disconnect from satiety signals.

Can breakfast be in the car? If breakfast needs to be in the car because you have to have your child to daycare at 6:45 a.m. for you to get to work by 7 a.m., then you bet breakfast can be in the car. And furthermore, breakfast or any meal can be in the car if that is what works best for you and that is what it takes to get your child fed at the right time. There are a lot of recommendations to parents that all meals should be eaten sitting down at the table—and although that sounds lovely and great, it's just not the reality for many families. Sit down for meals together when you can, and know the value of doing so, but also know the value of prioritizing getting your child fed when they need to be, getting to work on time, the help you're offering yourself by not having rigid rules about meals, all while keeping up with your busy life and your other commitments and maintaining your sanity. For kids and families who have early mornings, remember that it's important that your child is getting sufficient hours of sleep. The American Academy of Sleep Medicine states that the guidelines for sleep for kids are: nine to twelve hours of sleep for children aged six to twelve years, and eight to ten hours for those aged thirteen to seventeen years. So, if that means breakfast happens on the way to school or daycare to allow for sleeping twenty or thirty minutes longer, so be it!

What if dinner is late because we don't get home at the same time every day? If you aren't home, you can adjust dinner to a time that works for you. The important thing is that you're thinking about your individual child's day: Are they getting fed breakfast upon waking and before being asked to do anything (school, daycare, and so on)? From there, are they getting consistent meals and snacks throughout the day at reliable times? For example, if your child has nothing to eat between a 2 p.m. snack at daycare and 7 p.m. when dinner is on the table, they are going too long without food. Can you pack an extra snack so they have two snacks in the afternoon, or a dinner that someone who is caring for them can feed them? Then they can have a snack at the table with you when you're having your dinner. There is no "right" schedule—the goal is that you have thought about your child's day to prevent them from having to miss a meal or snack or them grazing on unsatisfying foods throughout a long period of time because there has been a lack of structured meals.

Dessert—with the meal or after? Why not a mix of both? How your family has dessert doesn't have to be rigid. In fact, we think that this is one area where you can be really flexible and relaxed. If you have never offered dessert with the meal, give it a try! When you stop pressuring kids—*Eat at least five bites* or *Finish your peas*—and relax with food, a lot of good can occur. Dessert isn't a reward for eating dinner. If your child is hungry, for the most part they will want dinner and probably dessert if it's available. If you're reintroducing desserts after not having had them available very often, you'll likely notice dessert will be *very* emotionally charged! This is a really predictable and common response—it's the exact reason why we don't recommend that parents make any foods off-limits or restricted: it has the opposite effect on the child's drive to eat once that food is offered. It's okay and natural for your child to be excited about desserts—culturally we are conditioned to be embarrassed by pleasure and enjoyment. Enjoying food, especially decadent or delicious foods—is so taboo and connected to being "unhealthy" or gaining weight that you might notice yourself being uncomfortable watching your child be excited about enjoying dessert. We suggest you just notice that feeling, reflect on where it might be stemming from, and then redirect your thinking to being grateful that your child is happy and is enjoying something. Be happy and enjoy it with them! It's really great for your child to witness you being relaxed around food, and supportive of their joy and pleasure.

TIPS FOR IMPLEMENTING YOUR FAMILY'S FEEDING ROUTINE

Communicate: Tell kids when meal- or snack time is coming up—this helps them know what to expect, and know that food is coming (no one likes to be in the dark about where their next meal is coming from). They won't develop a sense that they have to be responsible for that until it's age appropriate.

Offer a variety plate: Put fruits, vegetables, nuts, dips, anything, on a family-style plate in the middle of the table—they will feel less pressure with it not on their plate. Their curiosity (and the visual appeal of mixed plates like this) is likely to entice them to pick what looks good to them.

Plan for what is reasonable, then do more if you want to: The feeding routine, and planning for it, can feel really overwhelming in some cases. Maybe you're already there—the flexible feeding routine is something you've got down like a pro and you know your growth areas lie in breaking away from diet mentality or being more present with your kids. On the other hand, learning about the importance of the flexible feeding routine may be bringing up challenging thoughts: *But I haven't been prioritizing my kids' eating schedule and now I understand why they're snacking all afternoon and then not wanting to eat what I make for dinner!* You aren't alone. You're a busy parent, with a lot on your plate, and you may never have been told or modeled how to do this. You have been doing the best you can. You can do this. Approach the flexible feeding routine gradually. Start by thinking about what is most reasonable for you: Can you pre-make any meals? Buy precooked food? Ask your ten-year-old to get snacks for the younger sibling while you're in afternoon meetings? Whatever you need to do, keep it reasonable and realistic, and allow yourself to be imperfect and grow. As you and your family get into a new routine, and you repeatedly realign your focus on the feeding routine, this will get easier and you'll notice the benefits. People show up to the table with an appetite, there are fewer meltdowns before dinner, and you have confidence knowing what your role is in the feeding relationship and what your child's role is.

YOU WILL BE IMPERFECT AT THIS— AND WE ARE RIGHT THERE WITH YOU

Unless you're some super-parent, then you will have days or periods of time where the schedule is really difficult to make happen. Don't worry. In fact, the calmer you can be when you're off your routine, the more that will help your child with their own psychological flexibility down the line. Recall that flexibility is a core element of a positive relationship with food and body. You need to try to adjust your expectations of your child when the routine is off. It's their body's job to remember to seek out food that it needs, so when the schedule isn't happening, and the caregiver isn't fully implementing their role of the feeding routine, your child is going to have some type of response. It may be that they snack a lot more and then don't want dinner. It could be they notice the change in routine and, because they can't make sense of it, are having some outbursts, or a new attitude pops up. Kids will try to make sense of a change in routine, and as parents we have to be understanding that they will never fully know how hard or exhausting it can be to have to be the one planning and preparing meals every day, every week, for years. There is no way we can expect that our kids will be aware of the effort that goes into the schedule—*so we suggest you stop expecting that.*

Instead of beating yourself up for a floppy feeding routine, figure out what is getting in the way of you being able to provide the flexible and reliable routine. Are there small shifts you can make like setting an alarm to stop and fix lunch on the weekend? Can you start prepacking lunches, buy more quick-prep meals that just have to be heated up rather than cooked? What we're saying here is that the expectation isn't that this always feels easy, or that you can always do this feeding routine perfectly, but that when (*not if, but when*) something interrupts the routine you can have some self-compassion, notice what's happening, be understanding that your kid may also be acting differently as a result, and think of ways that you can realistically problem-solve to bring back the routine and structure of reliable meals and snacks so that your child can maintain trust.

- What is an ideal feeding routine that works for your family and life?
- What do you need in order to move toward this?
- Notice the next time you say no to your child's request for a food or snack: Why did you say no? What feelings came up for you around the food or the request for food?
- How are you practicing self-care in order to make sure your family is fed and you aren't putting too much pressure on yourself?

KEY 3

Develop and Use Your Intuitive Eating Voice

Using your Intuitive Eating voice is the embodied action you take. It's the way we help raise Intuitive Eaters. On the individual level for everyone, our inner Intuitive Eating voice directs our choices and behaviors. On the relational level with a child, the Intuitive Eating voice offers safety, trust, reassurance, attentiveness, attunement, and an example of what a positive relationship with food and body is.

This is what makes Key 3 so essential for raising an Intuitive Eater. The feeding routine isn't the same without the Intuitive Eating voice, and we rely on the Intuitive Eating voice to intentionally show unconditional love and support for our child's body. It's the vehicle we have to deliver the Intuitive Eating message to our kids, without having to sit them down and talk about "Intuitive Eating." You never even need to actually say those two words to make a difference. The difference is in your actions, your responsiveness, and the care with which you decide to slow down and use your words around food and body mindfully and with intention.

Your voice, what you communicate, both verbally and nonverbally, is what helps formulate your child's inner caregiver voice—and your voice can only function effectively when you have made sense of your past. In part 2 we offered suggestions for how you can make sense of your past experiences. The reactions you have and the words you use in response to your child's eating exist not at random, but because of what you heard—and what you've said to yourself—throughout your own life. This is why developing and using your own Intuitive Eating voice is so powerful.

It's fair to say that many, but not all, parents have the strong reactions to food and bodies that we do because of previous painful experiences with dieting, food deprivation, or body shame. According to Bessel van der Kolk, author of *The Body Keeps the Score: Brain, Mind, and Body in the Healing of Trauma*, "Trauma isn't the story of something that happened back then, it's the current imprint of that pain, horror, and fear living inside people."[1] Our pain doesn't just disappear simply because it's in the past.

When we have had the experience of feeling that our body is wrong, inadequate, or unworthy, or that we are bad for eating something, that feeling doesn't go away. That memory, that experience, becomes imprinted in our mind. The desire to escape, fix, or avoid that feeling also hangs around, and when something happens down the line—for example, years later when you witness your child sneaking a donut like one you were shamed for eating when you were ten—you could have a reaction that reflects your shame, your need to escape or avoid or fix, rather than a response that is neutral to the present situation. Dieting is traumatic. Food restriction, being weighed or criticized, and having your worthiness or potential evaluated based on your eating or weight is all traumatic.

Food and body shame are so rarely discussed openly, despite it being something the majority of people have experienced, that we suppress it, hold it inside, and hope to never cross paths with those demons again. What diet mentality shows us is that we carry these lessons along with us through life, and when we become parents, they end up becoming the patterns we re-create when feeding and raising our own kids. Unless we resolve them. Intuitive Eating helps us resolve our unhelpful thoughts and food-policing voice, so that we can neutralize food and enjoy eating again.

Give yourself permission to acknowledge and work through the trauma that you experienced, whether it was put on you by someone else or culturally inflicted via dieting. You thought dieting meant self-respect and healthy living. Give yourself all the permission you need to feel this disappointment, and how hard it can be to not react to your child's eating and body changes. If this were easy, we wouldn't have needed to write a book to support parents through this. It's not easy. It's painful, and you can move gently at your own pace.

The reason why highlighting past food and body trauma is so important is because for some readers, just learning about the Intuitive Eating voice will be all they need to model it. For others, it requires an unpacking of years—maybe decades—of memories and patterns in order to stop the cycle for your own child. We all have a different journey here. **Many of us have to create our Intuitive Eating voice, which takes time and practice.** What can't be ignored and what research repeatedly confirms is that what caregivers say about food, eating, and bodies has a significant impact on a child's attitude about body appreciation and on their Intuitive Eating skills.[2]

If you need to, spend some time back in part 2, reflecting on the way you were raised with food, the experiences that stayed with you, and your feeding legacy. Who do you need to talk to about the past? How can you process and grieve? What do you need to feel heard, seen, and cared for so that you can move forward and hear, see, and care for your own child the way you wished had been available to you?

INTUITIVE EATING PHRASES

As a parent, as you've learned, you have a number of different roles within your role as the caregiver. You're the cook, planner, shopper, treasurer, boundary setter, and role model. *Phew!* That's a lot of roles. It can be difficult to not only try to fulfill all your roles, but also help your child work through their own complex emotions and hunger states. In this chapter, we're giving you some examples of how you can use your voice to portray these different roles and model Intuitive Eating to help your child develop their inner IE voice.

SAYING YES TO FOOD REQUESTS

Picture the moment when your kid asks for something specific to eat. When you say yes, you're going to want to be aware that you're not saying yes because of any reward for good behavior or reward for eating something "healthy," but rather because they have permission, an appetite for it, and it's available. You don't always have to say yes (see "Ways to Say No" on the following page), but when you do, work toward it being about the present moment and permission, not because of how healthy the food is, as a reward, or because it's a special occasion.

Here are some neutral ways to say yes:

Sure.

Can you wash your hands and meet me at the table?

How much do you think you need?

How many/much would you like?

Yes, do you need any help with it?

Sure—I'll also get you ____ and put it all on the table for you.

The above are all phrases that neutralize the food when you say yes to a food request.

WAYS TO SAY NO

As the caregiver, you use your best judgment and decide what is available and when. It's to be expected that kids will ask for food between meals, and it's important that instead of just reacting, *you pay attention to why they are asking.* Are they bored? Hungry? Is the routine off? Is there a new or unusual food around that's sparking interest? Keeping in mind your parenting values, and the importance of flexibility, you will also have times when the right decision for your family is to say no. **If you notice that the desire to eat is coming from boredom, your role is to do what you can to work through or resolve the boredom, not blame them for wanting to entertain themselves with food. Really seeing your child's need for companionship, stimulation, play, and purpose is just as much an important part of the feeding relationship as the meal and snack routine.**

Does your child understand why you're saying no? Is it bedtime and they're trying to stall by asking for a snack? Communicate that it's bedtime and you're done having snacks for the night. If it's not bedtime and they ask for food, can you express permission and say *Sure?*

If it isn't a good time for them to eat for a specific reason—you're in the car, you don't have time, they're going to have a meal or snack soon, maybe you don't have the particular food they're requesting or can't afford it—be sure you're pausing to identify why you're saying no to help get out of the habit of diet-mentality thinking, and then communicate that reason clearly.

There are many valid reasons for saying no to a food request, just as you can't always play with your child, buy them the toy they want, or appease their every desire. Boundaries, responsibilities, and your family's meal and snack routine are just some reasons why you may need to say no. Here are some ways to say no that aren't about deprivation, fatphobia, or rigid thinking about food. **One thing to keep in mind is that you need to communicate to your child the reason for saying no. Assure them they will be given another eating opportunity soon, and that there is no shame in them ever asking for food—it's a completely human and understandable thing to ask for.** Saying yes and being flexible when it works for you gives balance to when you decide to say no. Saying yes really helps your child trust that they aren't bad for wanting something to eat.

Here are some neutral ways to say no:

Right now, we need to do _____, so let's come back and have that in a little while.

We just finished up breakfast, so this is something we can have later.

It's not snack/mealtime right now—but we're going to eat soon. Thanks for being patient.

I know these both look yummy. You need to pick one to have right now, and next time we'll have the other one.

I understand you're upset we're not having that right now—I'm so glad to know you like that and we can be sure to have it more often.

We need to save some of that. Can I get you something else?

This is what we have available tonight—you don't have to eat it if you don't want it.

It's okay if your child gets upset with you if you say no to a food request. Especially young kids: that is their way of expressing their disappointment, or testing boundaries. It doesn't mean you're a bad parent, you're depriving them, or restricting them. Kids will naturally try to gain control at times. The more you give them the appropriate level of control by letting them have some choice, letting them decide what and how much they eat, will help them over time to know what to expect. In the beginning, when creating the flexible feeding routine or setting some boundaries and saying no, there may be some hurt feelings. That's okay. Allow all the feelings to show up: your job isn't to make your child feel only positive feelings; it's to respond in ways that align with your values, hold boundaries, and show your child you will make sure they're going to have enough to eat and they're allowed to have pleasure and permission to eat.

EMOTIONAL ATTUNEMENT AND THE VOICES WE USE TO HELP KIDS TUNE IN

Our emotions are inextricably linked to our appetite and eating. Eating is emotional, but that doesn't mean food is always the solution when we experience uncomfortable emotions. A significant part of connecting or reconnecting to our inner Intuitive Eating wisdom is being able to tell the difference among the kinds of hunger we experience. In order to help a child differentiate these kinds of hunger, we get to gradually model doing it ourselves, as well as teach them ways of meeting their emotional needs that don't solely involve soothing with food. We get to show our kids the joy of loving and getting pleasure from food, which are emotional eating experiences, while also helping them know they can feel their feelings, trust they will survive, and develop a variety of skills to cope.

Emotional hunger can often feel like physical hunger when we have repeatedly used food to soothe uncomfortable emotions. Humans learn to associate emotional states with feelings (such as associating sadness or anxiety with an urge to eat). When eating to soothe becomes our primary coping response, we aren't practicing other really important ways of coping—including simply feeling and tolerating emotions, talking about them, asking for help, and receiving loving, caring support. In raising an Intuitive Eater, part of the process is guiding your child to know the difference—that when they are sad or scared, they can trust that there is support available from someone who cares about them, or even from their own self-care.

Physical hunger is our body's need for fuel and nourishment. The messages of physical hunger are often predictable, familiar, and the hunger is resolved when we've had a meal or snack. Emotional hunger may linger even after eating.

Kids may become reliant on food for emotional soothing when there is a gap in their emotional needs unfulfilled by a caregiver or as a response to trauma (food provides a temporary escape, numbing, distraction, and so on). This can become even more pronounced, on top of unmet emotional needs, when there is any level of food deprivation or dieting.

Even a less obvious case of food deprivation—such as Anna experienced with her parent's constant emphasis on healthy eating—is enough to leave a child feeling unsatisfied and in fear of deprivation, which makes food much more effective and powerful as a coping tool in times of distress. When restricted, ice cream becomes a very satisfying and soothing food, for example; however, when normalized and unrestricted, it's just ice cream and doesn't offer the same emotional value as far as a coping tool.

For many people, including many young people, food becomes lifesaving; we often overlook how protective it is that people have food to turn to when they feel they have nothing else available. Food can provide a real outlet for coping, pleasure, and a short-term escape from negative thoughts and emotions. For this reason, it's important to view emotional eating as something that is offering someone something they otherwise don't have. It may not be the ideal coping tool, and it may cause some unpleasant side effects (mainly an upset tummy), but it can be an essential survival tool to help people cope through distress, loss, and/or grief. Some people with binge eating disorder (BED) have survived through incredibly difficult life circumstances because they *did* have a coping mechanism—binge eating (this can be true for all eating disorders as adaptations and tools of self-protection). Ethical and effective BED treatment must never involve a goal of weight reduction or a dieting/restriction component, as this distracts from the true healing, which includes learning to offer oneself choices and options for coping with distress, while healing the relationship with food and body. BED is often also an eating disorder borne out of restriction, but unfortunately this is often overlooked in eating disorder treatment with providers being more focused on the perceived overeating. No one can recover from an eating disorder by way of more restriction.

Here's the gray area. *Showing your child that emotions are linked to eating is a great thing*—in fact, separating emotions and food is rooted in diet mentality. It's really valuable to model for your child that you *enjoy* and are attuned when eating. Can you help your child work through difficult emotions *and* notice that they may want some special food at the next meal to help feel extra comforted? *Yes.* Diet culture has created a false understanding that says any and all emotional eating is "bad." *That simply isn't true.* Sometimes, emotional eating is a healthy coping mechanism. Eating is safe, it's legal, often available, and it can be effective. The assessment we can make about the emotion behind the desire to soothe with food is one that comes with Intuitive Eating as well. If we are lonely and need a hug while our partner sits next to us on the couch, we can ask for a hug and have that need met directly. But if we are grieving the loss of a parent and aching for that connection, eating their favorite food on their birthday because that's what you always did together is not only a valid way to soothe, but also a way to experience connection when you need it.

FOOD ISN'T ALWAYS WHAT THEY NEED

It isn't your job as a parent to fix your child's difficult emotions, or to make their bad moods or sadness disappear (as understandable as it is to want to). Rather than trying to fix their negative emotions, *we can help them work through them.* Kids grow stronger from working through uncomfortable feelings. When we race to make negative feelings go away, especially by offering food to fix them, we aren't helping them to feel their feelings, or trusting that they can be okay and tolerate difficult experiences.

Examples of modeling emotion with food using your Intuitive Eating voice

I'm excited for a yummy dinner!

I want this meal to last forever.

I'm so sad I filled up already and I don't have room for dessert.

This lasagna is so amazing, I'll be excited to come back to this restaurant again and have it next time.

I'm really missing Grandpa. I think I'll make his chicken and dumplings recipe tonight.

The taste and smell of this makes me so happy.

I'm feeling blue today, I really want a comforting hot meal for dinner.

Examples of emotionally tuning in with your child

Do you need a hug?

You seem upset, do you want to talk?

I'm here for you.

What do you need right now?

Do you have big feelings you would like to talk about?

Using your Intuitive Eating voice to *support* body connection

What is your body telling you?

How does your tummy feel?

Did you get enough to eat?

How does _____ taste?

What do you love about it?

Do you like your cereal when it gets soft, or when it's still crunchy?

I trust you. I hear you.

I trust your body.

It looks like you're finished, did you get enough to eat?

What do you need right now? How can I help?

Using your Intuitive Eating voice to *model* body connection

I trust my body.

I'm still hungry.

I'm sad I don't have any more room—my tummy is all filled up!

I don't feel hungry, but I'll eat because I know I need energy for the day.

This doesn't taste how I expected it to.

This tastes exactly how I was hoping it would!

When I'm really upset, it's hard to want to eat.

I'm frustrated. I'm going to take a few minutes to reset and then try again.

Can I have some more?

May I take one home?

No, thank you, I'm not hungry right now. Maybe later.

Thank you for making this—that was so thoughtful, but I don't really like it.

If there's enough for everyone, I'd love another piece of pizza, please.

My body is none of your business.

IMPORTANT PHRASES WHEN STARTING TO USE INTUITIVE EATING WITH KIDS

How are you? A good friend of mine (Amee) was giving a talk at a conference and a parent asked, "What do we say to our kids when they keep asking for cookies?!" His answer? "How about 'How are you?'" Emotional and physical cues can both feel like hunger to all of us. Parents often ask us, "What do I do if I see my child eating in a way that I know isn't about physical hunger?" First, how do you really know it's not about physical hunger? Have they expressed that they're eating past the point of comfort? What assumptions are you making?

Next, we know that strong emotions can mask internal body signals, inflate appetite, and interrupt hunger and satiety cues. It's quite possible that although you think they're eating food they're not truly hungry for, their experience is quite different. Kids who have had restricted access to food can often seem to ask for these new and exciting foods *a lot*—especially at first. They may eat a large amount of a food that was previously unavailable or limited. There are two reasons for this: the first is that their brain is programmed to assume that it will be a limited-time offer, and the second is this new food is exciting, the novelty of it has a powerful draw. The more these new and exciting foods are available, the more you're encouraging habituation to them—the novelty and the appeal decreases. This gradually neutralizes the power of these foods.[3] If certain foods have been restricted, your child's conditioned response might be to believe this food will not be available regularly, and subsequently want to eat more (so they don't "miss out") until they trust that it will be. Your job is to accept that the process takes time, normalize the food, and have foods around regularly that your child enjoys (to the extent you're able)—particularly if you realize you have been restricting some foods.

Ask yourself: Could this pattern of eating a lot at one time be a response to restriction or undereating at an earlier point in the day? Not getting enough to eat during the school day is very common. There may be ways for you to help them eat more adequately, if that's the issue. Growth spurts, energy for activities, and puberty are all reasons many young people will eat more than they are used to, or eat more than you think they "should" be hungry for.

No matter the reason, our recommendation is to not focus on the food or eating at all. Check in with your child if you have any concerns, but focusing on their weight will send the message that you think they're eating too much. This will feel like judgment to them, *whether or not you intend it to,* and that judgment will be harmful. For some, judgment will elicit defiance: a subconscious desire to eat more either to assert their autonomy (part of their healthy ego), to passively communicate to you that they are in charge of their own body, or possibly to rebel against any threat of deprivation. Kids and adults are all psychologically wired to rebel against overcontrol.

Instead of approaching your child about their eating, we offer you the phrase *How are you?* You can authentically check in with your child; you can even sit down to have a snack with them. If you have a concern about your child's eating, really connecting, setting aside your assumptions and judgment, and just providing a space to connect with them is incredibly loving and healing. If they are worried about something with their eating, creating a space safe enough for them to feel comfortable sharing that with you can have a truly meaningful impact.

You can also try being really direct by saying, *Honey, I've noticed you're really hungry in the afternoon and I wanted to check in to see if you're getting enough to eat during the day. I want you to know you can always eat as much as you need or want, and you're always in charge of how much you need to eat. I'll never judge you for that.*

Is there anything going on that I can support you with? I could be totally wrong—and if so, never mind me!

GIVE YOUR KID SOME TIME TO REBUILD
TRUST IN THIS NEW APPROACH

As parents, we can allow space for our children to learn to trust when we tell them they aren't able to have a cookie right now; it's not "no" to cookies, it's no to *this cookie right now*. For instance, if the cookies are the holiday cookies you're gifting to friends and there is only a limited amount left over, you tell them they may not have one, while assuring them that you can make more or buy more soon. *Following through* on that statement allows them to trust that sometimes we say no to foods we want—not because the food is "bad" or unhealthy, but because it's not always the right time or available. It's okay to normalize that it can be disappointing to not have the thing we want. All parents realize the importance of helping our kids through feelings of disappointment. Sometimes we are disappointed about food. But making decisions separate from health, body, or food fears allows parents to set boundaries without enacting diet mentality. It's okay to say no: that's the boundary we have to hold as parents sometimes. We want you to be able to check yourself—*Why am I saying no?*—and communicate that to your child.

We often see kids come into our office who have stopped eating breakfast because of anxiety about things going on at school. Since emotional interruptions aren't about food, in order to help your child resolve the issue of not eating breakfast or whichever meal isn't happening, you need to be able to get to the root of the problem. Forcing your child to eat in the morning will likely cause them to add another layer of being upset at you, for not understanding or fully "seeing" them. They may feel they have to start being dishonest about their eating to take care of your feelings, all while not really helping them resolve the issue. It's really important to use a curious approach any time you're concerned or worried about an eating behavior. What is this really about? How are they feeling about going to school? What could be happening for them? For some kids in the early stages of development of an eating disorder, regularly skipping a meal is a dangerous sign. If you have an older child, talk to them and let them know you're worried, and you want to put your heads together to figure out how to make breakfast work for them. Trust your gut: if you sense there is disordered eating or an eating disorder, seek the support from a weight-inclusive registered dietitian or therapist.

Along with *How are you?*, we'll also offer a couple other ways to communicate that you see your child, you're there for them, you're not judging them, or you're worried about them.

WHAT DO YOU NEED FROM ME? WHAT DO YOU NEED RIGHT NOW? IS THERE ANYTHING I CAN DO TO SUPPORT YOU?

These phrases can be helpful for older kids and teens, when they are able to share and sense on a deeper level what they really need. Some young kids can be surprisingly aware and able to do this as well. Can you encourage your child to tell you how you can check in on them, both with reminding them to eat and with non-food-related issues, in a way that feels helpful to them instead of invasive, annoying, or unhelpful?

SURE.

"Sure" is a response that communicates the Intuitive Eating principle of *permission to eat*. When your child asks for food, your "autopilot" reaction (very likely rooted in diet mentality) might be something like, *No, that's not good for you, pick something healthy*. Realize how all-or-nothing this statement is. If it's not "healthy," why do you let them have it sometimes? Kids are very concrete thinkers, so this becomes confusing; it also makes that food more desirable. Restraint theory shows time and time again that having permission to eat something keeps it emotionally neutral, and that kids are much less likely to overeat it later when they finally do have it or when you're not around. If you want to say no to your child's request for a chocolate cupcake (that you have saved for a birthday party this afternoon) for a morning snack, you can say, *We're not having cupcakes right now, but here are two other options*. If the chocolate cupcakes aren't specifically for an occasion, you can say, *Sure*, and really deflate the power of that food and let them have a cupcake for a snack. It doesn't mean they will have a chocolate cupcake for a snack every day. It's your dieting mind that is so triggered by the thought of a cupcake for a snack. Even to a kid, a daily chocolate cupcake will lose its luster.

Often my (Sumner) husband will be giving our son a bath or putting him to bed and my daughter and I will be in the kitchen getting some dessert. One day, I happened to serve a slightly smaller amount of ice cream with whipped cream than she would normally have. When she finished the first serving she asked for more whipped cream. My brain said, *No! She's already had enough*. My Intuitive Eating voice said, *She wants it, and I can trust her body*. So I said, *Sure*. She finished the next serving of whipped cream and then said, *Mommy, can I have some more*, with some *chocolate syrup on it?* Again, my body tensed, and my old diet mind said, *She can't control herself, she'll never stop, what are you doing, you uninformed idiot?!* and my Intuitive Eating voice said, *Teaching her she can trust her body is the most valuable thing you can teach her with food.* I said, *Sure,* and gave her some more of what she wanted. I connected with my values to help ground me and stay the course: she had already eaten her last meal of the day (this food wasn't interrupting a meal), I didn't want her to feel that this food is restricted or limited, and I value body connection and building trust that her body can tell her when she's had enough. She ate the third serving of whipped cream with chocolate syrup, and walked away from the table with a ring of chocolate around her lips. She was satisfied. I worked through the diet talk in my head. I had shown her I trusted her, and she inherently has had another experience of Intuitive Eating and letting her body tell her when she has had enough: she didn't need me to step in and do that for her. We ended the evening with satisfied bellies and no unnecessary negative energy or fights about dessert.

MY BODY IS NONE OF YOUR BUSINESS.

Somewhere around the age of five or six, your child will begin to be ready to talk directly about how to handle comments or attention from other people. It's critical to teach your child how to respond rather than to *sit back and hope* they won't have to use this phrase. At one time or another, everyone will experience some act of uninvited attention, criticism, or cruelty regarding their appearance or body—and it's very likely to happen when you're not around to help them through it. When you feel your child is emotionally mature enough to hear you, you can start that vital lesson, teaching them explicitly that *their body isn't the business of anyone else.* Other than their parent or caregiver—and at times a medical professional—no one's opinions about their body are more important than their own. Empowering your child with what to say, when to speak up, and how to simply communicate a boundary will help them when something unexpected happens. I (Sumner) had this talk with my daughter just before she turned six, and I probably should have had it sooner, before she entered primary school. The summer between kindergarten and first grade, she became much more independent, spending considerably more time playing outside, at the neighbor's houses, and with friends in her room than she ever had before. I realized that my child was growing up, and there was no way I could control what people might say to her, but I could arm her with some words to build an internal sense of truth so that when anyone commented on her body in any way, she could turn to them, hold her ground, and confidently state: *My body is none of your business.* You will need to repeat this and work on it over time, but try to do it at a time when nothing specific has happened to prompt the conversation, and your child isn't distracted and can hear you, and then have them practice it. You might say something like: *So what can you say if anyone ever says anything to you about your body that you feel is unkind, rude, mean, or you just don't want them to say it? You can say, "My body is none of your business."*

YOU DON'T HAVE TO EAT IT.

This is a tried-and-true phrase for many dietitians and parents. This phrase conveys everything about the add-in, pressure-off approach. You decide what is served, but no one will be forced to eat it. It's especially helpful in the toddler stage, when your two- or three-year-old starts to naturally want to defy your every decision, and says no to just about everything you make for them. Stay calm, keep your cool, and just steadily state: *You don't have to eat it.*

SOON.

This is for all the times when your child is asking for snacks or milk, and the next meal is coming right around the corner. The goal is to support them coming to the table with an appetite. Dr. Katja Rowell, aka the Feeding Doctor, suggests using a phrase such as *Dinner is coming soon, thanks for your patience* as a way of helping them understand why you're saying no in the moment, and reassuring them that the next meal or snack is coming up. You'll have to use your best judgment to gauge if their hunger is so high that it's better to have something to nibble on before the meal or not, to prevent crossing over into extreme hunger. An appetizer can definitely be appropriate at times—go with your gut and don't overthink it.

WE NEED TO SAVE SOME OF THAT. CAN I GET YOU SOMETHING ELSE? HERE'S WHAT WE HAVE.

(This is a good one for budget restrictions and special foods.) Intuitive Eating isn't just a free-for-all where parents have no say in what is eaten. It's important to teach kids that some foods aren't available in unlimited amounts, and we need to be able to confront the feelings that are associated with that necessary limit. Only you can decide what you're able to offer in unlimited and limited amounts while modeling and supporting body connection and satisfaction. Your job is to try to separate diet mentality from other reasons why you may need to place limits.

WHEN YOUR CHILD ASKS FOR A SNACK
TWENTY MINUTES AFTER BREAKFAST

Although you're doing what you can do to set up a flexible and reliable feeding routine, that doesn't mean that your child will never ask for food between eating times. Do adults sometimes want to eat something a short time after a meal? Yes. Do we need to shame ourselves or feel like there's something wrong with that? No.

In this scenario: (1) expect it to happen, and know that there's nothing wrong, and (2) decide what feels right to you. Remember to keep your eye on the big picture of the feeding routine (is there a flexible routine in place?) and use your Intuitive Eating voice, which brings the focus to eating with permission and attunement.

When they ask for that snack and it's not snack time, ask yourself: Is a simple snack right now doable and reasonable?

You might say: *Sure, we can have it at the table. You can have _____ or _____. After that we'll wait until lunchtime, okay?* (No need to overthink why they are hungry.)

Are you getting coats and shoes on to head out the door to school? If so, a response might be: *Right now we need to get in the car, but you can have part of your snack from your lunch box on the way to school if you need it.* (Acknowledge their request, that it's okay to ask, and explain what you can do.)

Or: *We're not having anything right now because we finished breakfast and right now we need to go to school. Snack will come soon.* (You're not shaming or making them feel bad for asking, but letting them know that food will be available soon enough. You don't bend over backward or adjust the daily schedule. If they are hungrier they will eat more at snack time.)

For the future . . . if requests to eat again soon after a meal are happening frequently: Ask if they've had enough at the end of meal- and snack times: *It looks like you're finished, did you get enough to eat?* Are they being offered enough food they actually want to eat? Are they allowed to have a second helping?

MULTIPLE MOUTHS, MANY PREFERENCES

If you have multiple children and they all want something different to eat, the boundaries become even more important. In my (Sumner) house, one of my children likes to eat noodles or macaroni and cheese with nearly every meal. I check in with my values: I value offering variety, value letting her explore and try things, and value not catering to her all the time because that isn't what the world is going to do. I also value trust and want to build trust that she knows she can often have the food she wants; I know she enjoys it, it works for our family to offer it often, and so very often we will have plain noodles or macaroni and cheese offered with the other food we (the parents) have decided to make because that works for our family. I would not prepare numerous specific foods in response to requests. You get to decide how to balance and make decisions that are aligned with your values.

You may have already offered an afternoon snack, but thirty minutes later your child asks for a lollipop. Saying something like *Yes, sure, you can have that—let's have it at the table. After this one we'll wait for dinner, okay?* shows them you're making a decision that demonstrates permission and is neutral about the sweet. Responding in the same way you would to a banana or an apple—and a second banana or apple—allows both you and your child to know that the limiting is about the fact that dinner is coming, not about the food itself. In this instance, it's not restricting—it's setting a boundary. If the lollipops—or Halloween candy or bananas—are regularly available, your child won't feel deprived. You know that it's probably not going to affect their appetite in an hour or so, and you're communicating the plan and the fact that there won't be another one after this. When you can do this with sweet foods—foods that are commonly restricted or put on a pedestal in other environments that influence your child—it helps emotionally neutralize the food. If your child asks for a muffin, which may fill them up and affect their appetite for dinner, think about a response that isn't about the food, but about the goal of coming to the table hungry. You might say something like: *I hear you want that. You can have some of it, let me cut a piece off for you. You can have the rest later because we're going to eat dinner soon.* If they throw a fit and want the whole thing, your response is: *Throwing a fit doesn't change my answer. Would you like this piece of the muffin?* You, the parent, get to decide. If dinner is fifteen minutes away, you may really know your child and know that they won't be very hungry if they have some muffin and so you can say: *I know that looks good, doesn't it? We're not having any muffin right now, but would you like a piece with your dinner?* You can give your child a piece of a muffin with dinner if that's what they want. When you're able to, being flexible, while clearly communicating, helps. If you find yourself in this situation often, check in with your child the rest of the day to make sure that they're getting enough to eat and have the freedom to choose foods that excite them.

What these examples communicate to your child is: *I hear you. I can tell you're getting hungry and dinner is coming soon. I'm not saying no because of the food, I'm saying no because we're getting ready for dinner.*

When there is one and only one opportunity for a lollipop—such as being able to pick one after-dinner sweet, there is a lot of energy and excitement around that daily opportunity. We have worked with families who say, *I don't know why my child is so focused on sweets whenever they see some—we have a treat after dinner every night.* The answer here is that yes, you're allowing a daily sweet, but that may not be enough to neutralize it; it's still very special compared to other foods you encourage them to eat—it's still a "treat." It's very likely your child is hearing about "treats, sweets, desserts" in different ways all around them—from what other kids are eating from their lunch boxes, at friends' houses, at Grandma's . . . and they'll pick up on the situation at home, where sweets are really special, limited, and not allowed outside of that one time of day.

It's understandable that parents want to set a firm limit around "treats," given that they are so demonized by diet culture, but when something is treated differently from other foods, it actually makes your child more interested in it. When we can understand how limiting certain foods makes it close to impossible to feel neutral about them, we can see the benefit of relaxing and giving more permission around these foods, giving kids the chance to self-regulate. This is why, even when saying no is a practical choice, we have to follow through with actually removing the restrictions on those desired foods. Like in the lollipop example, remember when they asked for a second lollipop and offer it at the next eating time. This reinforces that they have permission to eat it. If the intention was to not spoil their appetite for dinner (your boundary), having it with dinner (or after) removes the threat of deprivation.

REFLECT ON KEY 3

WHEN YOU FEEL UNCOMFORTABLE WITH
YOUR NEW INTUITIVE EATING VOICE

You may experience that it feels really difficult to give your child permission to eat as much as they want, particularly with sweet or special foods. Your discomfort is completely understandable. You might think: *How in the hell is it really okay for me to let my child eat as many cookies as she wants?*

Think about your values, and think about these two important scientific truths:

1. The only way your child can get the information about why they wouldn't want to eat past comfortable fullness is to experience the discomfort of it if it happens. Kids experiment with eating just as much as they do with other things they learn. *Let them learn!* Then you don't have to play the role of the food police every time a delicious or novel food is around. Let them have the responsibility of knowing when to stop because they want to—not because you're forcing them to. Intrinsic motivation is real, and we need to let it support our children with self-regulation.

2. The deprivation or limits around food psychologically makes them want it more, and increases the drive to eat it no matter how they feel. Your policing will not help them have a peaceful relationship with food.

When your child eats too much chocolate because you didn't police it, and you notice they might not feel well, you can say, *What do you think happened?* You're likely to hear: *I think I ate too much chocolate.* Then you express compassion for them, empathy that that amount of chocolate doesn't feel good, and that their body will take care of it, it just might take a little time. Of course, none of us ever wants to see our child uncomfortable or feeling unwell, but you're teaching them that you're not the police, they have permission to eat, and their body communicates with them very clearly, all while reducing the power food has over them for the longer term.

Let your child eat as much as they want: they will learn you aren't their food police, and that it's their responsibility to decide when they've had enough.

Now, we know what you might be thinking: *I may give my child unrestricted permission to eat, but other parents don't do the same! How do I reconcile this?* **Here are some tips to help you feel grounded and confident about utilizing the 3 Keys, even when other adults around you don't:**

1. Many adults make "sugar" comments. Kids don't understand what sugar is—this confuses them (for example, they will also learn in school that fruit has sugar in it). Do you want to send the message that sugar is bad to a five-year-old? We recommend not colluding with the other parent, not bringing attention to the conversation, or saying something simple and clear, such as: *We don't have that rule in our house.* Or: *We don't worry about sugar in our house. Food is food.*

2. After reading this book, you will know more than most other parents about all the aspects of supporting your child to have a healthy relationship with food. Need something concrete? We hear that. Later, you'll learn more about how permission, pleasure, and satisfaction are all very real and very significant parts of your child's whole picture of nutrition and well-being.

3. Kids aren't motivated by cognitive information or future health consequences; if anything, they are motivated to rebel against the food police!

4. If you don't allow sweets when other parents don't allow sweets, consider this: you're raising a child who is going to live in a world that surrounds them with unlimited choices, including all kinds of sweets. If they have been deprived, they are likely to overcompensate when they have freedom, "like a kid in a candy store."

5. As soon as they are at their friend's house where food such as sweets and snacks are possibly readily accessible, a deprived or restricted child will be highly driven to eat the foods that have been off-limits and controlled at home. We see this all the time. Just because you don't see a behavior doesn't mean it's not happening.

GINA'S STORY

Gina grew up in Mexico with Lebanese and Syrian roots, as well as Sephardic Jewish roots. Her parents married when her mother was only sixteen, and Gina was born when her mother was only seventeen. When she was very young, the only stress Gina remembers around food came when her younger twin brothers were born prematurely and struggled to stay awake at mealtime. She fondly remembers coming home from school to a warm meal.

There was some natural body diversity in her family: her mother was tall and thin while her father was short and fat. Gina is the only girl in the family and, as a result, her body was quickly scrutinized. The majority of this came from her aunts. She had aunts who lived in Mexico and aunts who lived in Israel. The aunts in Mexico would often compare her body to theirs, or to her other aunts'. Gina was used to hearing the question

"Will you have your dad's body or your mom's?" This question came with a rather explicit message: *You'd better end up with our thinner body and not the fat bodies that are on your dad's side. You don't want to end up like those aunts.*

Gina remembers this body comparison really coming on when she was about nine years old. She recalls a time when she was eating a lollipop and one of her aunts physically took it from her mouth and threw it away. She then told a confused and heartbroken young Gina that she didn't need that—it was "fattening." This was the beginning of the body conversations for Gina.

The most pivotal moment in her relationship with food and body came when she was fourteen. There was a traditional monthlong visit to Israel at the end of middle school for the kids in her community. Gina, who had been a competitive diver for years, planned to go on the trip with her class, taking the first break in a long time from her five-hour daily training regimen. Her body was finally getting a break from intensive exercise, and at the same time she heard the common warning issued to the girls who went on this trip: don't come back fat.

Gina heard the message from her diving coaches loud and clear in preparation for her trip: don't get fat. She heard this from everyone around her: don't get fat. And she heard it from her mom: don't get fat (and don't come back with pimples). Going halfway across the world, to a country with an entirely different culture, and not engaging in the intense level of exercise and training that she was engaging in prior to leaving, Gina gained weight on the trip. (We also have to add here that she already had a delayed menstrual cycle and was likely weight suppressed, so gaining weight was her body's natural and healthy reaction to less activity and more food—especially around the time of puberty; as an eating disorder dietitian now, she knows this.) Returning home felt shameful for Gina, despite the wonderful experience of the trip.

The comments started quickly after she returned. Her trainers and coaches made more comments about how "heavy" her dives looked and grumbled when she would ask for help with a flip. The most impactful moment came when the boy she had had a relationship with prior to her trip to Israel returned from his trip (he was gone for six months to Europe) and he walked past her at school as if he hadn't seen her at all. His cousin, a good friend of Gina's, told her the reason he was ignoring her was "because she had gotten fat." She was gutted. She returned home that day and talked to her mom about what had happened. The problem, she felt, was that she had gained weight. Her mom's solution to this problem was a diet that her mother had followed. Gina followed the diet and lost weight. She now looks back and knows this was the start of her eating disorder. She was just fourteen.

She began restricting the types of foods she would eat and studiously avoided carbs for years. She was thinner, but she was so hungry. Her family was also going through a time of financial insecurity, so their ability to buy other types of food was limited. Her eating disorder prevented her from eating the affordable foods her family could provide, like rice and beans. So she would eat mostly fruits and vegetables. She also had a very visible side effect from this: she turned rather orange (a side effect from anorexia and eating a lot of foods with beta-carotene). Gina continued diving until she was eighteen, and her coaches noticed the changes in her. She was tired and sad; she was not who she used to be. Her coach recommended she see a dietitian. Her mother was overwhelmed and didn't know how to help. An eating disorder was something that, although dieting and changing appearance was common in her family, Gina's mother had never experienced herself because she was naturally thin and conventionally attractive, so she couldn't relate to Gina's suffering. Gina's father took her to a dietitian. They could only afford one session, so in the limited time they had together, this dietitian emphasized carbohydrates and their importance for athletes. One of the foods that this dietitian had written down as an example for Gina—bagels—actually became a "safe" food for Gina to eat, even in the midst of her eating disorder, simply because she was given professional advice that it was good for her. But despite the warning signs, most people didn't notice the red flags of her eating disorder.

In fact, Gina reflects back now and has even asked her now-husband, whom she met at sixteen, why he didn't say anything when she was so obviously sick. He knew she was not okay, but didn't know how to help. Around the age of twenty-one, Gina and her husband moved to Israel. There, Gina started studying nutrition. At the beginning of her education, she was still very disordered with her eating and felt very afraid to eat many different foods. She joined a research team and started working with some dietitian professors and researchers that she had a lot of respect for. She started to observe them eating—and enjoying their food. Croissants with Nutella, bread, rice. One even mentioned buying ketchup for her child. Gina was surprised and relieved to see these "experts in food" eating and savoring all kinds of foods. Seeing these experts in nutrition eating these foods and being comfortable, she trusted their opinions and started to have positive experiences—savoring warm bread with friends and croissants with people she looked up to. She started to let go of her eating disorder. She recalls the first bite of bread she'd had in years; she and her friends were driving and the car broke down. While waiting for help, they decided to eat the bread they had in the car. It was warm, delicious, and exactly what she needed in that moment.

Living in Israel also allowed her to develop a relationship with the aunts who had been demonized her whole life. She had been told, "Oh, you don't want to be like those aunts," but when she met them and spent time with them, she discovered they were actually warm and kind and loving. And they were fat. Those fat hands made food and gave hugs and spread warmth. Gina decided that she would rather be like *those* aunts. She had been told her whole life that she "hopefully wouldn't look like her dad," but now that she knows that those bodies, the bodies of her dad and her aunts, are full of love and life, she is quite grateful to look more like them.

Gina didn't grow up with excessive rules or fears about health. Her mom offered a diet as a solution to the problem she was presented with. It wasn't out of a desire to harm her daughter or even out of her own desire to change Gina's body. She was trying to help in the best way she could with what she knew. Thin privilege protected her mother in a very image-obsessed family. But Gina wasn't protected by that same privilege once she started to gain weight. What Gina really needed was for someone to tell her that her body never needed to be smaller.

Looking back, Gina notes that when she was a young teen with an eating disorder, she was afraid to give voice to her restrictions. She didn't want to tell people about the truth of her disorder and her fears of food. But now as a professional, she sees a shift. Young girls are actively voicing restrictions and rigid rules that Gina never would have because it's more acceptable to restrict things; disordered eating is glorified and normalized as dieting and pursuing health. As a dietitian now, Gina is working to change the messages for kids and young people in her community. She wants to change the messages of the fear of weight gain around that common trip—and wants to help parents know that kids need to be supported in whatever body they have here and now.

PART IV

THE INTUITIVE EATING APPROACH TO NUTRITION, MOVEMENT, AND MORE

GENTLE NUTRITION

Most parents are concerned at some point about *what* their kids are eating, as well as *how*. One of our jobs as parents is to provide our kids with food, and that includes nutritious food. But what is nutritious food? We believe it means providing foods that help them grow and be active, supporting things like functioning neurotransmitters, gut health, immunity, healthy bones, hormones, energy for growth and developmental changes through puberty, consuming adequate iron and other micronutrients, fiber and digestion, and supporting good sleep. *Phew—is that it?* Surely we've left something out. It's *so* easy to spin into overconcern or become a stress case about kids and food, isn't it?

You may genuinely feel confused about what a nourishing meal for your child that supports all their needs would look like. You've stuck with this book up to this point and read plenty about the dangers of dieting. You want to feed your kids tasty and also health-promoting foods—*without a side of diet mentality*. You likely have been exposed again and again to fear-based messaging that demonizes certain foods, or food groups, spiking your anxiety and worry. There might even be a voice inside your head that has already loaded up on all the armor available to you through diet culture, to question and prevent you from believing in Intuitive Eating. The defensiveness people have to protect diet culture and weight-centered health advice is completely understandable given the world we live in. We are (nearly) indoctrinated into believing that every bite of food we take is either *helping us or harming us.*

So, what is the truth? How do we take all that information that we've been given about what's "healthy" and what's "bad"? Well, we seek *gentle nutrition.* In Intuitive Eating, we use this term to talk about nutrition recommendations.

To seek a balance between understanding what a nourishing eating pattern looks like in real life and to not become overconcerned about nutritional minutia that can create problems for your child is completely justifiable. "Gentle" is actually a really important part of this phrase: gentle implies that there is awareness around giving your kids balanced and nourishing food, without overemphasizing "healthy" eating (*there is no definition of healthy eating anyway*). Gentle nutrition incorporates what we know about the importance of having a healthy feeding relationship, reducing stress around eating, and supporting a child's autonomy with what we know about nutrition. Nutrition isn't one-size-fits-all, nor is it a one-chance deal.

A main criticism of Intuitive Eating is that it must ignore nutrition science and health. But the truth is *that isn't the case.* Intuitive Eating doesn't go against nutrition science, *it adds to it*! With gentle nutrition, instead of just highlighting *what* we feed kids—and what we "shouldn't" be feeding kids—we acknowledge that *how* they eat, and *how they feel* about food and their bodies, are just as important for their health and well-being as nutrition facts are. Gentle nutrition and Intuitive Eating include and value the what, when, why, and how of eating, not just the what.

So much of what you may hear and read about feeding kids leaves out many of the components of gentle nutrition. The whole picture includes: macro- and micronutrients, the joy and pleasure from food, the satisfaction factor, body connection, autonomy, competence, and the feeding relationship. It's a great disservice to parents to oversimplify recommendations for feeding kids. If we do, we miss out on honoring and understanding these little people as whole humans. They are experiencing, learning, and building their own beliefs and values. If your only job were to be concerned about what to feed them and to tell them what and how much to eat, you would not be able to set them up for developing independence and confidence with food—something they will absolutely need when you're not around. As your child develops into an independent eater, they can learn to apply all the various factors that play a role in gentle nutrition.

CAN EATING ONE CERTAIN FOOD OR INGREDIENT REALLY BE A DEATH SENTENCE?

If you have a life-threatening food allergy, or if a food has been laced with poison—yes. In nearly all other circumstances, this isn't the case. Food influences health, but not as severely as we might think. Many things contribute to health, including things that we have no control over; even if we do "eat perfectly," we might not be as healthy as is promised by diet culture. We might never "achieve ideal health." We know that *stress is one of the biggest contributors to inflammation and impacts on our health.* The way we exist around food can be a stressor if we are putting that pressure on it.

We can be aware of nutrition while still aiming to emotionally neutralize food for our kids. We allow them to tap into that inner signaling, to eat the amount of food—be it dessert or dinner—that they are hungry for, and help them know they won't be deprived or restricted. Intuitive Eating respects their here-and-now body and lets them know we don't expect them to be anyone other than who they are. We don't need them to try to change their body to earn our approval. We value their mental health and their authentic selves.

You're free to make whatever choices leave you feeling your best, and you aren't morally obligated to follow any certain way of eating. However, we encourage you to be informed of what the research shows regarding the outcomes from dieting, restriction, and parental control so you can arm yourself with a critical view when you're faced with fear-based nutrition messaging.

Earlier, we shared Anna's story. Her parents were so focused on "being healthy" that they missed out on the importance of the whole picture of *gentle* nutrition. Anna believes that her parents were trying to do their best by encouraging "healthy eating," but she sees now how this narrow view of health created a harsh and distorted relationship with food. Anna's inner narrative and critic attached to the beliefs that food was going to dictate her health and future, and it did. It created deeply embedded patterns of restriction, guilt, and disordered eating. Anna's story is too common.

Choosing Your Path Forward:
Maintain the Status Quo or Foster Intuitive Eating?

These two paths to achieving the goal most parents and caregivers have for their children,
which is optimal and individualized well-being, likely have very different end points.

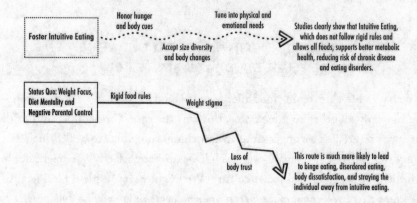

NOURISHING FOOD GROUPS

You may have picked up hundreds of diet rules throughout your life. An *add-in, pressure-off* approach supports you in including nourishing foods, while not stressing about every meal, or pressuring your child. Imagine completely wiping your mind clear of any food rules, and only thinking about nutrition from a gentle nutrition mindset and reframing how you define "healthy" for your family. It's absolutely okay to want to give your kids nourishing meals, fruits and vegetables, and other delicious and nutritious foods, but offering those foods is just an offering. Let the other rules go. Remember that the more permission your kids have, the more relaxed they (and you) can be around food, and the more they will maintain or relearn Intuitive Eating. For now, just think about preparing and providing meals that have variety and a balance of the main food groups, while prioritizing satiety and enjoyment. Your child was born with intrinsic motivation to thrive, to try new things, and to seek out enough nourishing food.

This needs to be emphasized again, as this is foundational to supporting your child's Intuitive Eating path: *no food in and of itself has the power to make your child healthy or unhealthy, or control things like disease, intellectual capacity, or performance.* There is a lot of good nutrition science out there, but we also still know *so little* when it comes to how food impacts the body. No single meal, single day, week, or even month makes or breaks anyone's health. Kids naturally eat various amounts, and will demonstrate various preferences day to day—that is completely normal and not a sign that there is anything wrong.

Nutrition science is imperfect. Unfortunately, every decade or so it seems that what was once claimed to be "the answer" to good health through nutrition is retracted and we learn new information. Some examples of this are the low-fat diet craze of the '90s (*how horrified the now "low-carbers" must be at the era of "fat-free" eating, which greatly increased the carbohydrate intake of a lot of dieters*); then the high-protein, low-carb craze (*still hanging on today, twenty years later*) from the early 2000s; and now the high-fat keto, super-"clean" Whole 30, "caveman-style" paleo, and, more recently, the intermittent fasting (IF) fad. Throughout all of this, calorie counting and "points" tracking from WW (previously Weight Watchers) has remained steadfast on our minds—reminding people everywhere that they should "eat cautiously," "earn their food," and "make up for cheat days." As soon as the current trendy diet fades, a new one replaces it, because diets have never helped us achieve what they promised. Dieting isn't benign. The body will fight against deprivation and do anything to protect itself from starvation—including adapting hormones, neurochemicals, and metabolic rate in order to defend against starvation-including diets. Being stuck in these trends and all the diets that go along with them is like being stuck on a carousel: it just keeps going on and on. But when we ditch the idea that we can't be in charge of our own eating, we get to walk away from the carousel.

It's normal to still feel unsettled after learning all of this diet history. Take a deep breath. Remember your priorities in your relationship with your child. Tuning in to your signals, your family's routine, and really seeing your child gives you a lot of information to help you and your child know what, when, and how much to eat as well as how to meet non-food-related needs.

Dieting and diet culture as an industry is the reason why you needed to pick up this book. People are struggling to make sense of how to eat. Therefore, we can't talk about nutrition without at least making sure you know that *fad dieting, even under the guise of "wellness" or "lifestyle change," if it involves policing or depriving yourself, isn't synonymous with healthy eating.* Dieting—restriction, elimination, eating in moderation, "making better choices," this list could go on and on—are all one and the same. They are a product of diet culture and exist in our mind as diet mentality.

That's why we encourage you to have awareness and intent to provide nourishing foods and varied food choices, without overemphasizing perfect eating, "healthy" eating, or "good" and "bad" foods. Your child will get more than enough of that influence (unfortunately) from diet culture all around them.

Gentle nutrition aims to offer a balance of food groups: starches and grain carbohydrate foods, protein, fats, fruits, and vegetables without perfectionist or all-or-nothing thinking about the meal. All parents can probably relate to the thought *Anything will do tonight, as long as it's food.* We support this. There have been many nights when I (Sumner) serve up a hot bowl of boxed cheddar shells for my kids or myself and call it a night. No shame.

Carbohydrates: Grains, Cereals, Starchy Vegetables, and Sugar

Cereal

Bread: bagel, cracker, pita, sandwich bread

Rice

Pasta

Tortilla

Potato

Corn

Beans and peas

Any grain (flour, quinoa, buckwheat, amaranth, barley, wheat, rye)

Sugar and sweets

Juice and milk

Protein

Eggs

Nuts and nut butter

Beans and soybeans

Milk and dairy

Fish and seafood

Tofu

Poultry

Meat

Pork

Lentils

Seeds

Fats

Oils

Butter

Ghee

Avocado

Nuts and nut butter

Cheese, milk, and yogurt

Animal fat in meat/fish/poultry/eggs

Fruits

Fresh: banana, melon, grapes (halved for small children), apples, berries, kiwi, pineapple, oranges and tangerines, mango, etc.

Frozen: frozen fruit of any kind

Canned: canned fruit of any kind

Dried fruit: apricots, cranberries, raisins, mango, apples, or any kind

Other: applesauce, fruit juice

Smoothies and blended juices

Vegetables

Fresh: carrots, asparagus, cucumber, bell peppers, spinach, lettuce, snap peas, etc.

Cooked: any cooked vegetable, roasted, sautéed, grilled, fried, in soup, casserole

Frozen: any frozen vegetable

Canned: Any canned vegetable such as corn, beets, spinach

Juice: Tomato juice, or mixed fruit and vegetable juice

SAMPLE MEAL IDEAS

These are simply suggestions for parents who get stuck with the daily thought, *What to serve?* You can serve kids any foods that you would prepare for yourself. This basic guidance is important to hold in your mind:

- Serve at least one food that they like and are familiar with at a meal.
- Offer new foods, preferably family style on the table, or on their plate even if they don't choose to eat them—but know that it can take twenty or more times of exposing kids to a new food for them to feel motivated to try it—and there may be foods they never want to try. Avoid pressuring.

- Try offering food in a self-serve/family-style way to support choice and competency with eating. It's fun and they have a job at the table, serving their food!
- Make food visually appealing if you can—kids often assess interest in a food based on how it looks.
- Serve safe (size/texture) foods to prevent choking.
- Remember that there is no need to get caught up in perfectionism—not every meal is going to have a fruit or a vegetable—and that is A-OK.

Sample Meals

Waffle with butter and syrup + yogurt + blueberries

Bagel + eggs + apple slices + milk

Banana bread + cottage cheese

Cereal bar + whole milk

Smoothie made with milk or yogurt + cereal bar

Falafel + pita + yogurt + cucumber

Apples + peanut butter + Goldfish crackers

Cheese sandwich + trail mix

Noodles with oil or butter + marinara sauce + mixed vegetable plate with dip + milk

Hummus + tortilla + cheese + orange slices

Fish + noodles with butter or olive oil + applesauce

Bean burrito + milk + chips and salsa

Fried chicken + biscuit + green beans + milk

Happy Meal + milk + cereal bar

Toast + avocado + veggie sausage + orange juice

Any food you have made + something your kid likes!

WHAT INFLUENCES SATIETY, ENERGY, AND FULLNESS?

It's commonly recommended to offer a mix of foods from different food groups (carbohydrate + protein + fat) at each meal. (*Remember: you decide what to offer, they decide what they'll eat and how much.*) The reasoning behind the combination of these nutrient groups has to do with blood sugar and satiety—which is influenced by what and how much we eat. Simply put, when you eat something, your body has a natural hormonal response to digest the food, break it down, and extract energy to use and store. One hormone that is released is *insulin*. Insulin helps to move carbohydrate (sugar) from our blood into our cells (muscles and brain) for fuel. Blood sugar (glucose) is necessary: it keeps us alive! If blood sugar drops too low, we don't feel well, can't think as efficiently, may get nauseous, and in very extreme circumstances (after completely using up all the body's stored carbohydrate) we can become very ill or even die (this usually is the result of a severe health condition like insulin-dependent diabetes). In most normal circumstances, when blood sugar drops, we experience hunger, then move on to more uncomfortable and serious signs of low blood sugar such as dizziness, headaches, sleepiness, shaking, or confusion. There is a common misunderstanding that "blood sugar" is a bad thing. It isn't. Everyone has blood sugar (blood glucose) in their blood at all times—it's the molecule that keeps our brain fueled and our body alive. A well-nourished, reliably fed body will strive to remain in *homeostasis*, or a stable state. This includes a relatively flat wave of blood glucose levels—rising and falling throughout the day in response to how we eat, how we move, and even things like illness and stress.

The hormonal response to eating is part of what dictates that communication from your body to your mind that you're satisfied and that it's time to finish eating. Ghrelin, leptin, insulin, and neuropeptide Y are some of the many hormones that influence our complex biological system of appetite regulation. The vagus nerve is another key player in this communication pathway. Your body is built to sense information from within, both from fullness receptors in the stomach itself, and from signals sent to the brain after eating to adjust your appetite. This internal sense of satiety is one example of *interoceptive awareness*. Interoceptive awareness may sound complicated, but it's actually simple: when attuned, we can sense signals from our body. These signals are things like needing to go to the bathroom or feeling your heart rate rise when you're anxious. Receiving these signals gives us the information we need in order to know the next right step. This process is key to how Intuitive Eating works. When we sense this information about hunger, satiety, and fullness from our body, and combine it with awareness of our thoughts and emotional state, we're accessing the dynamic interplay that is Intuitive Eating. With Intuitive Eating—including gentle nutrition—we have the opportunity to eat nourishing and satisfying foods, while not losing sight of the whole picture and the factors that influence well-being.

Blood sugar is a common topic of conversation in our household (Amee). My partner has type 1 diabetes, so our daughter has learned from a young age that Daddy needs sugar when his blood sugar gets too low. She's learned what sugar is best for him to have and she'll gladly offer to share her Halloween candy with him. We have also used this nutrient and blood sugar and energy dynamic to talk about foods that are most helpful before she goes to her various activities. She's learned, through trial and error, that having a pack of gummy candy right before a dance class won't keep her energy as high as a granola bar or a yogurt. She's never been hurt by trying the gummies before dance class, but she will leave the class looking a bit sweatier, simply because the energy from that snack was used up a lot more quickly than from another, more energy-dense snack.

Thinking about it from an Intuitive Eating view, the body's response to dropping blood sugar is yet another sign of how wise and accurately it directs us when to eat. Bodies generally feel hungry when blood sugar drops. Body signals such as feeling hunger sensations or a growling stomach, salivating at the thought of food, and mood or concentration changes are all messages from our body that we need to make it a priority to stop what we're doing and get something to eat. Some people experience interruptions, or difficulty in noticing early signs of hunger—they may be easily distracted, or highly focused on work or other tasks, and forget to eat. We actually have worked with many people who describe this. It's not unusual to need to set an alarm, or a reminder to check in after two to four hours from your previous meal or snack, and assess your hunger. Other people simply are less sensitive to early signs of hunger, and will benefit from deciding to eat at regular intervals, as a way of implementing self-care and preventing getting overly hungry. The flexible and reliable feeding routine, Key 2, is how you as a caregiver can support your child in eating at regular and consistent intervals throughout the day.

Various things can impact our ability to notice early hunger signals. Certain medications, stress, being distracted by external events, a history of dieting and silencing hunger signals, and certain compensations (like drinking too much fluid or caffeine) can blunt hunger signals. Focusing on feeding yourself—and your child— regularly and reliably can often help bring these signals back online and help them to be easier to notice, even when there are obstacles.

FEEDING KIDS—KEY NUTRIENTS

The best chance for optimal nutrition, for anyone, is getting a variety of foods. Not everyone has the same financial privilege to be able to afford a wide variety of foods, or can access fresh foods based on where they live and the impact of food apartheids. Food apartheids are areas where there is systemic inability to access fresh food. There may be a marked lack of grocery stores or other food sources that aren't gas stations or fast food restaurants. This means residents of these areas are often reliant on vehicles or public transportation to access resources. These food apartheids also disproportionately impact communities of color, leading to even further health disparities. Thank goodness there are many lower-cost foods offered in nearly every grocery store that are fortified with essential nutrients kids need, such as iron. Fortification is a huge public health benefit of processed foods in the United States that often goes unnoticed.[1]

Although this isn't an exhaustive list, some key nutrients that are considered vital for proper growth and development for kids are iron, calcium, vitamin D, fiber, vitamin C, and essential fats.

IRON

Why it's important: Adequate iron from food helps prevent iron-deficiency anemia. In iron-deficiency anemia, there is a reduced amount of red blood cells in the body. Red blood cells carry oxygen from the lungs to the body organs and muscles. Iron deficiency can impact growth and brain development and, in the case of severe or prolonged deficiency, can interrupt your child's learning ability. Iron status is routinely assessed at pediatric visits, so be sure your child attends all pediatric checkups and include iron-rich foods in your child's meals and snacks. If a child has a too-low intake of iron, a too-high calcium intake can compete with absorption of high-iron foods. This is only an issue when calcium intake is very high and iron intake is very low. Additionally, if your child is low or deficient in iron, they may be recommended to take iron supplements. These do not taste good, and forcing or hiding these supplements can have a negative impact on your child's relationship with food (creating fear or aversion to eating) or a negative impact on the feeding relationship between you and your child; for instance, they may worry you're hiding something yucky in their food. You can certainly give supplements a try, but don't lose sight of the importance of having positive feeding experiences for their long-term health. If they are very averse to supplements, instead try reducing milk to no more than three eight-ounce cups per day and increasing iron-fortified foods like iron-fortified breakfast cereal in their routine along with vitamin C–rich foods (see below).

Food sources

Iron-fortified baby cereal (babies should be at least four months old)
Fortified breakfast cereals (check the box label)
Beans

Fish

Chicken

Red meat

Spinach

Vitamin C helps iron absorption: consider serving iron-rich foods with vitamin C–rich foods such as tomatoes, citrus, orange juice, strawberries, bell peppers, and melon.

Iron from animal sources (heme-iron) is generally more bioavailable, or easily absorbable, than iron from plant sources (non-heme iron). Combining vitamin C sources and non-heme iron sources can help remedy that difficulty.

CALCIUM + VITAMIN D

Why they're important: Calcium and vitamin D work together to help build and strengthen bones. Calcium is a mineral required for bone development. Inadequate calcium intake can lead to soft or weak bones, poor growth, muscle pain, and weakness. Vitamin D is a fat-soluble vitamin (technically, a steroid hormone). Fat soluble means it requires fat in the diet to function optimally. Vitamin D, in addition to helping support bone mineral density, is also associated with preventing health problems such as heart disease, diabetes, and osteoporosis. Bone density builds during childhood and adolescence and peaks around the late twenties. Babies who are exclusively breastfed are encouraged to have a vitamin D supplement, which your pediatrician should recommend for you. Too much vitamin D can be toxic, so talk to your doctor about the recommended dose of a supplement.

Calcium needs

1–3 years: 700 mg daily

4–8 years: 1000 mg daily

9–18 years: 1300 mg daily

Vitamin D needs

Under 1 year: 400 IU daily

1 year or older: 600 IU daily

Some kids may need more than the recommended 600 IU per day of vitamin D. Always check with your doctor for personalized recommendations.

Those located above northern latitude 37 or below southern latitude 37—areas with very little sunshine during large parts of the year—may be more likely to have low vitamin D stores due to the angle of the sun on the atmosphere. They are literally unable to manufacture it from the sun for half of the year. In these locations, it can be even more important to talk to your doctor about what they recommend.

Vitamin D insufficiency is more prevalent for those with darker skin tones due to the fact that pigmentation reduces vitamin D production in the skin.[2]

Food sources
Vitamin D–fortified milk and yogurt
Cooked fatty fish
Portobello mushrooms
Tuna
Vitamin D–fortified orange juice
Egg yolk

FIBER

Why it's important: One of the key reasons why fiber is emphasized for kids is because the foods that provide fiber also provide a variety of important micronutrients and antioxidants. Colorful fruits and vegetables, grains, root vegetables, beans, and legumes are great sources of fiber. Kids need fiber to help aid in healthy digestion, prevent constipation, and support blood sugar regulation. Fiber is also important for healthy gut bacteria—aka our gut microbiota. In and along our digestive tract, we harbor trillions of microbes. We are reliant on these microbes to survive. They maintain our immune system, and we have what is referred to as a "symbiotic relationship" with them—we need these microbes as much as they need us. Without adequate fiber and carbohydrate intake, the balance of gut microbiota can suffer. Imbalance of certain strains of gut bacteria may play a role in conditions such as irritable bowel syndrome (IBS), irritable bowel disease (IBD), and chronic constipation.[3] What we know about fiber, carbohydrates, and microbiota is still emerging with new literature and science; however, at this point, there is strong evidence to support the notion that low-carb, high-fat diets (such as the ketogenic or "keto" diet) harm the integrity of the gut microbiome, which can lead to disruptions in health in both the short term and the long term.[4,5]

Fiber needs

1–3 years: 19 g daily
4–8 years: 25 g daily
8 years and up: 25–40 g daily

Food sources

Popcorn
Carrots
Oat-based cereal
Bananas
Whole grain pasta
Barley
Berries
Potatoes and sweet potatoes
Bean dip or bean burrito
Peas
Lentils and legumes
Fruit salad
Bran or wheat germ added to homemade baked goods
Salad/greens
Apples or applesauce
Pears
Nuts and seeds (or nut/seed butter)
Various fruit, vegetables, and plant foods—the list is endless!

There is definitely such a thing as having too much fiber. We recommend you steer clear, for yourself and your kids, of foods that have been fortified with added fiber—*look out for ingredients like chicory root, inulin, oligosaccharide, oligofructose*. These ingredients can cause stomach aches, gas, and indigestion. Fiber has become such a buzz word, thanks to diet culture, that food manufacturers have jumped on the opportunity to market their packaged foods as "high fiber" by using added fiber. We recommend that you and your family aim to eat fiber from naturally occurring food sources and avoid supplements unless otherwise recommended by your doctor. There is a time and a place for fiber supplements—but do get individualized advice from a doctor or dietitian before you go there.

VITAMIN C

Why it's important: Vitamin C is an essential ingredient for healthy teeth and bones, muscle and tissue development, and, because vitamin C is an antioxidant, it plays a role in maintaining your child's immune system. It isn't something their body can produce internally, so it's considered *essential* for their diet, making this one of the key nutrients to keep your eye on when preparing and planning meals and snacks. As mentioned above, vitamin C helps boost the absorption of iron, an additional bonus!

Vitamin C needs
1–3 years: 15 mg daily
4–8 years: 25 mg daily
9–13 years: 45 mg daily

Food sources
Red, yellow, and green bell peppers
Tomatoes
Melons
Citrus fruits, citrus juice
Tomatoes
Tomato sauce
Kiwi
Strawberries
Brussels sprouts
Cherries
Guavas
Persimmons
Papaya
Watermelon

Many supplements are marketed as cold-busters and immune promoters. But when we take in too much vitamin C at one time—say, from a mega-dose in powder form—we actually absorb less and end up filtering a significant amount out through our kidneys. This is another case where food sources are the best bet.

ESSENTIAL FATS

Why they're important: There are many different types of fat in foods. Essential fats, *omega-3 and omega-6 fats,* are required for the health and development of brain tissue and other delicate tissues such as the retina in our eyes as well as for building cells that form the central nervous system and cardiovascular system. Intake of omega-3 and omega-6 fatty acids in early life years has been shown to affect growth and cognitive performance later in childhood.

OMEGA-3 (EPA, DHA, AND ALA)

Children are less likely to be achieving the recommended intake of this kind of fat, compared to other fats from food. Inadequate intake is likely related to low seafood intake for many families. This is an opportunity for you, as a parent, to take advantage of the ability you have to use that neocortex area of your brain, the one that allows us to access logic and reason. It's in line with an Intuitive Eating approach to serve and offer foods and fortified foods that contain omega-3 fats to your child (and to decide to include more of any nourishing foods for your child, for that matter). Remember, coercing or forcing them to eat it isn't helpful, but offering it without pressure is! You may even talk to your doctor about recommending a supplement, although an omega-3 supplement is likely too expensive for many families who need to prioritize food before supplements. To increase omega-3 intake, you can consider intermittently buying omega-3-fortified milk when you're able to or cook with omega-3-fortified eggs. It could be a while before omega-3-rich seafood is readily accepted by your child—seafood is a strong flavor and often rejected by many kids, while others enjoy it from a young age.

Omega-3 needs

0–12 months: 0.5 g daily

1–3 years: 0.7 g daily

4 to 8 years: 0.9 g daily

9–13 years (boys): 1.2 g daily

9–13 years (girls): 1.0 g daily

14–18 years (boys): 1.6 g daily

14–18 years (girls): 1.1 g daily

Omega-6 needs: Data from a 2018 study found that most children are likely to be consuming at least the recommended amount of omega-6 fats daily.[6]

Food sources of omega-3

There are three kinds of omega-3 fats: EPA, DHA, ALA

Fish, especially fatty fish such as salmon, mackerel, sardines, and cod
Canned light tuna
Shrimp
Oysters
Walnuts
Flaxseed
Some brands of fortified eggs (in the yolk only)
Lesser amounts in grass-fed meat, milk, and eggs
Chia seeds

Food sources of omega-6

Canola oil*
Soybean oil* (frequently used as an ingredient in many foods)
Soybeans

Also contains the omega-3 fat ALA.

The above-listed nutrients do not represent an exhaustive list of all nutrients a child needs. Additional key nutrients that support neurodevelopment and are especially important for the first two years of life include protein, zinc, choline, folate, iodine, and vitamins A, B6, and B12.

LAST BUT NOT LEAST:
THE NUTRIENT OF "POSITIVE MEALTIME EXPERIENCES"

Most of all, don't forget to emphasize *positive experiences* with meal- and snack times. Kids don't always want to eat the same thing, and they don't have the same appetite every day, just like adults. They will not develop a growth or a nutrient deficiency from a few days, or even a few weeks, of low-variety eating. In cases where there is extreme picky eating, we recommend that you work with a health provider who can assess if your child's diet is meeting their nutritional needs. Some children, particularly very selective eaters, may eat only around twenty different foods, and can be healthy. Individualized assessment by a pediatric feeding specialist or registered dietitian is optimal if you observe your child having long-term selective or very picky eating, or consistently not consuming the groups of key nutrients listed above. Your child may benefit from a supplement in order to adequately meet their needs for one or more of the food groups they tend not to eat. **It's more important to maintain a peaceful and positive association with food and meals than it is to force your child to eat something they don't like or to which they have an aversion.**

HYDRATION AND BEVERAGES

Hydration is a part of gentle nutrition and it's a vital contributor to how kids feel and function. Tummy troubles and specifically constipation can result from not drinking enough fluids. Reminders to drink water throughout the day can be very helpful to little minds that are captivated by the world around them and just aren't thinking about thirst. Keep their favorite water bottle handy and filled up when out of the house, and serve water with meals and snacks. School-age children can do well with a little responsibility around this; you can tell them: *Remember to try to drink from your water bottle throughout the day!*

BEVERAGES BETWEEN MEALS CAN DECREASE APPETITE

Kids who drink milk and juice between meals may experience an interruption of their hunger cues—*but it's not really an interruption,* it's their wise body being really clear that they are no longer as hungry for that meal because they drank milk or juice. Their body knows it has had some nutrients and energy from the beverage they drank not long ago. This is the primary reason why it's okay to say no to drinks other than water in between meals and snacks. Tell your child, *Right now there is water if you're thirsty. You can have _____ with lunch.* The impact juice or milk or soda has on a child on their appetite for their next meal can vary from child to child, because different kids have different energy needs, different metabolic rates, and different-sized bodies. My (Sumner) daughter will usually not be very hungry, possibly even uninterested in food at all, if she's had a cup of milk within about an hour before her meal, while my son is still generally ready to eat even after drinking milk. He might adjust his total food intake to his appetite if needed. My (Amee) daughter is unfazed by drinking milk or juice in between meals or with snacks. You *do not* need to coach your child through this adjustment by saying something like *Rex, you had milk, so you probably don't need to eat as much dinner as you usually do, okay?* That would be pressure and judgment. **Let your child make their adjustments on their own.**

So, what do you do with the child who requests milk or juice between meals, but their pattern shows they won't be hungry for the next meal? We suggest you support them with some boundaries to help them show up to their meal with some comfortable hunger. If they aren't hungry, saying something to the effect of *You wanted milk, so now you have to eat your dinner, too. You're not allowed to have milk and then not eat your dinner* is *pressuring* them to eat beyond what *their* body is asking. The decision around whether your child can have milk between meals is a *boundary* for you to set. If you know your child will likely not be hungry for their next meal soon after drinking something, and you're okay with them not eating much dinner when dinner is served, then it's up to you to decide if you want to serve them milk between meals. Understandably, many parents want to use boundaries in a supportive way, to facilitate the feeding routine—which can mean saying no to milk or juice between meals. When you place a boundary, it will not always be accepted. There could be whining or crying, but it's important to be as consistent as you can. Communicate the why: *We're having dinner soon, so no milk right now, thanks for being patient!* (This isn't meant to be rigid. If you know they are very hungry, you always get to make the call and perhaps give them an appetizer to hold them over and count it as part of their dinner.) Perhaps you have a child you feel isn't eating enough, and your natural reaction is to give them any food or beverage any time they ask as a result of your worry about their low intake. However, a responsive feeding approach would suggest to not serve the milk, in order to support them to have a comfortable hunger signal, which helps them feel their internal drive to eat, at the next meal.

REFRESHING AND SATISFYING

Beverages aren't just about hydration, although it's certainly the biggest reason why we drink, but diet culture has really demonized beverages that contain sugar and calories. Beverages are satisfying, delicious, and not "bad" just because they have calories. The simple example we talked about above proves that beverages do impact satiety signals and we can trust those signals. With that, without any fiber, protein, or fat, juice and soda do digest very quickly, and impact blood sugar with a quick spike, but this doesn't mean they are unhealthy or bad.

There's no firm nutritional reason to avoid juice—in fact, there is evidence that including juice regularly as part of a child's eating routine can help boost vitamin intake and provides them a serving of fruit.[7] Juice offers some really valuable benefits: fruit juice with vitamin C can help increase iron absorption, and some juices are fortified with calcium, which can be helpful for kids who aren't milk drinkers. Juice also provides carbohydrates—something kids need! But juice isn't advised for children under two and should not ever be provided in a bottle, as it may cause dental cavities. Waiting until they are around two or older to introduce juice helps your child get used to drinking water for thirst instead of sweetened beverages. It helps set them up to enjoy and establish a preference for water. Also, very young kids have tiny tummies! They can fill up quickly, and yet they are growing and developing at such a rapid pace that they need to be eating food to nourish their body; if they fill up on juice or milk, they may not have room for the meal (because they are so attuned with their fullness signals at this age). Their meal is where they'll get most of the nutrition they need, such as protein, starch, micronutrients, fiber, and fat. Juice can complement a meal or snack. Juice that's 100 percent fruit juice has the most real fruit nutrition compared to artificially flavored juice, and you'll maximize the nutrients in what they drink—which, for kids who have a very limited intake of fruits or vegetables, could be a helpful part of an add-in approach.

REMEMBER TO STAY NEUTRAL

We suggest keeping a neutral attitude around juice. If you're somewhere juice is available and your child asks for juice, stay neutral. Say, *Sure*, and let them have some—they may or may not like it. For the most part, juice is best offered with meals or snacks and not in between for the reasons mentioned above: kids may fill up and not want to eat later, missing out on the food they need. Once in a while this isn't a big deal, but if it becomes a pattern, you will likely notice a struggle at mealtime if they don't have interest in eating.

Kids will become increasingly interested and captivated by juice, soda, or any other food or beverage that you place off-limits if they sense you have a strong reaction to it. Allow it to become something that is no big deal. You can always keep some juice stocked in the fridge, or you don't have to buy any juice at all—it's up to you. (Although buying it occasionally can be a way to show you're neutral about it and it's not "bad.") If your child doesn't like juice or if they don't drink it because you don't buy it, that doesn't mean you're depriving them of anything. If early in their life they have become accustomed to drinking water, they will tend to hold on to that preference because they know how good and refreshing water is. In their first two years of life, kids generally aren't asking for things—they eat from what you make available. This is a time to establish some foundational preferences, including preferences around what they drink. Just as offering variety is helpful early on, so is setting some family standards around beverages. If juice isn't offered, they don't know to ask for it, and do well with just milk and water. Then they can enjoy the taste and pleasure of juice when they're a little older, without having adopted a pattern of drinking juice, or expecting it, from a young age. This isn't an all-or-nothing recommendation. For some kids, who may struggle to get enough to eat for any reason, having juice available, if it's accepted by them, can be very nourishing.

Your attitude and what you model matter the most. How does your child observe you drinking beverages? Do you ever enjoy a glass of orange juice or lemonade? Do you regularly model drinking water with meals? Do they observe you feeling anxious and irritated when they want a juice box at a birthday party? How do you respond at the grocery store when they ask if you can put some juice in the cart? If you have a history of dieting, are you drinking colorful "diet" drinks or diet soda often as a way of avoiding eating—and are they confused as to why you get to drink various interesting beverages often but they are limited to milk and water? What can you do to help support your child to have a healthy relationship with juice or soda or any other beverage through modeling and through neutrality?

WHAT ABOUT SUGAR?

Humans love sugar. Adults, kids, and babies love sugar (breast milk is around 7 percent sugar). Some people don't feel good eating past a certain amount of sugar—that is their body communicating to them, *We're good, we've had enough.* The rebound effect of restricting sugar is that you may feel incredibly strong urges to keep eating it as a result of *deprivation*, not as a result of having eaten some. **The research on sugar addiction is flawed: it doesn't control for, or acknowledge, how restriction (aka dieting) fuels the feeling of being out of control.**

Yes, sugar processing has changed. Yes, there is more sugar in our food supply than before. *And* that doesn't change the biological wiring the human body has to detect hunger and satiety. It's likely the way we have come to *relate to sugar* that causes people to eat in a way that they feel they can't control.

THE VERY COMMON FEAR OF SUGAR

We will not ignore that among some groups there are nutrition-related health problems involving sugar intake—but these aren't because kids can't control themselves, or because parents are trying to hurt their kids by giving them too much juice. It's because of other factors, many of which are out of their control, that create an environment where eating balanced, adequate, and nourishing meals is challenging. There is an imbalance of accessibility to healthful eating in our society, which has led to some underserved areas and groups having to rely on inexpensive convenience foods that also happen to be higher in sugar. Our food supply does have a significantly higher amount of sugar in it than it did fifty years ago—we don't ignore this. However, *this fact doesn't change the premise of the importance of Intuitive Eating.* Nor does it mean that these foods are bad or need to be avoided. Families and communities who have no or low access to fresh, nourishing foods are disproportionately affected by the changes that have taken place in our food supply. These families are more reliant on fast food restaurants (in many places these are the only restaurants and, in some cases, the primary food source), convenience foods, and packaged foods, and have a higher intake of sugary beverages such as juice and soda. Calorie for calorie, processed foods are often much more affordable than fresh foods, and when trying to get as much food in your budget as you can to stay as full as you can, you will likely eat the more calorie-dense, processed food. When you look at health differences between zip codes of higher socioeconomic levels and those with lower average socioeconomic levels, it's clear that there is more to the story than how much sugar has been added to the food supply. **Access to nutritionally adequate foods is fundamental to maintaining health, and in communities where access has been interrupted we see significant health disparities.**

The story that is often told is that sugar is the culprit, the dangerous ingredient to avoid, but the science on sugar doesn't back this up. When all factors are considered, it isn't wholly the sugar to blame for negative health impacts such as diabetes, metabolic syndrome, or fatty liver. We aren't really getting to the root of the concerns we need to tackle about childhood health unless we look at a combination of factors, including: food access and affordability, racism and economic inequity, disordered eating, weight stigma, and psychological and emotional health, to name a few. These are the major players in public health "emergencies," yet the majority of funding and resources continue to be poured into "obesity" research. *Science is missing the boat,* and the outcomes of "childhood obesity" interventions show this to be true. If we are truly worried about kids' health and nutrition, we need to see more interventions and more resources pointed at social justice, food justice, mental health, weight stigma and size discrimination in healthcare, and prevention of eating disorders.

Many health experts emphasize the potential risks of eating certain foods or ingredients, like sugar. The topic of sugar and sugar addiction is complicated. When talking about the "dangers of sugar" and refined carbohydrates, many "experts" repeatedly leave out scientific facts that show there is more to the equation of health and disease risk than nutrition alone. Eating sugar, on its own, isn't responsible for causing anyone to develop type 2 diabetes—there are many other factors involved, particularly genetics. When one ingredient or food is demonized and important facts about how nutrition-related conditions develop are left out of the conversation (the influence of genes on developing diabetes is usually not part of the wellness dialogue), then the actual impact of the demonized food on the body is skewed. Who is most easily influenced by "fear-based" nutrition messaging like this? You, the health-conscious consumer, and subsequently your kids. Those who aren't fully versed in reading scientific studies (*and who really can be, if it's not your job?*) and aren't as informed about the science of how social determinants of health, systemic oppression, and mental health impact a person's disease risk are understandably quickly moved to embrace these scary beliefs about food as truth. *In the human mind, it often is more appealing to believe something that isn't in fact true than to live with the uncertainty of something more flexible and nuanced.*

THE SOCIAL DETERMINANTS OF HEALTH

Social and psychological health factors, such as being able to get to medical appointments, having depression, generational trauma, experiencing weight stigma, and racial discrimination, are all significant factors that impact chronic disease risk and allostatic load (chronic stress levels). Claims like "Sugar causes type 2 diabetes" are enormously popular, oversimplified, and part of diet culture. Those claims put the responsibility on the individual to manage every aspect of their health, largely through diet and exercise. This form of individualism has its own negative impact on mental health, which impacts physical health. Studies have shown that in populations that are disproportionately impacted by type 2 diabetes and poverty, like Indigenous communities, the most effective intervention to lower blood sugar levels (a1c) was to provide affordable and safe housing.[8]

Over and over again, "experts" make the case that eating sugar is comparable to a death sentence. You may have heard doctors, researchers, naturopathic providers, and nutritionists attempt to convince people that the "simple shift" of cutting out sugar is an essential step for health. What is missing from these quite convincing displays of diet culture jumbled with medical advice is that an estimated 20 to 40 percent of households in the United States don't have enough money to even buy enough food for their families every month or cannot access a store that sells produce. The predictable effect dieting has on binge eating, depression, weight cycling, and metabolic health over time is also not discussed. They simply recommend, "Just cut out sugar, eat protein for breakfast, it's that simple." In researching this, we didn't hear or see anyone acknowledge what happens to the majority of people who attempt low-carb dieting (bingeing and weight gain later on), or those who try to completely omit sugar from their diet (this is rarely sustainable). They don't discuss the cravings, binges, shame, eating disorders, negative GI health effects, and all the other consequences we know are directly tied to restrictive eating patterns. It's very easy to claim that there is a "simple solution to change your life and your health" when you fail to include all the facts. Next time you're watching, reading, or listening to someone who uses fear-based nutrition messaging, you might recognize how quickly this triggers your internal diet mentality. You might feel like you have to "fix" your eating (picture your cortisol rising, stress response on deck). *Now, imagine what this does to kids when they hear it.*

Even if we ignore the way these recommendations completely deny the existence of poverty, we are still skipping over the fact that *it's okay to enjoy sugar*. We live in a culture that demonizes the things that bring us pleasure. Here in the United States, a large part of our culture is the descendants of Puritans—and it shows. Two of the things that we need to continue the species—and meet our basic human needs—are regularly demonized and looked at as gluttonous. Sex and food. Both give us pleasure, both are demonized. Food has even been created in order to prevent us from wanting to be gluttonous or "sinful"! For example, the graham cracker and corn flakes were invented to be so boring and bland that they could stop Americans from masturbating.[9] We use words like "decadent" to describe chocolate cake; the definition of decadent is "characterized by a state of moral decline." Wow. It's a cake, not a ritual sacrifice. Food is allowed to be enjoyable, and having a "sweet tooth" isn't something you need to overcome.

What we do hear sprinkled into these convincing talks demonizing sugar or pleasure are testimonials about how people "feel better, more energized, more alive" when they have made a diet change. *What's the hidden gem here?* The hidden gem that we agree with is that when you *tune in to your own body*—when you notice how you feel physically—you have a powerful amount of information to guide you to know how to eat, what feels best for your unique body, and you don't need to follow diet rules to dictate your decisions. You're allowed to eat as much or as little sugar or any other food or ingredient as you want. We hope you will find it beneficial to have all the facts in order to make the best decision for you.

SUGAR AND ADHD

It has been a pretty mainstream "fact" that "sugar causes or worsens ADHD symptoms" (this same myth persists for food dyes and additives). Although there may be valid reasons for some individuals to avoid certain ingredients, this shouldn't be applied generally for all kids. Children, in general, may show increased signs of hyperactivity after consuming sugar, but studies show that this is more likely related to the excitement of eating sugar as a rare treat instead of an actual medical interaction. We do have some evidence that individuals with ADHD are more likely to eat more sugar than a neurotypical person, but this is more likely due to the craving for dopamine that their brain is lacking. If you find yourself in this situation and fear the act of eating sugar, truly ask yourself why. If you, as the parent, help maintain the boundaries and help your child—or yourself—find various ways to get dopamine bursts into that deprived brain, then the occasional sugar dopamine burst is A-OK. Other ways to get a dopamine burst are listening to music, achieving a small goal, playing video games, getting a hug from someone you love, or watching a short funny video (laughter is hugely effective).

No dietary recommendation is delivered in a vacuum: nearly everyone has been influenced by diet mentality in some way, and many people have been significantly hijacked by it. So, when an "expert" writes an article, or delivers a TED Talk that says, "It's simple, just eat protein like eggs for breakfast instead of carbs—it will change your life," a person hears that in the context of thinking, I thought eggs were bad for me, *or* I just read an article about eating a plant-based diet, *or* I don't like eggs, *or* I have an egg allergy, *or some other piece of nutrition or diet advice. People are extremely confused; there isn't one simple solution, and there isn't one way of eating that is going to work well for everyone. Therein lies the beauty of Intuitive Eating: you get to choose what feels best, what feels like permission, what way of eating is truly a decision you're making based on wanting to feel great, enjoy food, be flexible, and take care of yourself.*

In 2016, the American Heart Association (AHA) took sugar restriction to a new level, stating that children and teens (ages two to eighteen) should limit their added sugars to less than 6 teaspoons per day and no more than 8 fluid ounces of sugary beverages per week.[10] So, let's break this down. If my child has a waffle for breakfast, with 2 tablespoons of maple syrup, he is maxed out on his "allowed" sugar for the day according to this recommendation. That means no jelly on that PB&J for lunch (and "natural" peanut butter only), no honey on the cornbread with dinner, certainly no scoop of ice cream later on. Only one 8-ounce cup of juice or chocolate milk per week—that limit is actually quite rigid. When your child notices this rigidity, it impacts how they relate to that food or ingredient, and will likely create some type of charged response to those foods once they have more autonomy and choice (when you're not around).

It's no one's place to tell you how to define your experiences: if you personally feel like you're addicted to sugar, *then that is your lived experience.* But we want to ask the question: Is it possible that this feeling of being addicted to sugar is related to a long history of dieting that may have involved sugar restriction or a belief in your mind that you're out of control with sugar? Have you been told (or read) that you're addicted to sugar? Quite often that is the case. We can be significantly influenced by what people in positions of power tell us, and get hooked into these beliefs as absolute truths. One of the major problems with the research on food addiction and sugar that researchers have not controlled for (and this makes it very different from other substance and process addictions) is how much dieting is a factor in the eating experience—even though the vast majority of people who struggle with food addiction are recurrent dieters. Are you eating spoonfuls of sugar out of the bag? Probably not—you're probably eating things that have a mix of ingredients, with particular textures, that are *soothing and pleasurable* for a complex set of reasons—not for the sugar itself.

We didn't include this to stir up an argument about whether or not sugar is addictive. However, we do feel that it's unfortunate so many parents are feeling that they need to place strict limits on their child's sugar consumption—for reasons that are unwarranted, and that can often have the opposite effect for their child—sugar becomes powerful, emotionally charged, and they end up overeating it, bingeing, or hiding their sugar consumption to avoid your disappointment. Shame becomes very tied up in their eating when a child feels they are disappointing you, or doing something wrong.

The AHA recommendations were put in place without really considering how restrictive they can be and feel for parents and for kids. Recommendations often come out of interventions or studies conducted in a lab setting, not real-life settings or with regard for the long-term effects. A rigid rule about how much sugar to consume per day isn't helpful unless researchers are also looking at the result of what happens when flexible, gentle nutrition turns into rigid, restrictive rules. We aren't suggesting that there be no awareness of sugar intake, or to serve soda with every meal, but we do feel that it's important to help parents have realistic expectations, and to understand the value of not giving sugar or any other foods a lot of power or attention. Letting go of our fears around sugar will allow it to become more neutral and to reduce the overall anxiety and excitement around it.

Sugar, just like any other ingredient—in excess—can and may have a health consequence over time. Eating spoonfuls of olive oil can also make you sick, but that's not because olive oil is toxic. Drinking alcohol is technically drinking poison, but we haven't banned it yet—despite it being deadly and addictive. Anything in excess may have harmful effects—including dieting, overcontrol, and restriction.

You can't talk about nutrition-related health concerns—for example, nonalcoholic fatty liver disease (NAFLD), which occurs at a much higher rate among low-income communities—without addressing the lack of access and affordability of food and systemic racism barriers. Getting a balanced meal on the table—getting *any* meal on the table—is something parents in those communities often have to work much harder at than families in middle- and higher-income communities do, and this has an impact on what is offered, what is affordable, and how food is being consumed at home, even for the very youngest of children. In these communities, we see a lack of fresh food, sometimes no grocery stores at all, and high numbers of fast food establishments and corner stores. Growing up or raising kids in that environment, along with incredibly high stress and limited healthcare access, has a huge impact on health outcomes and diet patterns. When you look at the surface it appears true that sugar must be the primary culprit in causing these problems. Researchers see higher sugar intake and higher rates of diabetes and NAFLD. These things are correlated. However, when you go beneath the surface, and really see what contributes to health problems, you find deeply unjust disparities and historical effects of trauma that cannot be overlooked if we truly want to help improve the health of our communities.

YOUR KIDS CAN SENSE YOUR FOOD POLICE ANXIETY

When your tone changes, you get that certain look on your face, or you show even slight frustration at your child's desire to eat something, your child will pick up on it. (*Pause: when this happens, is that you projecting your diet beliefs onto them? Is it that you care so much what other people think about your child's eating, because you have been conditioned to think that what they eat reflects your ability to be a good parent?*) It's just in their beautiful, curious nature to want to push the buttons they see in you. Janet Lansbury, bestselling author and host of the podcast *Respectful Parenting: Janet Lansbury Unruffled*, frequently talks to her listeners about this key piece of insight about young children: **their curiosity drives nearly everything they do.**[11] They are curious about why you react to these foods. What is it about them wanting another serving of cake that causes you so much distress? They are built to pick up on these signals.

PARENTAL STRESS AND CHILD NUTRITION

There is evidence to show that parental stress levels impact the health of the household—particularly the health of children. An increase in parental stress can directly lead to a stressed child. Parents' stress levels influence parenting style and can alter the feeding relationship.[12] When a parent is under significant stress, such as working multiple jobs or night shifts, or isn't able to be around to prepare meals, all of this will undoubtedly influence the eating, physical activity, mental health, and overall health of the child. Much of the research investigating sugar consumption as it relates to "childhood obesity" actually looks specifically at underserved populations, because these are the groups who are experiencing relatively higher rates of negative health outcomes and who happen to be consuming more sugar relative to communities with more financial means and more access to food. What isn't made clear to you via flashy headlines and media articles claiming sugar is toxic and addictive is the complexity of these issues. These health concerns are a result of many different health determinants, lifestyle factors, stressors, and social injustices combined.

GENTLE NUTRITION EDUCATION CAN BE HELPFUL

There are groups that benefit from gentle nutrition education—for example, community health education programs that help teach parents about things like waiting to introduce juice until after two years of age—and these programs are important, but our communities also need support across many different areas of mental health and healthcare access. Providing diet-centric, weight-focused nutrition education to these groups of already stressed-out parents is like providing financial counseling and education on "how to save money" to families who are living paycheck to paycheck: it's completely missing the point. The weight stigma and food restriction that comes along with most nutrition "interventions" to tackle "childhood obesity" often contribute to worsening the problem.

SUMMARIZE AND REFLECT

Whew. You made it through the chapter on nutrition. This one could have been a whole book. There is so much out there—so much to *unlearn*.

- *What beliefs do you have about nutrition that have been challenged by this chapter?*

- *What emotions are coming up for you after reading this chapter?*
- *How has your own history of dieting impacted the way you view nutrition now?*
- *What do you need to move toward gentle nutrition for you and your family—if you want to?*
- *Thinking about an add-in, pressure-off approach, what kinds of foods would you like to add in for your child? How might those meals look?*

KIDS, MOVEMENT, AND SPORTS

Movement and its relation to our body and health is the cousin of nutrition. It can be so deeply rooted in diet culture, yet is an important part of our lives, and likely an aspect of some of your children's favorite activities. Movement for kids and adults is ideally about having fun and developing new skills—never about losing weight or burning calories. When it's not fun—it won't be for everyone—it may be an intentional choice to support physical strength, rehabilitation, mental health, or skill-building. The key difference with our approach to movement is that the choice is based in body appreciation; it's not a mandate from diet culture. We need to be aware that in our culture, even when you say it's "to stay healthy," kids are conditioned to know and subconsciously associate "healthy" with "thin." "Staying healthy" is an association we should question and would be best unassociated with movement.

WHEN YOUR CHILD GETS INTO SPORTS

Of course, we know that for many kids, participating in sports is positive: it builds social connection, grows self-esteem, it's fulfilling, and it's fun! Some kids can develop an interest early on, and become passionate and dedicated athletes by grade school or middle school. This immerses them into sports culture from a young age. If your child is one of these passionate athletes, we want you to be informed about the ways this may impact their risk of developing disordered eating.

We often see kids get into a certain sport because they love it. Then, as they get older and approach middle and high school years, there becomes more and more pressure on athletes to have an "athletic," trim, lean, or thin build. The sports culture all on its own comes with increased risks for eating and exercise disorder development. Actually, if you have a child who is very into sports, you'll want to be extra aware of what they're being told about food, eating, and weight control in the setting of their sport, from teammates, other parents, and coaches.

It's estimated that disordered eating affects around 62 percent of female and 33 percent of male athletes, specifically athletes that compete in sports that place a high emphasis on aesthetics, appearance, size, and weight such as bodybuilding, wrestling, gymnastics, figure skating, dancing, rowing, running, cheerleading, and horse racing, to name a few.[1] Among female high school athletes, 41 percent reported disordered eating, and they were eight times more likely to experience an injury than their teammates who didn't report disordered eating.[2]

Further down the line, one study found that for college athletes the risk of developing anorexia nervosa was 25 percent (female) and 10 percent (male) and bulimia nervosa 58 percent (female) and 38 percent (male). These numbers are extremely high, and show that if your child is involved in competitive sports, just by being a part of the sports culture, they are at high risk.[3]

MOVEMENT AND FUEL

Body changes that come with puberty, combined with the increased food needed for their sport *and* more attention on weight, shape, and appearance, is a recipe for body dissatisfaction and increased attention on food and weight. It's common to find adolescents and young adults, with their newfound freedom of eating away from their parents more often than ever before, taking it upon themselves to start dieting without anyone noticing. *That is, until you do notice.* This can be really scary for parents, but it highlights the importance of talking about bodies and normalizing body diversity and body fat from a young age—so that your child is more equipped to say no to the temptation of dieting when it's presented as a potentially necessary step to help them excel in their sport.

The more movement in their life, the more your child will naturally be hungry. It's not unusual if you notice your middle-schooler or teen eating what appear to be large amounts of food at one time—their bodies are hungry for this! Your natural reaction might be to encourage them to eat less, to wait until dinner, or to choose something "healthier," which can feel really shaming and imply that you don't approve of the way they are eating. Ask yourself: Do you know how much they've had to eat that day? (No, you don't—unless you actually do, but you probably don't.) Is it possible they are really hungry and need to have permission to eat as much as they need without feeling guilty or embarrassed? Maybe they are eating emotionally; if that is the case, what they need is support, space, permission, and love—*not to be shamed for eating.*

Explicitly stating something like *Are you really hungry for that?* or *Are you listening to your body? You've had two bowls of cereal* will not help them feel supported; it will likely produce a shame spiral and cause them to want to eat apart from you, in private. Support them by reminding them to have meals and snacks, having food available, and asking for their input on what foods they want to have around for breakfast, easy lunches, and after-school snacks. Involve them and show them you want to support them in getting enough to eat and feeling satisfied. **Home should never be a place where someone feels bad about what they eat.**

If your child is eating a lot of "light" or diet foods—particularly in the high school age range and even more so among high school athletes who are growing and very active—they will likely not be getting enough calories to meet their needs, and their body will eventually register that. When the body and brain begin to recognize there is a calorie deficit, neurochemicals and hormones shift to protect their body, often causing noticeable surges in appetite and cravings. For some people, the pattern that ensues is binge eating, alternating with restriction, and on it goes. Many young athletes and active people who have high calorie needs but make it a priority to "eat healthy" (which to them may mean eating fewer calories) will begin to experience urges to binge. This isn't a "normal" part of being a teenager. Despite being common, binge eating is a direct outcome of undereating or being unintentionally underfueled. So, although your child or teen may complain to you that they feel "out of control" or "eating too much"—and they may be gaining weight, too—the problem lies in the undereating, not the binges. *Restriction is never the road to peace with food.* Eating large portions can be normal, but when the feelings of guilt and shame, or compensation like exercise, vomiting, using laxatives or diuretics, or restricting food occur, these are signs of a more serious disorder. Eating disorders require professional treatment as well as a compassionate and supportive home environment that allows a child to recover from disordered thoughts and behaviors. Placing limits on food, regardless of how much they are eating, is never the answer. Eating disorder behaviors can also be a coping mechanism that your child develops to survive difficult circumstances. (You'll have a chance to learn more about eating disorders coming up soon.)

HOW MUCH MOVEMENT IS IDEAL?

Physical activity guidelines for youth in the United States and Canada say our kids need an average of sixty minutes or more of physical activity per day.[4] It's true, there is a lot of consistent evidence that associates more physical activity with improved health. Generally, the more physical activity the better *is the thinking*. When we investigated where this target of sixty-plus minutes per day is coming from, we found that sixty minutes is higher than where benefits are actually seen in studies. The reason why it's higher than what is shown to actually be beneficial is to encourage more pronounced health benefits (*hey, if they're healthy with twenty minutes, why not tell them to do sixty?*) and to encourage more activity for kids who are already pretty active. It's an overshoot to make sure they didn't recommend too few minutes for some people. For some kids, this sixty-minute daily goal may be no problem, but for others it's not realistic. This is a form of *monotonic thinking*—basically, thinking that if a little of something is good for us, then a lot of it must be really good. Americans in particular think this way.

Keep in mind . . .

- Not every child is going to benefit in the same way from the same amount of exercise.
- Hardly any studies examine symptoms of disordered eating or eating disorders among kids with high levels of physical activity over time

(we know it isn't always the more the better, and we'll talk about this more in the next section).

- As parents we can't think about movement as an all-or-nothing thing—in fact, "From a behavior modification perspective, having a target that seems out of reach may actually undermine physical activity participation."[5]
- Movement doesn't have to be *exercise*. Active play, walking, *movement* is the important part.

Too much pressure, or too much emphasis on the need to exercise for health, can backfire just the same way pressure to eat can. Instead, pay attention to what movement activities are enjoyable to your child. Don't shame them about being sedentary or "lazy" or make them worry that they'll gain weight unless they exercise. Offer to do things with them, and if they say no—accept it. More importantly, if you notice your child's movement has significantly changed (increased or decreased) or they are no longer interested in doing things with friends or teammates, find out why. Really help them feel seen, and allow for the reality that they may not be feeling like moving much, which could be a sign of something more important at its core or it could be as simple as having more interest in other things like art, music, creating, or reading.

BENEFITS OF MOVEMENT

We asked you to start to let go of "getting healthy" as an expectation of exercise. So, what should the focus of movement be? Well, joy for one. But there are various benefits to exercise *independent of body size or composition change*. You're more likely to experience these benefits if movement is a joyful experience instead of just another stressor or thing on the to-do list. It's unlikely to be a joyful experience for kids when we put the pressure on them to do it when they don't want to.

MOVEMENT AND ITS RELATIONSHIP TO MENTAL HEALTH

The impact of movement on depression is striking. Getting outside and moving can be a potent "antidepressant" (note: we support the use of medication if needed and don't think that outdoor time is a replacement for medication). Studies do show that even modest movement can significantly improve at least one depressive symptom. The "modest" part of that is very important. As little as sixty minutes a week can show this improvement. Not a day, a *week*. That seems pretty manageable.[6,7,8] There is significant reduction of risk when kids engage in some sort of movement and extracurricular activities throughout the week. This benefit is shown in kids as young as six. Again, this doesn't have to happen to the extent that we are often told that we have to engage in movement. Anything from one to six days with movement have shown these benefits.

BLOOD PRESSURE

A review that included eight experimental studies looked at the effect of physical activity on children's blood pressure and found that for kids who had high blood pressure, adding just 9 to 30 minutes per day (60 to 180 minutes per week) resulted in significant reductions in blood pressure in response to aerobic movement—this is considerably less than the guidelines of sixty-plus minutes per day, yet it was enough to have a significant health benefit—unrelated to weight change or BMI.

INSULIN

A review of another eight studies looked at the effect of physical activity on fasting insulin and insulin resistance. The average amount of exercise in the interventions was ten to thirty minutes per day; much like the previous studies that found a benefit to blood pressure, these found significant improvement on at least one marker of insulin associated with an increase in aerobic movement—again these interventions were nowhere near sixty-plus minutes per day, but nonetheless showed a positive difference when looking exclusively at insulin.[9]

BMI AND BODY FAT

In a review of twenty-four intervention studies that ranged in time from four weeks to two years with an average of seventeen to twenty minutes of exercise prescribed daily, only six of the twenty-four studies found any significant (albeit small) changes in BMI or body fat (significant was half of one percent decrease in body fat and 0.07-point reduction in BMI). To sum it up, the children involved in these exercise interventions were found to experience improvements in blood pressure and metabolic markers, without a change in weight or body fat. Let's emphasize: **there are lots of benefits kids get from movement—it doesn't have to be rigid, and according to these results it doesn't have to be vigorous, and it doesn't have to be an hour a day every day.** A large systematic review of over 162 studies looking at physical activity and youth showed that all types and intensities—all levels, low, moderate, and high intensity of movement—are beneficial to physical health, mental health, and cardiometabolic markers.

The more kids are enjoying and choosing to do things that bring them joy, the more they will naturally want to be moving around in ways that feel good to them. We really need to support kids to find things that they like, without making them feel shamed if they aren't interested.

PROBLEMATIC EXERCISE OR ACTIVITY

Although we are constantly hearing the message "the more exercise the better," we rarely get a glimpse of the other side of the story—the story of a significant number of people of all ages with eating and/or exercise disorders who experience a problematic, unhealthy relationship with movement. This can start as young as nine or ten, and is common among teens and young adults. Even as recently as 2020, there was no consensus among researchers in the field of how to define problematic exercise. This is likely because so many of the behaviors and signs of problematic, excessive, or compulsive exercise are normalized as "healthy" behaviors in our culture. From the time kids start kindergarten, they begin to hear the message: *If you don't exercise, you'll be unhealthy. If you don't exercise, you'll get diabetes, or be obese.*

Eating disorders and exercise disorders are so stigmatized, private, and secretive that unless you work in a treatment setting, or have personally experienced an exercise or eating disorder yourself or in someone you care about, you'd probably never think twice about the people all around us exercising. But do we really ever think that someone is out for their morning jog because they have a problem, or their eating disorder is controlling their thoughts, forcing them to exercise to avoid the guilt and panic of missing a workout? No, we assume everyone who is exercising is getting "healthier" from it. That's the picture that is painted for us everywhere we look, no one ever stopping to say, *Hey, you know what? One out of every five of those women on their morning run is suffering with an eating disorder that may be impacting her hormones, her heart, her digestion, her mental health, and it could kill her. I wonder if she needs help.* The problem is, by the time someone with a problematic relationship with exercise is approached by a concerned friend or family member, or realizes the problem and wants to get help—they have heard the message that "more is better" reinforced so many times it's incredibly difficult to reverse the belief that it's okay to cut back, or to stop. It's okay to not exercise. Your body won't fall apart. Your health won't deteriorate overnight or in a week. Feeling guilt or shame because you didn't exercise is the problem.

Problematic exercise behaviors pose a significant health risk to your child and may or may not be part of an eating disorder. It's important to take these concerns seriously and to understand how much they are exercising, if they are hiding exercise, and what the motivation behind the exercise is. If you're concerned that your child is engaging in problematic exercise behavior, we encourage you to seek professional help with an eating disorder–informed psychotherapist or medical professional.

SIGNS AND SYMPTOMS OF PROBLEMATIC EXERCISE

- Sudden change in the amount of exercise.
- Irritation or emotional outbursts if they are unable to exercise.
- Changing plans or avoiding social activities in order to exercise.
- Exercising alone in their room.
- Secretly exercising or hiding the amount (time, intensity, duration) they are exercising.
- Openly sharing with you that they can't stop or it's causing distress.
- Weight loss associated with exercise.
- Overuse injuries—like stress fractures.
- Loss of period.

SUMMARIZE AND REFLECT

Movement and exercise are inextricably linked to how we relate to food and body. So ensuring we have a positive relationship with movement is critical to raising Intuitive Eaters. We want to reflect on how your relationship with exercise or movement is *right now*. We know how important your own relationship with exercise or movement is, so we are going to start with you. If you can relate at all to the thought that you feel like you *have to exercise* (rather than you want to move simply because it feels good, you need to in your daily life, or you want to), then think about these two questions:

1. *If you never made yourself exercise again—what do you think would happen?*

Seriously imagine: How long would you sit and lie down, before you naturally felt a desire to get up and move your body? Can you recall how you feel after a long plane ride, or sitting in a lecture or conference all day? What is your body's natural desire to move; what does your body crave? How would it feel to move if you were making sure that you put sleeping and eating higher on the priority list, above exercise?

If your answer is *I would choose to sleep and never get up for intentional physical activity again*, why do you think that may be? Is it possible you're tired? Need a break? Could it be you're naturally moving enough throughout your day-to-day life, and more exercise isn't what you actually need?

2. *If you only moved in ways that brought you joy or an internal sense of well-being, how would you choose to move?*

If your answer feels out of reach, what does that tell you? Could it be that the type of movement you're doing is more prescriptive than optional? Can you find ways to explore new physical activities and see how they feel? Can you commit to stopping doing any exercise that doesn't feel truly like a choice you want to be making?

Body appreciation through movement enhances the joy of moving. Find the benefits of the movement itself, and the benefits that you experience after the movement has ended. Let movement be a tool that supports you to live the life you want, rather than a rule, a punishment, or a requirement. When you as a parent have a relationship with movement that nourishes your life, your children are able to see that positive relationship in action. And when your child is free to build a relationship with movement on their own terms, without pressure or guilt, they will be more likely to view movement as a positive part of their lifestyle.

IF YOU'RE CONCERNED ABOUT YOUR CHILD'S LEVEL OF MOVEMENT

Concerned they aren't getting enough activity? When did you notice this concern? If you're feeling concerned about their weight, put that to the side and look again at their patterns and movement. If you didn't have the weight concern, would you still think they weren't moving enough? Where is your concern coming from? Are you comparing your child to someone else? The goal here is to unpack if you're judging their weight/shape/size and that is leading you to think they need more activity, or if their size isn't related at all to your concern. If size is related, remember that weight loss isn't ever indicated for a growing and developing child, and physical activity isn't likely to cause weight loss in general (we shared all those studies in this chapter about how exercise benefits kids without significant weight loss). It's associated with health markers, reduced depression and anxiety, and better sleep, but as a parent it's critical you don't judge your child regarding their movement and activity. There may be a reason why they aren't interested in much physical activity: find out from their perspective—or say nothing at all—and just continue to offer doing enjoyable activities together. If you realize your concern is tied to their weight, the vast majority of the time your child will be able to sense your disappointment about their body and will be able to sense that you're wanting them to move to lose weight. This is incredibly shame-promoting for your child, will not encourage them to be active, and will possibly even create more of a sense of hopelessness and loneliness. Your child needs to know that you love and support and respect them no matter their body size. We highly encourage you to not pressure them to exercise, or unintentionally shame them by focusing on how little they move. Instead, aim to connect authentically with them, be on the lookout for signs of depression, understand what is going on in their life, and invite them to do things with you when it's natural. Not every child is going to be naturally motivated to be very active or involved in sports—and that is just fine.

Concerned they are overexercising? When did you first notice this? Was it a sudden shift, out of line with their usual drive to move or be active? Did anything else stressful happen for your child at the time you noticed them moving or exercising more? How do they respond when you bring up exercise? Do they want to avoid talking about it? One of the earliest behaviors parents might notice when a child is struggling with an eating disorder is a sudden increase or decrease in exercise. Even what may appear to be a justified *I just like to run now with my friends, it's no big deal* should at least prompt you to take closer notice of what happens when they don't run (*Surprise! You wake up early and make them waffles, and they need to put off the run—how do they respond?*). If they need to keep adding more time, workouts, or distance, or if you notice they are moving a lot more and not eating more to meet their energy needs for the increased activity, they may have a problem. These things could be nothing more than an interest in a new hobby, or could be concerning signs of an eating disorder. If you notice anything that raises a red flag for you (*listen to your gut!*), consult with a specialist, talk to your child, be persistent, and let them know you're concerned.

COMMON MEDICAL AND
HEALTH CONCERNS

The possible situations and struggles you may face on your parenting journey related to feeding your child are endless. We could never even attempt to cover them all in just this one book, and we can't predict what you will actually face. If you're facing down this challenge of fostering a positive relationship with food and body for your child while simultaneously navigating a medical or psychological diagnosis or condition, you have to be gentle with yourself and your children.

Intuitive Eating, for the most part, is an approach that many children will respond well to, and their future adult Intuitive Eater will grow more secure and trusting as time goes on. In other cases, feeding and eating difficulties are much more complex, and the 3 Keys alone may be only part of what you need to consider to keep your child well, fed, and safe from harm. While we believe that the 3 Keys—and Intuitive Eating—can be applied to most individuals, it's ultimately your decision to determine what parts of this are relevant to your child and what parts aren't. The flexibility of the keys includes the ability to make these decisions.

We also wanted to show you how Intuitive Eating can apply to a few different medical and mental health conditions. There are all kinds of diet recommendations for so many different health conditions—and a significant number of them are based on very little science. While we understand that some people may be finding relief from some of these diets, we can't in good faith recommend that anyone follow restrictive diets when there is little to no evidence to support them. Because, while some people may find a bit of relief, we know the risks of dieting are high.

DEPRESSION AND ANXIETY

Depression is something that more and more people are talking about these days. The openness with which we talk about depression and suicidality means that more young people are going to be able to get the help that they need. One in five young people suffer from some sort of mental illness.[1] This is a significant enough problem that it needs to be talked about and normalized.

Depression and anxiety (and medications to treat these conditions) can impact appetite. Some individuals will have an increase in appetite and others will have a decrease. Some may even experience an increase in gastrointestinal symptoms (having a "nervous stomach"). This can be a difficult experience as an adult, but when we are trying to provide a positive food experience for our kids, we want to ensure that they are consistently getting enough to eat. That may mean aiding them with additional external cues.

When appetite changes related to mental (or physical) health happen, we do advocate for following external cues, like the clock, as reminders to eat. Because *even if the side effect of the condition is eating less, eating enough is the most important thing.* Eating less or weight changes related to mental or physical health conditions aren't desirable outcomes, even though many times weight loss will automatically be considered a "healthy" thing, may be praised, or will not be addressed as a sign of a problem at all by doctors.

These external cues, such as setting an alarm to eat a snack, or communicating with your child that you're going to help them by reminding them when it's time to eat can be really important. Because, in this situation, it's not that they are less hungry because the body needs less food, it's that they can't feel the cues as strongly. Making logical and rational decisions to eat based on knowing what your child has eaten in the past and their activity level is caring. Depression is one of many examples of when appetite, hunger, and fullness can be interrupted and, as parents, we can really step in here and help support our kids to eat enough.

Eating enough will also help medications work properly, help mitigate anxiety, prevent the development of an eating disorder secondary to the depression, and support continued growth and development during this important time. Eating enough can also support increased neuroplasticity—meaning it can be easier for therapy to be effective and for any person to be more able to use logical thinking, even in times of distress.

EATING DISORDERS

In some respects, it's pretty incredible that there aren't more eating disorders among youth and teens than we currently see given the immense pressure, social comparison, and appearance-based standards in Western culture, for everyone, but particularly for transgender folx and girls and women. Our culture objectifies bodies and places an incredibly high value on appearance. Harm is experienced across the gender spectrum, with particular harm focused on female bodies—experiences of sexualization, and unrealistic expectations of beauty, body shape, size, muscle tone, and even personality. All of these factors have direct or related negative effects on how girls and women experience the world in their bodies.[2]

Additionally, any child who identifies as nonbinary or trans, or who doesn't yet have words or awareness to describe their experience of feeling misgendered, has an increased risk for developing eating disorder behaviors—particularly to numb, escape, self-harm, or avoid the difficult experiences they have being in their body as a result of a society that is as a whole not accepting of or welcoming to nondominant identities. Eating disorders are highly associated with the body dissatisfaction, gender dysphoria, and distress that is widely experienced by the LGBTQIA+ community.

Healing and preventing eating disorders isn't the responsibility of the individual; we need to change our culture. What we hope you have learned at this point is that Intuitive Eating is one protective measure against the development of disordered eating and eating disorders, *and* that eating disorders don't discriminate. They can happen to anyone. Just as weight doesn't define a person's health, weight isn't a way to assess if someone has an eating disorder.

Close your eyes and picture a person with an eating disorder. Who do you see?

If you visualized a thin, young, white, cis-gender female, then stereotypes and myths have done their job: you have been led to think that that is the profile of who develops an eating disorder. Because of these harmful stereotypes, there is stigma and shame for most people who don't fit that profile, keeping the majority of people who have eating disorder struggles from seeking treatment, or from even telling a loved one or a doctor that they need help. Many people will never get the treatment they need. They think that you have to be "too thin" or "underweight," or that eating disorders are only a white people problem, or only happen to teenage girls.

The onset of eating disorders commonly occurs at life transitions. That includes early adolescence and puberty, which can start as early as age eight or nine, periods directly following traumatic events, starting college, getting married, having a child, and the onset of menopause (and others—these are just a few examples). If you're reading this book, the most likely upcoming event for your child is the onset of puberty. This can be a particularly difficult time. Middle school is generally a rough time for everyone, with hormones and changes all around. This is another time to notice if you're having different feelings toward your children's bodies based on their gender or size. Boys (or those assigned male at birth) can often be encouraged to eat more, and weight gain and eating falls more into the "boys will be boys" school of thought. (Although this isn't an all-or-nothing thing; more and more boys and men are experiencing eating disorders and the same pressure as girls and women do.) Girls (or those assigned female at birth) are often pressured to not gain too much, to not eat too much, to maintain the prepubertal shape that is, oddly, close to our cultural beauty standards. According to the growth charts used for pediatric growth tracking, it's normal for girls to gain twenty to forty pounds or more over the course of puberty, but this is often viewed with apprehension by parents and medical providers.

Dieting or intentional weight loss at this age is never encouraged and should always be viewed as a red flag for disordered eating (subclinical eating disorders), if not an eating disorder. Excessive exercise, body checking (excessive touching and viewing of the body to monitor body size and shape), weight loss, loss of menstrual cycle once begun, distress over body shape or size, and overconcern about appearance and eating healthy are all warning signs of an eating disorder. This is, again, a time to use the questions *How are you?* and *What do you need right now?* and to listen. *Really listen.*

We said intentional weight loss can be a warning sign, but unintentional weight loss can directly trigger the development of an eating disorder, even one that isn't spurred by body dissatisfaction. Unintentional weight loss can happen for a variety of reasons: health problems, medication, new activity and sports participation, or things like depression or anxiety disrupting the internal cues. Unintentional weight loss can lead to the experience of comments about body changes, which can trigger the desire to continue to hear those compliments.

THE SPECTRUM OF EATING DISORDERS

When you think of an eating disorder, *anorexia nervosa* (AN) is probably one of the first you think of. AN is generally thought of as the primary eating disorder, although it comprises only about 10 percent of diagnosed eating disorder cases. Other eating disorder diagnoses include *binge eating disorder* (BED), *bulimia nervosa* (BN), *avoidant/restrictive food intake disorder* (ARFID), and ED-T1DM, which is also sometimes called "diabulimia." ED-T1DM occurs when someone who has type 1 diabetes manipulates their insulin use to cause weight loss. Lastly, the most common diagnosis is called *other specified feeding and eating disorders* (OSFED).

OSFED is the diagnosis used when someone's signs, symptoms, and behaviors don't fit the diagnostic criteria of the other disorders for various reasons. Someone with OSFED may restrict their calories, but not have a low enough body weight to be diagnosed with anorexia nervosa, may overexercise, or vomit (purge) after eating, but not regularly or frequently enough to meet bulimia nervosa criteria. An OSFED diagnosis may also comprise a combination of binge eating, restricting, and/or purging, and a person's weight may still be considered "normal" or "overweight." The thinking is often *If a child isn't underweight, they must not be malnourished.* This is harmful because kids and teens who are struggling with an eating disorder are often assumed to be fine if their weight has not changed much, or (dangerously) assumed to be eating "too much" if they live in a larger body. The case can often be that they are restricting calories to dangerously low daily amounts, binge eating, abusing laxatives, vomiting after eating, taking dangerous diet pills, overexercising, or engaging in a number of other risky behaviors.

One of the diagnoses for someone who is severely restricting their intake but is not underweight is *atypical anorexia*. It's a misnomer, because it's far more prevalent than AN. But when people in larger bodies are losing weight or restricting food—even to extremes—it can commonly be interpreted as positive. **But studies show that the physical, medical, and mental side effects and risks from *atypical anorexia* are *just as dangerous as anorexia nervosa.***[3] Meaning that missing this diagnosis—or not taking it seriously—can be a deadly mistake. All because of weight stigma and the assumptions that thinner is better, and that you can't possibly have a dangerous eating disorder if you aren't "too thin." We encourage you to learn more from the resources we share in the back of this book.

CHILDHOOD WEIGHT CONCERNS

It might feel okay to move your child toward Intuitive Eating and worry less about their eating if your child is in a body with a "normal" BMI. If you and your child are constantly being told that their body is at risk, gaining weight too quickly, or that they need to lower their BMI, this conversation can be a lot more difficult. Hearing doctors and other authority figures give advice on how to curb weight gain or hearing your child's pediatrician ask about their eating habits while sounding concerned at every annual visit can make it difficult to not feel concerned about your child's weight. Your child doesn't have to be at a certain weight to be an Intuitive Eater. In fact, we firmly believe that a person's weight—including a child's weight—isn't part of the problem. We've already talked about the damaging history behind BMI and why we believe body diversity isn't only acceptable, but expected, normal, and perfectly okay. This is the extension of that belief. Even though people might be telling you that weight is a problem that needs to be fixed, we believe that the most critical thing you can do for the health of your child is help them foster a positive relationship with food and body and avoid reproducing or reinforcing stigmatizing and shame-inducing messages.

Even the American Academy of Pediatrics recommends *against* dieting and weight-loss attempts in children. They are very aware of the risks. But many parents will continue to hear from pediatricians and other doctors about the risks of their child's weight or diet. When children hear medical professionals constantly criticizing their body size, they begin to view their body as a problem. There are so many different forms of weight stigma, and this is one where we can begin to stick up for our children. You can make it known that you do not want them to make comments about your child's body or food in front of them. If you're comfortable having conversations about your child's body in private, you can request a private conversation at the end of the appointment between you and the doctor. But you can help ensure that medical encounters are safe for your child.

On top of the weight stigma that children can experience in a doctor's office, there is also bullying they can experience in school. *This is a systemic problem.* Weight-based bullying is the most prevalent type of bullying in school. In an online survey of over 350 higher-weight or previously higher-weight adolescents between the ages of fourteen and eighteen, it was found that 64 percent of those who responded had experienced weight-based bullying at school from peers and friends, including verbal teasing, exclusion, cyberbullying, and physical aggression. Thirty-six percent of those who experienced bullying reported experiencing it for five years. This wasn't limited to bullying from other students. The participants also reported that teachers, other parents, and coaches were routine perpetrators as well.[4] This bullying from both adolescents and the adults who are supposed to protect them is directly related to the messages that come from diet culture about the "goodness" of bodies. The comments and criticisms, as well as messages in health class (and science, math, and so on) about the ways to achieve thinness and health, are *microaggressions*—subtle or indirect acts of discrimination or criticism toward a marginalized person. These microaggressions are forms of bullying.

This doesn't exist in a vacuum. Just like beauty standards, bullying comes from the standards we pass down. Kids hear from adults around them that weight-based bullying is okay. They hear coaches putting down the kids who aren't as athletic, they hear parents talking about other people (adults and children), they get laughs from peers when they make fun of someone else. They hear it from the media, doctors, social media, and five hundred years of misinformation passed down that has taught us that thinner is better. They hear fatphobic jokes in the movies and TV shows they watch. Children's shows are just as bad as adult shows for fatphobia. Think of a Disney villain. Chances are, they're fat. Or the only fat character in the show is a joke. The goofy friend who is always eating. Even news media doesn't get out of this one—mudslinging in politics is often reduced to fatphobic or appearance-based remarks about the opposing candidate. (And this kind of public bullying exists even in "woke" spaces.) Diversity in weight, ability, race, gender, and sexuality aren't represented in the portrayals we see in the media. Only a very small percentage of the media messages we take in actually portray diverse bodies and intersecting identities. We have all been duped, and now we are seeing the effects of it on our youth.

In addition to this, when a parent supports their child or adolescent in pursuing weight loss or feeling negative about living in a larger body—even if it's "for health"—the internalized weight stigma is reinforced, and leads to the child concluding that, yes, pursuit of weight loss is the right thing to do. As opposed to you, the parent, showing up to witness their pain, support them emotionally, and be the voice that tells them no one has the right to bully them. Kids need to hear that their body isn't the problem, and that the problem is weight stigma.

WE AREN'T TRYING TO ERADICATE SHORT PEOPLE, SO WHY ARE WE TRYING TO ERADICATE FAT PEOPLE?

Malnutrition can stunt growth, affecting height, but it doesn't mean that all short people are short because of malnutrition. There is no stigma about being short, or a belief that it's a person's personal and individual responsibility to prevent shortness. So even though undernutrition can stunt growth, we don't fight to end world hunger to end shortness, we fight to end world hunger because we believe it's every human's right to have access to enough food.

The "childhood obesity epidemic" is amplified by the misinterpretation and generalization that weight is "the problem" when, while weight may be a side effect or symptom for some underlying health concerns, the weight itself isn't where the attention is needed. **You don't help a child to feel and be well by pointing out their weight as problematic; you help a child feel and be well by helping them respect and care for their body, ensuring they have enough to eat consistently, have enjoyable and safe ways to move, and that they have reliable ways of coping and getting their needs met.**

So far, public policy has attempted to "fight childhood obesity" by educating kids and parents about nutrition, yet we are completely missing the mark on the health problems and disparities causing concern, while also worsening rates of eating disorders among kids and young people. In reality, the factors that contribute to nutrition and weight-related health concerns are things like lack of variety in foods that are available and affordable, dieting and weight stigma, lack of safe play spaces, and disparities in healthcare.

Efforts need to stay focused on getting kids enough nutritious foods to eat, having safe places to play outside, mental healthcare, transportation to grocery stores, caregivers around to prepare food, social support for parents, and policies that support all families having access to the food they need.

There are some wonderful programs in place to help support educating mothers on the importance of good nutrition during pregnancy and early childhood and also provide some financial support for purchasing food. These programs are important, and there is a difference between educating people about what their kids need and promoting fatphobia, fear of weight gain, and restrictive eating practices under the guise of health.

Another thing to consider when we are placing additional attention on a child's weight is what the result of that emphasis will be. The child will be more focused on their own body and more likely to perceive their body in a negative light. The actual impacts of increased focus on weight are things like more weight stigma, nearly endless recommendations to diet, and increasing rates of eating disorders for younger and younger kids.

GROWING UP WITH A DISABLED BODY

Some kids don't eat by mouth—they may have a feeding tube that is sustaining them. Others don't walk—they move through their world with movement aids, or a wheelchair. Blind children don't "eat with their eyes," as we often say kids do, but they develop keen awareness in other ways. If a child eats in a different way, because of how they were born, or something that happened to them, then that is the right way of eating for them. The idea that there is one right way, that some version of Intuitive Eating could be "the way," is far too limiting. A child with a feeding tube has a different experience of eating and what it means to eat than a child who doesn't have that experience. One isn't better than the other; different children learn important things in different ways—and their experiences are real, valid, and vital. We aren't parents of a child who had the experiences mentioned above. What we'd like to say here is that whatever a parent or a child needs to do to adapt to their needs, or to their environment, to promote a way of nourishing their body that feels necessary, or right to them, is their right version of Intuitive Eating. How a child eats isn't their identity; it doesn't define them.

The purpose is to allow children, all of us really, to eat without the rules of diet culture or restriction. This means that when your child's health is involved and you have found something that is actually working for your family, you've achieved the goal. We are here to support you in raising a child with as positive a relationship to their food and body as we can.

HOW CAN WE BEST SUPPORT AUTISTIC KIDS?

All children deserve to have a healthy relationship with food and their bodies, regardless of their neurotype. Neurological differences may impact your child's feeding skills, behavior and food preferences. For example, your child might be more limited when it comes to food choices or might present some form of "food rigidity." However, it's essential not to pathologize these behaviors and understand what are they trying to communicate. Accepting that your child's eating may look different than expected and prioritizing parent-child

relationships should be at the forefront when supporting autistic children. How
we feed our children is more important than what we feed them. Honoring
your child's bodily autonomy and letting go of diet culture is key to
raising body confident children.

—NAUREEN HUNANI, RD

There is currently research under way investigating the link observed between autism spectrum disorder (ASD) and eating disorders. Some evidence suggests a higher prevalence of ASD among youth with eating disorders, although this link is still being investigated and we need further understanding. There are estimates indicating the prevalence of ASD among those with eating disorders is around 20 percent.[5,6]

(We are aware of the diversity of perspectives regarding language. In real life, we would use either person-first language [person with autism] or identity-first language [autistic, or autistic person] based on the preference of who we are interacting with. In our effort to use deliberately respectful language here, we have chosen to write this section using identity-first language, as we have learned that many autistic adults and their allies prefer to use this as a way of expressing and understanding autism to be an inherent part of their identity.)

Your role in supporting your child to maintain or rediscover a positive relationship with food and their body is to understand and support them as their unique self. Autistic individuals may have eating challenges related to having hypo- or hyper-sensitivity to sensations such as hunger, fullness, thirst, or aversions to foods with certain smells, textures, or flavors. They may experience sensory overload from their environment (noise, distraction, crowded spaces, and so on), all of which can make it difficult to regulate their emotions and be calm enough to eat their meal. If these children were ever pressured or punished, or experienced trauma related to feeding therapy such as being forced to eat something, their relationship to food may have suffered more than it would have otherwise had there been no pressure, or no harmful intervention. It's critical that parents understand how problematic pressuring and/or forcing their child to eat or drink something they are highly averse to can be in causing further eating difficulties down the line. Respect your child's preferences. Getting enough food for health and developmental reasons is the priority over eating a wide variety of foods, along with having a positive, open, and supportive parent-child relationship, which is the foundation of building trust.

We aren't specialists in this area, however; we highly recommend the work of

Montreal-based pediatric and family nutritionist Naureen Hunani. She works with families to support positive feeding experiences through a responsive feeding therapy approach.

A few notes about feeding and autism spectrum disorder (ASD):

- Be understanding of potential stress from sensory overload. Help create a calm environment and support your child with emotion regulation so they can eat their meal.
- Autistic individuals may have sensory processing challenges, and foods that are stronger in smell, different in texture, or spicy or complex in flavor may be avoided. It's critical to see these aversions as not something they are choosing to have, but rather about how they are built. Never force-feed or punish an autistic child for having what may appear to be extreme or limited preferences.
- Some simpler foods such as crackers, chips, bread, French fries, and other highly processed foods are often demonized by diet culture for being "too processed," "kid food," or "junk food." These labels can be shaming and harmful for someone who has food aversions, and they aren't helpful in promoting competent, adequate, or calm eating.
- Supporting an autistic child from a foundation of trust with food and body can help them to gradually increase their range of preferred foods over time without using pressure or negative control.
- Many autistic children with feeding challenges have undergone feeding therapies that used forced feeding, restriction, and punishment around food. These traumatic experiences can further disrupt trust in caregivers with feeding, and create disordered eating or potentially an eating disorder.
- Support autistic individuals from a strengths-based approach: assume they will be able to self-regulate and eat adequately, even if that looks different from the ways other kids eat, when they are supported by their environment.
- Many autistic kids will need external structure and timing for meals, cues, and reminders to eat. These are supportive tools for them and for you as their caregiver, particularly if they don't identify with always being able to feel hunger and fullness, or forget to eat until it's too late.

- Unanticipated changes or skipping a meal could be anxiety-provoking and lead to eating less than they need or more than feels comfortable.
- Misinformation given to parents of autistic children may lead to the development of rigid, all-or-nothing thinking about "healthy" eating and health in general. This thinking can fuel the development of an eating disorder. All the more reason not to use food rules or fear-mongering with food.

MEDICATIONS AND EATING

If your child loses weight as a side effect from a medication, take it seriously and don't assume the weight loss is "healthy." Be sure they are eating at least three complete meals a day, in reasonable and adequate portions for growth and energy, plus two or three snacks daily. For any child who may have struggled socially, weight loss could be the match that lights a flame of attention, and approval-seeking dieting behavior, alongside compliments about their new, slimmer body. This can be a very dangerous time in terms of the development of an eating disorder.

Even a child who had no prior disordered eating or body image concerns can be triggered to develop an eating disorder as a result of unintentional weight loss. If your child's weight goes up, do not initiate any restrictive eating rules, dieting, or weight-loss attempts, as these are at best likely to be ineffective, and at worst, exacerbate existing eating difficulties, leading to rebound or compensatory eating, and further disconnecting the child from their hunger and fullness cues. If your child becomes fixated on body size, appearance, or food, seek support from a therapist, doctor, or dietitian who specializes in your child's medical diagnosis or condition.

Certain medications may blunt appetite, like medications for ADHD, and it can be difficult for a child to get enough to eat when they aren't feeling hungry. There may be times of the day when they have more of an appetite, and that can be a good time to encourage them to eat; however, this can happen at inconvenient times—like bedtime. Optimize each meal or snack by offering higher-calorie, nutrient-dense foods (with fat, protein, and carbohydrates) to meet their daily energy needs and prevent disruption in growth and development. Praising or encouraging weight loss as a medication side effect is harmful because it reinforces the message that your child's body is better when it's smaller. That belief will stay long after this one instance and have a lasting impact.

ALLERGIES AND INTOLERANCES

One of your primary roles is to create safety. If there is a medical reason, such as a true allergy or intolerance, for your child to avoid any foods, of course, honor that. One way to look at this from an Intuitive Eating perspective is that every body is unique. *Not all foods work for everyone—and that's okay.* An allergic response or sensitivity is a real reason (assuming you're coming to this conclusion from an actual diagnosis from a doctor and not from diet culture, fatphobia, or media influence) to need to restrict a food. You modeling the boundary that no, your child cannot have it, helps them honor that boundary for themselves. Find other alternatives that are enjoyable and satisfying and make sure to have those available often. There are very real and significant emotions that accompany the experience of having to avoid a food you like due to an allergy. We commonly see people who have grief or sadness or anger surrounding their experience of having an allergy. We also see this for parents who face living with the anxiety, fear, and extra attention required to keep a child with food allergies safe.

There is a lot of confusion around food allergies, intolerances, and sensitivities. One of the reasons underlying this confusion is that the science is still emerging. We don't know exactly what causes some people to have food allergies or intolerances and why others don't. We do have some promising theories and science, but we are still learning. Here's a very basic overview to help you understand some of the differences between allergies and intolerances.

ALLERGIES	INTOLERANCES
An immune system overreaction which produces antibodies (IgE) to an allergen, food, or other substance. The body thinks the allergen is an invader.	Cause uncomfortable symptoms but are not life threatening. Mainly involve the digestive system. Can be due to trouble breaking down food, related to enzyme deficiencies or sensitivity to food additives.
May be confirmed by a doctor with an IgE test.	IgG tests given for food sensitivity testing (not the same as IgE tests) aren't scientifically valid, according to the American Academy of Allergy, Asthma and Immunology.
Allergic reactions range from mild to life threatening.	Common symptoms are gas, bloating, abdominal pain, and diarrhea, but symptoms can vary and include other non-GI symptoms. Unlike allergies, these do not cause immediate life-threatening reactions; response/reaction may be delayed.

If it's a slight intolerance, where the symptoms are gas or a slight upset tummy, you might also have some flexibility around this as they age and are able to assert some autonomy. Don't shame or punish if they want to try something, but do allow them to be curious and get to know how their body responds. If they are lactose intolerant, can they tolerate a small amount of ice cream or milk or cheese, but not large amounts? There could be a huge benefit to them getting to know their body's unique needs and limits, without having all-or-nothing thinking around foods that they may be somewhat sensitive to, without having a true allergy with a very real health risk.

IRRITABLE BOWEL SYNDROME

Irritable bowel syndrome (IBS) is a very common diagnosis. It can look very similar to intolerances and is closely related to them. Basically, when you eat certain foods or are feeling particularly stressed out, you may experience gastrointestinal upset, usually in the form of diarrhea and/or constipation. (There are other symptoms that can be related to IBS, like bloating, burping, acid reflux, flatulence, and so on.) There is even a medical diet related to treating IBS, a low-FODMAP diet. However, this diet is extremely restrictive and only recommended to be followed for about six weeks. This protocol is best done under the guidance of a registered dietitian who is well versed in low-FODMAP diets and is aware of the need to screen for disordered eating. While there is this particular medical diet that can be done in the short term, we actually know that one of the most effective things one can do to reduce IBS symptoms is . . . yoga.[7] Yoga and other enjoyable physical activity help the nervous system and reduce stress, which is likely a huge contributor to IBS symptoms. For lactose intolerance or sensitivity (related to IBS or not), over-the-counter lactase enzymes can help alleviate symptoms and allow someone to include more dairy and lactose in their daily lives.

The gastrointestinal system is full of nerve endings and experiences emotions rather like our brain does. Which means it's highly susceptible to changes in our normal states. If your child isn't sleeping well, not getting enough fluids, or has had a recent change in stress or activity level, these factors can contribute to IBS. Pressuring to eat is likely to backfire, even though you know they need more food, fiber, or fluids. Coming back to the add-in, pressure-off approach can be helpful. If your child isn't having bowel movements, they will avoid eating further, which can exacerbate the problem, as digestion slows when eating slows. Remember that if symptoms become too intense—like your child is experiencing chronic diarrhea or constipation—talk with your doctor.

Diabetes is often very connected to diet culture for us. Which is unfortunate, because diabetes is a legitimate medical condition that should be taken seriously, with no blame placed on the individual. Type 1 diabetes is an autoimmune condition, meaning that the body's immune system attacks its own healthy tissue, destroying it. People with type 1 diabetes are insulin-dependent for the rest of their lives. Type 2 diabetes has a slower progression and also has an element of insulin resistance (anyone can have insulin resistance, however; this isn't limited to those with type 2 diabetes). People with type 2 diabetes may not need insulin, or as much insulin. There are multiple other types of medications to help manage symptoms, and they may even be manageable for some with non-medication interventions. However, both types of diabetes are lifelong and chronic.

Diabetes has a relationship to carbohydrates, which is one of the reasons diet culture gets brought up in the conversation on diabetes. Most individuals with diabetes either need to know the carbohydrate content of the food they are eating or need to eat under a certain amount at any one meal or snack in order to manage medications and blood sugar. A sugar-free, carbohydrate-free diet isn't commonly indicated for a person with diabetes, despite it being one of the most pervasive myths out there for this population. Eating at regular intervals (every three to four hours) is generally recommended for people with diabetes, as is eating carbohydrates regularly (not excluding or avoiding them altogether). It's also recommended to pair those carbs with a fat, fiber, or a protein in order to slow down the rise in blood sugar. Remember when we talked about sugar? Sugar can usually be tolerated by people with diabetes, and the information from Key 2 can be really helpful for managing blood sugar and serving meals with combinations of food groups, like including protein and fat with grains. Restriction and rigid diet rules are often recommended, yet for many people who attempt to follow them, they aren't supportive of overall health or for diabetes management. In fact, binge eating may be one of the most harmful disordered eating symptoms for a person with diabetes, and it's worsened by restriction. Generally speaking, it would be better for someone with diabetes to eat a piece of cake than to avoid cake and binge on sugary foods later. The flexible feeding routine helps prevent blood sugar lows (by not skipping meals), and also helps by encouraging balanced nutrients (carbohydrates paired with protein and/or fat) in meals and snacks. When considering how to best manage blood sugar, know that many things can affect it. Movement can lower it. Being sick makes it higher. Stress of any kind can raise blood sugar significantly. And any physical activity beyond what is normal for you can cause a significant drop in blood sugar.

One of the most important things we can share is: diabetes is never the fault of the person who has it. Even having type 2 diabetes, which we often inaccurately associate with judgments like eating too much sugar, being fat, and being lazy, isn't the fault of the person who has it. Type 2 diabetes is actually more genetically linked than type 1 diabetes, meaning that if you have a strong family history of type 2 diabetes, you might not be able to avoid it. Yet again, stress plays a significant factor in the development and intensity of diabetes.

TO MEAT OR NOT TO MEAT

What about eating a plant-based diet, or going vegetarian? If you or your child is choosing to be vegetarian or eat only plant-based food out of ethical concerns regarding animal welfare or the environment, great. We aren't here to argue ethics. We're here with the facts. As you have read, allowing an individual to develop and maintain trust in their body is the foundation here. Many cultures support or encourage vegetarianism and veganism. And many do not. Having the sensitivity to note that we shouldn't be recommending these ways of eating to everyone is important.

If you see your child go vegetarian or vegan, understanding the "why" for this change is important. Unfortunately, cutting out meat or animal products can be the sign of a burgeoning eating disorder, as it easily removes main food groups from allowable choices and can justify restricting as a behavior. Due both to its inherently restrictive nature and the fact that there are copious resources on the "healthiness" of a plant-based diet, vegetarian or vegan diets can sometimes be a way to eat less, or can spark the obsession that we see in eating disorders and orthorexia.

Aiming to eliminate rigid thinking no matter what your food choices are and continuing to promote a healthy relationship with the food you *do* eat is the most important thing. We generally encourage a flexible attitude for those who want to eat a plant-based diet. We also acknowledge that some cultures place high value on following these ways of eating—and cultural reasons are generally less likely to lead to eating disorders than new-onset rigid plans.

SUMMARIZE AND REFLECT

There are many different medical conditions that can impact your child's body or their ability to eat intuitively. More than we can address here. We encourage you to step back and notice if the recommendations you have been given to follow about certain health conditions are about the condition itself or about diet rules. Recognizing when to seek out medical care, if you haven't already, is extremely important.

- *How has diet culture infiltrated your beliefs about medical conditions?*
- *What medical conditions do you or your children have that have impacted your food beliefs?*
- *Do your existing beliefs about "health" and eating feel in line with your new priorities to support a healthy relationship with food and body for your child?*

PART V

DEVELOPMENTAL STAGES AND WORKING THROUGH CHALLENGES

DEVELOPMENTAL STAGES OF RAISING AN INTUITIVE EATER

WHERE IS THE INSTRUCTION MANUAL FOR THIS JOB?

It's completely understandable to yearn for a way to "do parenting better" in each new phase of your child's development, but, as you know, the past does influence the present and we just don't get a fresh start no matter how badly we may want one. We have to learn from our experiences, our successes and our mistakes (we all make them), and move forward with our child as we all grow.

THE WINDOW OF OPPORTUNITY

Our children are astounding to observe. One minute you're captivated by their soft, fuzzy newborn head, buttery skin, and magical baby scent in their first weeks of life, and before you know it, they've outgrown the high chair, are practically running up the stairs, and ready to start preschool. As you witness the unbelievable pace of development and growth throughout their early years with gratitude and love, you're also thrown into scenarios you don't feel ready for and tested in ways you never could have imagined. Feeding challenges and questions vary based on the developmental stage of your child, and just when you think you've got it down, you're confronted with something new to figure out. With each of these stages, one thing is true: we always want to be able to give our child what they need to succeed and thrive.

As you read in Gina's story, when she turned fourteen and returned home from her summer class trip, her emerging eating disorder was on the verge of taking her hostage inside her own head. Yet her eating disorder thoughts weren't new; the seeds had actually been planted much earlier, and in waiting for years prior. Incidents and experiences that happened to her throughout childhood didn't cause her eating disorder (no one causes someone to get an eating disorder), but they did set in motion some of the social and emotional conditions that were ideal for promoting the swift development of her eating disorder to take off in adolescence.

THE FIRST TEN YEARS

The first ten years or so of a child's life are a window of opportunity. In this window of time when they spend the majority of their meals with you lies an opportunity to support Intuitive Eating. After the first ten years, yes, you still may have influence and remain tuned in to their eating and mental health, but they will begin to eat fewer and fewer meals with you, eventually becoming close to totally independent with food by their late teens.

In this chapter, we're talking about the different developmental phases as they relate to eating and feeding. We want to help normalize your struggles, let you know you can do this, and that we don't start building body confidence and peace with food in adolescence, when eating disorders and body struggles most commonly appear. We can and need to do this *from day one*, or from wherever you are today: your day one with Intuitive Eating.

THREE DEVELOPMENTAL STAGES

From newborn to your child's early teen years, successfully arriving at the completion of the first four stages of psychosocial development described by E. H. Erikson[1] supports our kids in achieving four virtues: *hope, will, purpose,* and *competency*. According to Erikson's theory, these are character strengths that we use later in life, to help us survive and grow through difficult circumstances and challenges. When we haven't achieved one of these virtues, we may feel mistrusting, hopeless, unwilling, incompetent, or empty of drive or purpose. Erikson's theory of psychosocial development is one of the key theoretical foundations of Intuitive Eating. Erikson's stages correlate with a child's developmental feeding stages, which are all crucial times to foster the autonomy that aids in raising an Intuitive Eater.

The developmental stages we are referring to in this chapter are: Birth to Wobblers (birth to two years), Toddlers and Early Childhood (two to five years), and School Age to Early Adolescence (five to twelve years). The information provided for each developmental stage is specific to supporting their Intuitive Eating abilities at that age. There will be some things you notice we miss or don't talk about; the reason for that is simple: we just don't have enough space to go into intense detail for every one of these stages. However, we provide additional resources, should you want them, at the back of this book. You will see certain developmental tasks highlighted that your child is working on in each stage for you to tune in to. Along with the child's developmental tasks are important caregiver tasks for each stage related to the 3 Keys. The caregiver tasks nurture the psychological, physical, and emotional development of the child, including the development of their relationship with food and body.

BIRTH TO WOBBLERS (BIRTH TO TWO YEARS)

This stage is all about two big things: establishing trust in the environment and building attachment with a primary caregiver. From what you've already learned, it's clear how these tasks are related to Intuitive Eating. A caring and responsive feeding relationship between caregiver and baby establishes a sense of *trust,* and promotes *satisfaction* and the importance of physical and emotional *comfort.* Trust comes from being fed consistently, adequately, and safely by the primary caregiver. Satisfaction is a result of allowing your infant to eat as much as they need to fulfill natural hunger cues, and comfort comes from having their physical and emotional needs met (such as soothing). Soothing and comfort are initially provided by a caregiver followed by the development of your baby's increasing ability to self-soothe, all within the first two years of life. During this stage, three important elements of the Intuitive Food and Body Relationship Model are emphasized and fostered: trust, comfort, and satisfaction.

Because so much development—physical and psychological—happens in the first two years of life, we've broken down this developmental stage into two parts: birth to six months, and six months to two years.

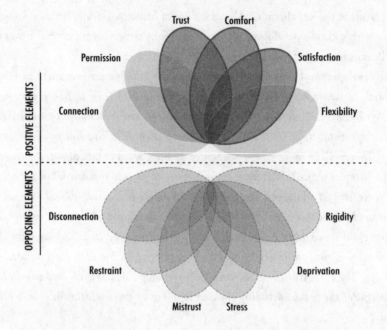

Your child's developmental tasks: Birth to six months

Build attachment to primary caretaker(s).

Form trust in the environment around them.

Your child's developmental tasks: Six months to two years

Continue to build attachment to primary caretaker(s).

Continue to form trust in the environment around them.

Develop self-awareness through movement and emerging language skills.

Develop a sense of independence.

Grow their ability to comfort themselves—use blankets, toys, songs, self-play.

BIRTH TO SIX MONTHS

The moment a baby is born, they are ready for food. Eating is the most basic survival instinct. Feeding an infant in the first four to six months is reliant on responding to their early cues (fussiness or cries) for milk or formula in a timely manner. Without needing to learn anything, an infant knows to find the breast or bottle when it's offered, and they know to turn their head away when full. (*In some cases, there may be a disruption in an infant's ability to latch, suck, or swallow, among other developing oral motor skills, or they may not have an adequate drive to eat. These problems require individualized support from a trained medical provider such as a speech-language pathologist or lactation consultant.)* Building a healthy bond between caregiver and child happens as trust is established through this feeding response: a hungry baby is fed when they "ask" for it. In many cases, your infant's eating schedule will match up fairly closely with the example feeding schedule you see below. You'll probably learn from your doctor, doula, or midwife about this suggested general schedule (this isn't individualized; it's more of a general idea) for feedings, which states that newborns eat about every two to three hours and will gradually sleep for longer periods of time, and eat less frequently as they develop and age. In other cases, it may be slightly different. Because this book isn't intended to provide individual medical care, we are unable to go into detail. If you're concerned, please talk to a doctor.

At birth a baby's stomach is just the size of a marble and able to hold only one to two teaspoons of liquid and will gradually increase to hold about four to eight ounces per feeding by the time they are four to six months old. Three reputable sources, the American Academy of Pediatrics (AAP), La Leche League International, and Fed Is Best, all recommend on-demand feeding of breastmilk or formula. Not every parent will choose (or be able) to breastfeed, nor should they feel pressured to. Between the ages of two and four months, babies will fall into a pattern of eating that will allow you to have more of a predictable schedule that has been directed by their Intuitive Eating capabilities, yet this pattern will change every few weeks and months as your baby continues to be able to eat more at each feeding time, and can sleep for longer periods of time. The amount an infant consumes at each feeding will vary based on age, weight, and development.

TYPICAL FEEDING PATTERN FOR BREASTFED BABIES FROM LA LECHE LEAGUE

Babies will have unique feeding and sleeping patterns that impact their daily routine. La Leche League International is a resource for parents who want to breastfeed and may have questions or face challenges.

Example feeding patterns

First few weeks of life: 8 to 12 feedings in 24 hours
1 to 3 months: 7 to 9 feedings in 24 hours
3 months: 6 to 8 feedings in 24 hours

6 months: 6 feedings per day

12 months: Nursing may drop to about 4 times a day. The introduction of solids at about 6 months helps to fuel your baby's additional nutritional needs.

Sometimes a parent may feel strongly about doing everything they can to choose breastfeeding over bottle feeding, but for medical or other reasons, the infant isn't receiving adequate nutrition. In this case, we support all parents, first of all by knowing how overwhelming and disappointing this can feel, and second, by wanting you to know that your most important job is to make sure your baby is getting fed enough. If you chose to try breastfeeding, but realize it isn't the route to get your child fed, you can move on to the next option of formula feeding or tube feeding if medically necessary. Fed Is Best "provides safe, infant feeding education for breastfeeding, mixed-feeding, formula-feeding, pumped-milk-feeding, and tube-feeding mothers and families to prevent feeding complications to babies that have become too common from the pressure to exclusively breast-feed at all costs."[2]

The bottom line is that from day one, adequacy and consistency in feeding for your child is the most important thing, and, whether it comes from breast or bottle or both, will help build trust in the feeding relationship.

CAREGIVER FOCUS: ATTACHMENT AND TRUST

The tasks of building healthy attachment to a primary caregiver and forming trust with the environment in the first year of life cannot be completed without the responsiveness during feeding from you, the caregiver. Babies are completely dependent on you for eating. They can poop, pee, and sleep on their own—*but they absolutely need you in order to eat.*

Attachment, also known as attachment bond, is generally described as the way that babies learn to organize their feelings about their relationship with you, their caregiver. Attachment is thought to be the foundation for the rest of a person's life, and doesn't just have impacts on their emotional development. Attachment can set the stage for social, intellectual, and physical development as well. **To develop a secure attachment bond, an infant needs their parent or caregiver to be consistently looking and listening for their emotional cues in order to understand their needs, which a responsive feeding approach offers.**

HOW ATTACHMENT AND THE THREE PARTS OF THE BRAIN IMPACT COPING

We know there are three distinct parts of the human brain; this is what differentiates us from most other animals. These parts are where our abilities to be Intuitive Eaters come from: each part plays a role in the dynamics of Intuitive Eating.

1. Our instincts are derived from the *reptilian* complex part of our brain, which controls basic bodily functions that serve survival and reproduction, including hunger.
2. Our emotions reside in the limbic system, otherwise known as the *mammalian* center of our brain.
3. Our thoughts come from the *neocortex*, which is what makes the evolved human brain unique. The neocortex is how we are able to think abstractly, and utilize logic and reason—like choosing to eat before a long meeting starts because we know we'll have to miss lunch.

YOU'RE NOT CREATING A "SPOILED" CHILD

On-demand feeding is sometimes criticized as "creating a spoiled child"; however, the data is convincing: infants who have secure attachment tend to fare much better with independence as they grow. If their needs aren't consistently met, confusion about how safe they are or how much they can trust their environment can occur. Food is a primary need that must be attended to consistently and repeatedly, yet it's not the only need that impacts the way their brain is organized. Soothing, comforting, and tending to a baby's physical needs offers them the opportunity to not only receive your attention, touch, and care, but to begin to *respond* to your cues as well, which all help create secure attachment.

HOW THIS AFFECTS INTUITIVE EATING

When an infant's physical and emotional needs repeatedly go unmet, and there isn't a secure emotional connection with their primary caregiver, their brain-to-body signaling can change. (*Repeatedly having unmet needs can be severely stressful, and we're not talking about how you let your child cry in the bassinet for a few minutes because you desperately needed a shower.*) Humans rely on signaling in the brain to guide Intuitive Eating, just as we rely on signaling to guide emotional processing and responsiveness. Inner signals that come from the reptilian brain, such as hunger signals, in someone with a secure attachment bond, will be sent up to the emotional center, the limbic system, for processing. When signals for basic needs are repeatedly not met, the brain shuts down the signaling from reptilian brain to limbic brain, because it's rather traumatic to have to live with the information that our needs aren't going to be met. There is some incredible research around this, and it's one of the very first things I (Sumner) learned from Elyse Resch under her mentorship: often adults who are seeking help with disordered eating learned a very long time ago that it's easier to ignore their needs (emotional and physical) than to acknowledge them and feel the deep disappointment and lack of safety over and over again of needs not being met. *Ignoring our needs can develop from an unconscious adaptation to avoid feeling the things that are hardest to feel. This development can start early.*

Secure attachment lays the groundwork for the settling in of the six core elements of the Intuitive Food and Body Relationship Model: comfort, permission, trust, flexibility, satisfaction, and connection. All six elements begin in the earliest months and years, some possibly even the earliest few days of our life. In the cases when they aren't established (which is, honestly, for a lot of us), we believe that we can mend the broken connections, and heal our inner child—or possibly in your case as you read this, the child right in front of you.

So, what are some real solid tasks that you can do *now*?

Caregiver tasks: Birth to six months

- Feeding promptly and in a loving, warm manner in response to hunger cries and feeding until the infant turns their head away from breast or bottle.
- Self-care and mental health support as needed for the mother or primary caregiver.
- Adequate hydration and nourishment for the breastfeeding mother to support milk supply.
- Introduction of solids between four and six months using a responsive feeding approach.
- Communication with other caregivers about responding to signs of hunger and fullness so the baby is getting consistent caregiver messages about feeding.
- Don't force or pressure the baby to eat more. Respond to their fullness cues.

- As they approach readiness for solids, respond to the baby's curiosity about the food you're eating—let them touch, taste, and smell, whether it's a cupcake or a carrot; this is where neutrality with food starts to become important.
- Follow safety guidelines to prevent choking.
- Follow pediatrician recommendations for breastmilk or formula ounces daily, ultimately dictated by the baby's hunger and satiety cues.

BEYOND MILK AND FORMULA

Somewhere around an average of four to six months of age, your child will be ready for the introduction of complementary (food other than formula or breast-milk) foods! This is an exciting time: that first seated eating experience, complete with bib and photo ops. It's a big topic all on its own—all that is involved in how you support your baby to embrace the complicated journey of learning to self-feed. It captures everything from safety (*what is gagging versus choking?*), to decisions on approach (*spoon-feeding or baby-led weaning?*), to the structure (*single food introductions or preparing mixed meals?*), to getting familiar with their cues, and so much more.

SIX MONTHS TO ONE YEAR

Baby-led weaning (BLW), or self-feeding, is an alternative to or can be combined with spoon-feeding pureed food. I (Sumner) was learning more about BLW when my first child was a baby, and essentially ended up using a combination of feeding styles. The potential benefits of BLW are that it encourages the baby to practice the skills of self-feeding all on their own, with little intervention from spoon-feeding by their caregiver, who is there to facilitate it and provide safe foods, but not to actually put food in their mouth.

Research tells us that around seven months is a critical period where responsive feeding should be fostered, including self-feeding and self-regulation.[3] Baby-led weaning is a self-feeding approach, and *instead of or alongside* spoon-feeding, both are ways of approaching responsive feeding at this stage. Babies and wobblers who transition into eating complementary and eventually solid foods can be so fun to feed. Their natural curiosity, and motivation to taste, feel, and try a variety of foods is often so prominent in this life phase—and they haven't yet entered the "no" phase of being a toddler, where it can feel like almost overnight their preferences change. In this stage, babies are often excited about food, interested in the moment-to-moment experience of the sensory delights, and they are truly forming their core associations with eating and mealtime. Taking advantage of this transition, learning about, and using a responsive approach has the potential for lifelong benefits around eating and acceptance.

As parents, we tend to think it ought to be easy and straightforward. You pick a jar of baby food, get a nice little baby-size spoon, and you feed your eager, interested, hungry child. It may turn out that way for some, but in reality, for many of us, the story unfolds in a different way. This is why responsiveness and attentiveness to your child's unique signals is so important.

Caregiver tasks: Six months to two years

- You may choose to promote self-feeding by encouraging your baby to feed themselves with their hands with safe and developmentally appropriate food, and eventually learn to use utensils.
- With any style of feeding you choose, spoon-feeding or BLW or a mix, encourage your child to self-regulate how much and what they choose to eat from what is offered by not pressuring them to eat any food.
- Bring the high chair or baby seat up to the table, and situate the baby as a part of the family meal whenever possible.
- Focus on responsiveness, eat with your child, and stay attentive to them with eye contact and engagement.
- Trust their hunger and satiety signals: if they are doing more playing than eating, or turning their head away, they are likely finished.
- Don't force them to eat a certain amount; their portions will vary from meal to meal.
- Around the eighteen-month to two-year mark, begin establishing the structure of meal- and snack time, where eating is done in your home (table, dining room, and so on), and for the most part do not provide milk or juice between meals, which can interrupt their appetite pattern.

COMMON BARRIERS PARENTS FACE TO RESPONSIVE FEEDING WITH BABIES AND WOBBLERS

Time: If you're a busy parent, you may find it challenging to slow down and allow for a child-centered, responsive feeding approach all the time. But remember, this doesn't need to be perfect. Try to allow for feeding experiences that aren't rushed when you're able to. Allow twenty to thirty minutes for a meal, and when it's time to clean up, it's perfectly healthy and appropriate for the meal to end if you need it to.

Mess: Babies are messy! Although for some this is truly hard to handle, try to focus on your parenting values, and know that the experiences babies have with self-feeding—including touching, smelling, and playing with food—are all part of their natural curiosity. Keep things positive, and know that you can create the boundaries. If a child repeatedly throws a bowl of food or their sippy cup on the floor, they may be entertained by watching you respond by picking it up over and over again. Tell them, after the first couple of entertaining drops, *When it drops on the floor again, we will leave it there.* Let them observe your boundaries by not picking it back up. It's helpful for them, and necessary for them, to know you have those boundaries. If they don't get the entertaining reaction from you, they won't be as motivated to keep throwing things. Additionally, when they aren't getting enough of your attention—when there isn't eye contact, or responsive verbal or nonverbal interaction—they may try to do things that will get your attention. Consider both of these potential activators when your child may be doing something repeatedly that contributes to the mess (and the stress). Remember, to them, you're the most interesting person in the room.

Juggling multiple kids: There's nothing wrong or shameful about using store-bought pureed food or on-the-go pouches of purees if you need or want to. See if you can intentionally incorporate aspects of baby-led weaning into your feeding routine when you're able and when you feel comfortable.

You perceive your child to be "overweight": Weight bias is real. We have all been conditioned to fear higher weight. If you experience this with your infant, you'll need to work hard to overcome what you may have been told about their weight being a problem, or your feelings about their body. Honor your feelings, process them, talk about them with a trusted person who knows Intuitive Eating, or who doesn't feel your child's weight is a problem. Keep your center of focus on feeding them adequately and appropriately, not on managing their weight. Know that restricting or depriving your child, or pressuring or coercing them to eat or not eat something, will likely be harmful and interrupt their natural Intuitive Eating ability.

You perceive your child to be "underweight": In some cases, with children who have failure to thrive, or have lost weight, or are truly not eating enough, you need the guidance and individualized care of a pediatric feeding specialist or registered dietitian. Even in this case, be cautious of how pressure or force-feeding could potentially worsen your child's undereating. Responsive feeding is ideal as a therapeutic approach.

KATIE AND JACK'S ADVENTURE WITH RICE CEREAL

Katie was a first-time mom, eager and excited to finally make the move to introducing solids. When she was told by the pediatrician that her son Jack was ready for rice cereal, she was so excited for his first adventure into something beyond breast milk, she immediately sent her husband to the store, with a specific request. She told him it didn't matter if he got a particular brand, any rice cereal would do. He gave her an inquisitive look about what she was requesting him to buy, but knowing better than to question her, he headed off to the store. When he returned Katie took out the baby bowl, put a small amount of the cereal with some breast milk in it to soften it. She began by giving Jack a spoonful, and he immediately rejected it, spitting it out. When she called her mom to tell her what happened, concerned about why he wasn't interested, her mom nearly died laughing. Katie had attempted to give Jack Rice Krispies—not infant rice cereal. To this day she still talks about how she'll never live it down.

Jack intuitively knew that he wasn't ready for the texture of the Rice Krispies, and his instincts worked perfectly. He didn't yet possess oral motor skills needed to eat cereal with milk, or something crunchy. He refused to eat it. Katie is an incredible mom, now raising two little boys, and never made the same mistake again. However, this story is important because all of us, no matter how informed or tuned in we are to our parenting responsibilities, have made mistakes, misunderstood directions, or just simply screwed up. We all need to be able to laugh at ourselves and move on, while knowing that in a lot of cases, we can trust our kid's instincts, even when they're just a few months old. Also, Jack, and for the most part all babies, know so much, and they are quite competent in many areas of eating. We just need to be responsive, attentive, and know our role. Pressuring or forcing him to eat the bigger, crunchy pieces of Rice

Krispies could have been a really negative early feeding experience for him, and his mom did her job of noticing his response and not pressuring him to continue.

TODDLERS AND EARLY CHILDHOOD (TWO TO FIVE YEARS)

There's no way around it, each of these three phases is as important as the next. In this second phase, we enter a time in a child's life when their emotional awareness about the world expands from being just about them and their needs, environment, daycare, or schedule 24/7 to something so much bigger. *Other people come into view.* Children in this phase aren't only learning to eat in different ways—learning how to eat in a chair, watching you prepare meals, developing more likes and dislikes, developing new and effective ways of communicating with you about hunger—but they are also learning to interact with the world in a whole new way. Who do you think they're looking at for how to do that? You guessed it: you! Remember that spongelike mind they possess. By watching you, they're learning all about how to treat others, and beyond watching, they're *listening*, even when you may think they can't understand. You might think, *What does how they treat others have to do with their Intuitive Eating process?*

THIS IS WHEN KIDS LEARN TO JUDGE BODIES

We know that as young as three years old, kids start to develop awareness around preferences and societal opinions about bodies, influenced by hundreds if not thousands of messages a day, not counting the messages they get from you. Every one of us lives with implicit bias—racial bias, size bias, cultural bias. It's partly the way our brains are constructed from an evolutionary standpoint, and partly learned from our environment.

One of the things that we can focus on as parents is to prepare our children to understand the diversity of humans. Not just body diversity and normalizing different bodies, but also teaching them about skin color, ethnicities, religions, and diversity as a whole. Kids at this age already understand societal expectations and will begin to question things they see out of that "norm." Even if you and your family exist in privileged bodies (or have privilege that has made your lives fit societally normal expectations), you can work to normalize bodies that are different from yours. We have to actively normalize and talk about bodies and identities that we don't frequently see portrayed on TV or in movies, books, and billboards. This is an age where the beliefs that society has started to instill aren't yet so deeply ingrained. This doesn't mean that we can't continue to teach our kids about diversity as they age—we just might have to undo more sociocultural expectations when they are older. At this age, they are still developing their sense of the world. We can make it a more inclusive world.

THE *ME, MINE,* AND *NO* PHASE

For toddlers, autonomy is *the* driving force behind nearly everything they do. They are wired to seek out and act out their autonomy. And while we love these kiddos for everything they are (these years are some of the most memorable, fun, and exciting times of parenting), this stage of feeding can become really tricky and complicated.

They are set up to challenge you, to be interested in pushing your buttons, and to say no simply because you want them to say yes. So, in the moments when you're most frustrated or confused by their eating, just remember: this is demonstrating a good sign that they are on the right track developmentally. It shows they are developing a healthy ego, which doesn't want to do everything it's told to do. *Saying no, for a toddler, is something they have to do; they are designed to do this.* Having opinions, boundaries, and speaking your truth are all things we want to foster in our children, while teaching them respectful interaction with us as parents and others around them (not an easy feat!).

FIRST EXPERIENCES OF GUILT AND SHAME

As children develop increased self-awareness, feelings of guilt and shame can arise as their world becomes larger than just their individual self: for the first time in their life, they start forming more social relationships, *and start understanding that what they do can impact someone else.*

As parents and caregivers, we can be especially aware in this stage that how we respond to food- and body-related events can intentionally or unintentionally elicit feelings of confidence and competence, or less ideal feelings of guilt or shame. Guilt and shame, although similar, have very different end states. When humans feel guilt, we believe something we've done—our *action*—is bad. When we feel shame, we believe our *core self* is bad. Our broader patterns in caregiving to kids, how we repeatedly respond to a child, may cement these beliefs for the long term. We need to be particularly aware with toddlers not to send a message that they are wrong or bad for anything they want to eat, or for eating something. This takes us back to being present, choosing our response instead of reacting out of habit. It also highlights how necessary that work from part 2 is, about getting to know your inner child. When you have made sense of your own past, and understand your own relationship with food and body, you can avoid repeating things that perhaps you were conditioned to say or do around your young child.

FROM ON-DEMAND FEEDING TO A FLEXIBLE AND RELIABLE FEEDING ROUTINE

When your child enters into toddlerhood and early childhood, you're ready to teach (and your child is ready to learn) patience, boundaries, and limits. With food, this moves you from the essential focus of on-demand feeding (remember, patience and boundaries were not the focus; establishing trust was) to a slightly different focus, supporting them to understand that food will always be available and they will have what they need, *and* that there are times when we need to work on patience (*Food is coming soon*), boundaries (*No, you can't have another cup of milk because the last one you poured on your head, and we don't do that with our milk*), and understanding limits (such as when we need to save the last cookie for someone else, or there isn't enough to have as much as they want, or that their parent has set a boundary and negotiating isn't an option).

What happens during toddlerhood and early childhood? What does your child focus on and what do you focus on?

Your child's developmental tasks: toddlerhood and early childhood

- Continued growth of individuality.
- Gain verbal and communication skills for expressing feelings and needs.
- Emotional regulation and body function regulation.
- Increasing awareness of gender identity.
- Testing boundaries and limits with caregivers.
- Increasing interest in building relationships with peers and group activities.

Caregiver tasks in feeding

- Providing a flexible and reliable feeding routine as well as a sleep routine.
- Reading books that teach body appreciation and body diversity.
- Using your Intuitive Eating voice using words your child understands

to model listening to your body and communicating about things like pleasure, permission, and limits around food.

- Normalize talking about bodies neutrally without judgment. Show appreciation and curiosity.
- Give kids some choice: *Do you want bananas or oranges this morning?*
- Promote positive mealtime experiences.
- Begin to ask kids for assistance when they are ready: they can help with cleaning up, putting dishes away, and setting the table.
- Understand and ready yourself for a possible drop in variety of preferred foods.
- Talk with other caregivers, medical providers, and grandparents to communicate the harm of diet talk around your child.

According to Erikson, the two stages of psychosocial development in these years are autonomy versus shame to achieve the virtue of will, and initiative versus guilt to achieve the virtue of purpose.

When kids are given the opportunity to make the decision for themselves about what food they choose to eat and how much they choose to eat from what is available, they start to develop a sense of autonomy. They are also doing this with many other non-food behaviors in their life, but food is a big one, with many chances to practice each and every day. By developing autonomy, and continuing to build up the belief that their choices are allowed and trusted, they develop a sense of will. A parent can support the development of this virtue by allowing their child to make more independent choices—and to learn from their experiences, both positive and negative. Because you're the parent, you're also encouraged to provide a supportive environment, where they aren't punished for their eating or for making a mess, for example, or by helping them with new tasks if they need it as they gain more independence. If we apply this to food, support comes in the form of letting kids determine their preferences and tastes without judgment. It can also be the independence of choosing how much cake to eat at a party or pie to eat at a holiday. There is a chance they could eat so much they get a tummy ache. (This isn't a failure, it's simply learning how their body communicates and how to listen. It's actually a key experience for them, requiring little to no intervention on our part other than a gentle *Are you okay? What do you think happened? Your body will take care of it with a little time*.) By experiencing this discomfort without criticism or punishment, they are able to learn the internal cues they need to develop autonomy around eating. When food is emotionally neutral, they are more likely to experience the experiments with autonomy around food similarly to walking or playing a game. They naturally will choose what feels best for them most of the time when Intuitive Eating remains intact.

The development of initiative is similar to autonomy, in the sense that it builds up your child's ability and confidence in making choices. This might present in the form of asking multiple questions or trying to direct situations as much as possible. There is a balance in developing this virtue because we don't want our kids to be so invested in always being in charge that they can't share or allow others to make choices too. Squashing their desire to make choices or ask questions leads to guilt and fear of making choices. That's why it's important to understand and expect some of this behavior in the toddler stage, and see the benefit of it. Allowing your child to participate in the process of preparing, choosing, and planning food enables them to have some initiative without being in charge of every decision. You're still the parent, but we can definitely acknowledge that they can have opinions and make choices too! Finding this balance allows your child to successfully develop a sense of purpose.

SETTING EXPECTATIONS AND MEALTIME BASICS WITH TODDLERS

As with everything, it comes down to how we set expectations and use thoughtful ways of communicating around food that help us create positive mealtime experiences. Let's be honest: at times, it's pretty darn hard to keep your cool and not yell out your frustrations when there's whining, complaining about food, or reluctance to sit . . . particularly at the end of the day. But we can sure try, and following through with our boundaries and the consequences becomes important for supporting our toddlers to learn what is involved at mealtimes. At mealtimes, there is more to consider than just what your child eats. Just like every other part of their day, you have your own set of family expectations for things like how people are treated, what is an acceptable way to accept or reject a food that's offered, when it's okay to leave the table, talking with your mouth full, and so on. These are *behaviors and expectations* that you, the parent, establish. We won't attempt to tell you what your family behavior boundaries are, but the following is one piece of advice.

When you're setting a behavior boundary with a young child, the most important thing you can do for them is to be consistent. In the case when a toddler is throwing food on the ground because they enjoy the noises and the fascinating display of splattering sauce on the floor, it's a sign they are no longer hungry for their food (they'd be eating it if they were hungry) but rather they are playing with their food. Accidental spills and messes also come naturally with eating when you're a toddler, but playing or intentional spilling may be a behavioral boundary for you. How you respond to behavior boundaries matters because it impacts *your* experience in eating with your kids. *And your experience, your feelings, your attitude all impact their experience. You're an important part of this equation.* In many ways, you're the centerpiece at a young child's table. Remember, you're modeling for them, and that is a lot to ask of someone every day, year after year. And not only are you modeling for them, you and your experience matters independently from theirs. You do not exist purely to be a model figure for your child; you exist to live your life, according to your values, and you deserve to parent in a way that meets you at those values. How you feel matters. Setting the boundaries you need, so that joining your child at the table, or wherever you may be eating, is enjoyable and fosters connection, helps you.

You might say to a toddler repeatedly creating spills or throwing food: *It looks like you're all done. Have you had enough?* as you're moving in to remove the food or plate from in front of them. If they are still hungry, they will stop the behavior and return to eating. In her book *No Bad Kids: Toddler Discipline Without Shame,* Janet Lansbury goes into incredibly helpful and relatable detail in these issues. You may give them a moment to change the behavior, but if they continue, it's your time to be clear and end the meal for them. They will learn that it's not an expected or tolerated behavior, and will be driven to do what works for them next time so they can get enough to eat. The same boundary can be used for getting up from the table, using a loving, non-shaming, non-threatening voice indicating that the meal is done unless they can join you at the table.

Even with kids as young as two you may begin to notice them trying to use food as a way to assert some power; for example, asking for more milk or snacks instead of going to bed. Or saying no to the foods you prepare. These aren't personal digs, they are attempts to test the waters, find some control. A child asking for food to avoid going to bed isn't about food, it's about what they're trying to control or that they want something more (like time with you). When you can see that, your response can address the underlying issue; it doesn't need to shame them or punish them for wanting food. That may sound like: *It's bedtime now, my dear, so we're done having snacks.* Another way you can address this, if it's repeatedly coming up, is to communicate clearly earlier on in the day or night what they can expect in order to minimize any uncertainty or anxiety they may have: *After dinner we're going to play outside for a bit, and then take a bath and get pajamas on.*

Then we can have our evening snack and then watch a short show before storytime. Sound good? That way your child knows there will be an opportunity to eat a snack or drink something if they want to. But it's not up to them and it's not a mystery when it will happen. Ensuring that they have adequate food in their belly to go to bed is something you can do, and can help to assure you that the request for food at bedtime isn't about the food. Not giving up being in charge of bedtime is often important for parents, but allowing them to eat as much as they need is important for them. Children will often respond positively to knowing what the plan is, whether it's the routine before school, what needs to happen before you can go to the park, or before bedtime. Communicating the plan gives them structure and a sense of security.

It's the moments when kids try to get creative around the boundaries that parents often find themselves going to their default of what was modeled for them. These old, embedded phrases and responses are waiting for us on the tip of our tongue to use when we don't know what else to do. If you find yourself saying just the thing that was said to you even though you don't think it's right, try to notice it and pause. Even if you do say it, if it's not what you intended to say or do, have self-compassion and move on. You can try again next time (and there will be a next time!). Use mindfulness, take a few breaths before responding to the whining, the no's, or the attempts to use food by your toddler to assert some healthy power!

DWINDLING FOOD PREFERENCES IN THE TODDLER YEARS

When my older child was nearly three, I (Sumner) started to really notice her list of preferred foods dwindling. This is totally normal, but hard not to worry about. As a baby, she would gobble up almost anything she was served, but this changed in a relatively short amount of time. Every child is a unique eater. So much of how they eat is just part of who they are, how they are wired. It's another reminder to release the control you want to have over their eating, and to move away from the impulse to compare your child to their sibling or to another child.

Concern and guilt can start arising in parents when you believe your child is a fussy or picky eater, or not eating enough to be healthy. Kids' intake at meals will vary a lot and be unpredictable at times. However, research has repeatedly demonstrated that kids naturally eat more to make up for calories they missed earlier, and eat less when they have eaten more calories at an earlier meal.[4] It's understandable to worry if your child's appetite or food intake variety seems low, but remember that they aren't a machine, turn to your parenting values and the 3 Keys, and avoid pressuring or bribing them.

HELP FOR PICKY EATING

As we begin this section, in places we will use the terms "picky" or "fussy" to describe an eating style. Keep in mind it's *never helpful* for you to label your child as "hard to feed" or as a "picky" or "fussy," "bad" or "good" eater. Be aware to not use these labels when they are around, even if you think they're not listening. They may have limited preferences, or may have some unique likes and dislikes, but when they hear a label attached, it can become hard to get rid of. Instead of saying, *Thomas is a picky eater,* try *He may eat that, or he may not, but if he wants to he will.* We invite you to consider the idea that, despite how it's often portrayed, picky eating isn't a deviant behavior. We know the reality—*it's hard to deal with, and at times may make you want to scream*—but for many kids, this change in likes and dislikes is a natural part of this stage, and it is likely not at all about being difficult. It's about wanting to have a say in what goes in their body, along with a slowed rate of growth compared to the first two years of life. There is also evidence to support that how "picky" a child may be isn't just on them; parental feeding practices and child feeding behaviors are in relationship with each other, each influencing the other.[5] Remember how we talked in chapter 6 about how there is a bidirectional interaction in the feeding dynamics? Let's revisit this and see how pressure in response to worry can create more aversive eating, causing more worry and more pressure.

WHY YOUR RESPONSE MATTERS SO MUCH FOR PICKY EATING

We have good evidence to support the bidirectional relationship: parents worry about a behavior, which may create a counterproductive feeding practice, causing parents to pressure children and worry more. We see a parallel process for parents of larger-bodied children. Parents of kids who have a higher weight often, thanks to societal standards, feel more pressure to control their child's eating, food, and weight, which causes the child to react by eating *more* in response. Often, a child who senses pressure to lose weight or eat less will gain more weight over time from compensatory or emotionally driven eating in the absence of hunger, causing parents to deprive or judge the child even more, and so on.

THE WORRY CYCLE

The Worry Cycle, developed by Dr. Katja Rowell in her book *Love Me, Feed Me: The Adoptive Parent's Guide to Ending the Worry About Weight, Picky Eating, Power Struggles, and More,* interrupts the main goal of being able to have calm, positive

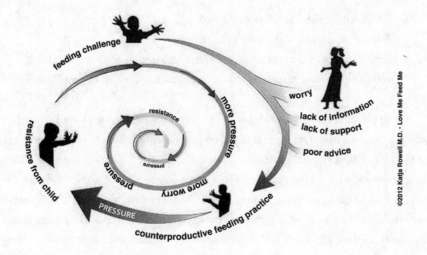

family meal experiences.[6] When parents can enter into potentially worrisome food exchanges, armed with the reminders that pressure and control aren't going to help their child feel calm, relaxed, or trusting enough to be able to do the best they can, parents can seek support outside of those moments, and turn back to the 3 Keys.

When you hear "Picky eating is totally normal," what does that really mean? How normal? How do you know if your kids are just enacting regular old preschooler pickiness—or a truly problematic fear of food? Parents' concerns are completely understandable and valid; after all, you're very invested in your child eating enough. We don't think any parent is overreacting when they worry about picky eating, especially when they see their child reject foods, both new and familiar.

Measures of picky eating vary: some studies cite 5 percent of kids are picky, while others cite a much higher prevalence of nearly 60 percent. We don't know exactly the trajectory of fussy eating at this point, but we do know that lots of kids, especially from the age of about two and a half up to five or six, develop preferences and often appear uninterested or completely unwilling to eat foods they quickly devoured as an eighteen-month-old. We see why parents reach their wits' end when it comes to fussy eating—it isn't easy, emotionally or logistically, to feed your kid when they refuse to eat what you're offering.

According to a 2020 review of ten studies, fussy eating is associated with:[7]

- Family stress and conflict at mealtime.
- High levels of parental concern and frustration.

- Child anxiety and feelings of disgust.
- A low association with health risks.
- Lower intake of certain vitamins and nutrients: including vitamins E and C, folate, and fiber (which can contribute to digestive complaints).

However, there is good news on the horizon for parents who are invested in raising Intuitive Eaters: research focused on fussy eating, which has increased since 2008, shows that a responsive feeding approach, like the 3 Keys, is associated with lower levels of fussy eating compared to a more controlling or non-responsive approach, such as using pressure, reward, or punishment with food. *This doesn't mean your child won't be a fussy eater if they are eating intuitively,* but it does indicate that a responsive feeding approach is the most helpful response you can have when they are fussy to prevent it from worsening in response to your reaction.

What happens when a child goes from adventurous "easy" eater to "fussy" overnight? Research has shown that a significant number of families grapple with the sudden pickiness in toddler years. "Fussy" can mean one or more of the following characteristics: not wanting to try new foods, needing food served a specific way (for example, in separate dishes), limited intake of food, disinterest in a certain food group, and frequent changes in preference requiring a particular way of preparing or presenting food. Kids may eat differently depending on who they are with when eating—grandparents, teachers, other kids, or their parents, for example.

Key 2—the flexible feeding routine—is the recommended approach for children to prevent some of the common difficulties you might face when it comes to fussy eating. If you can focus on the structure of meals and snack timing in their day, it will help you by creating space between eating times to develop comfortable hunger and appetite for mealtime, encouraging them to eat from their internal drive for food, versus you needing to "get them" to eat. Remember to include one or two foods that they like at meal- or snack time, so you're not expecting them to eat something they may feel averse to—that would be a negative feeding experience. Mealtime screaming matches, total food refusal, feeling like you should make multiple meals to cater to each child, or wasted food getting thrown out night after night cause immense stress on you as a parent, and can cause a significant rift in your relationship with your child. If you picked up this book because you're feeling confused, stressed, or overwhelmed about fussy eating, remember that even though it's not a quick fix, you can do this.

YOU CAN'T CHANGE YOUR CHILD, BUT YOU CAN
CHANGE HOW YOU RESPOND TO YOUR CHILD

One of the most important things to learn when shifting to an add-in, pressure-off approach is realizing that you can't change your child—you can only change *how you respond* to your child. This is the root of a responsive feeding approach. Although we trust it isn't intentional, parent feeding practices can directly relate to fussy eating, and also directly relate to the emotional climate at the table. Remember in chapter 6 when we talked about why parental control backfires? And how important the emotional connection and experience between a caregiver and a child (relatedness) is to create the environment where that natural, internal drive to eat and explore foods can thrive? When you have a child who is picky for whatever reason (genetic predisposition, texture aversions, sensory concerns, it's a part of their global personality, or out of reaction to pressure), it's naturally going to elicit an emotional response from you, and your internal beliefs may drive you to try controlling their food, offering rewards, or punishing them to solve the problem. Rewarding and pressuring around food is more likely to predict fussiness years after it first shows up, often around age two or three. If you can be prepared to stay the course with the 3 Keys, when your child first begins to show early signs of fussy eating, you're more likely to prevent the issues from worsening over time.[8] If you have been reacting to your child's picky eating, and it becomes a pattern, your child's emotional state will become activated or defensive around mealtime—no matter what the food is, it's more about the emotional energy and that two-way relationship between the parental feeding approach and fussy behavior. They feed off each other, and until there is a change in one (and you can bet it's not going to be in your child) they will continue to be reinforced due to your child's will to assert their autonomy and feed their body in a way that feels safe for them, and your will to get your child to eat a meal. Try to redirect your will to understanding that they will be more capable of relaxing with food, eating adequately, and gradually expanding their preferences in the long term when you remove pressure, coercion, punishment, reward, or detectable overconcern.

WHEN TO SEEK HELP

The following is an excerpt from the blog post "How to Help Toddlers with Texture Aversions" on *Yummy Toddler Food*, created by writer and recipe developer Amy Palanjian, with advice by Jenny McGlothlin, coauthor of *Helping Your Child with Extreme Picky Eating*:[9]

According to Jenny, these are signs that you may want to reach out to your pediatrician and/or a feeding therapist for help. (A small amount of texture aversions can be normal, but if some or all of these things are happening or you just feel it in your gut that something isn't quite right, do reach out for help.)

- Child regularly gags or vomits at each meal (with consideration for transitions to textured food).
- Child isn't eating enough in terms of quantity or variety to support healthy emotional, physical or social development.
- Parent reports significantly different mealtime behaviors than you see at school.
- Child isn't chewing well, spits out food after chewing, or can't keep food in their mouth.
- Child swallows food whole. (Here's how to tell if your child isn't chewing: Child younger than 3, but "chews" with mouth closed; Child chokes or gags while eating; Child winces during swallowing; You can identify whole pieces of food in diaper or vomit; Child is constipated; Child fails to maintain weight despite eating age-appropriate amounts of food; Child stuffs mouth full of food while eating and often needs reminders to slow down and take smaller bites.)

General tips for feeding toddlers:
- Try to stay calm: the greater emotional response you have toward your child's eating, the worse it's likely to be. If they say *I don't want it* or *I don't like it!*, say, *Okay. It's here if you change your mind.*
- Think to yourself: *I value letting my child's appetite direct what they eat, not my thoughts or feelings.*
- If they're not hungry at a meal, that can show up as being fussy or picky, when what you're probably seeing is low appetite. See if there are snacks or beverages (other than water) too close to mealtime and readjust the routine.
- Set the boundary early on that for the most part, eating is done when they're done with sitting. Playing or moving around out of their chair isn't only dangerous as a choking hazard, but blurs the lines between the start and ending of a meal or snack.

- Keep meal- and snack times positive: emotions are a huge component for most children to feel competent and capable with eating, and especially important for sensitive children.
- Avoid using food as a reward (a form of pressure) to motivate your child to eat, such as *You can have a cookie if you have a few bites of your chicken.*
- Remember they won't easily or quickly develop a nutrient deficiency. Try to relax. If they do, it can be addressed. If you are concerned, talk to their doctor.
- *Your value and worth as a parent don't rest on how your child eats.*

What does it sound or look like to offer food without pressure, using your Intuitive Eating voice?

- *You're welcome to have any of these—here they are.*
- *We made _____. Help yourself if you'd like some!*
- *You don't have to eat it.*
- Say nothing, but place it family style on the table.
- Place a small amount on their plate, but say nothing.

INVOLVING YOUR YOUNG CHILD IN FOOD DECISIONS

With this age group we recommend a mix of you deciding what is available, as well as giving two or three choices of what to eat at a meal or snack. Young children can become overwhelmed by too many choices, so limiting options is part of supporting them in a way that is developmentally appropriate. You also get to decide when there are no alternative options; it's perfectly understandable that sometimes you just need to decide what to serve and go with it.

We'll end this stage with reminding you to rest assured that you're not a bad parent for being frustrated. In the moments when you just want to throw your hands up and threaten to put them to bed with nothing else to eat, try taking a breath, using the pause between stimulus and response, and use self-compassion to remember that you aren't alone in this.

In this second half of that ten-or-so-year window, you begin to notice children's independence with food and eating growing. This is a good thing, a sign of capability and confidence! It's also hard to see your child not need you, and even harder to see them doing things that you may not want for them or not agree with—such as eating in a way you might find objectionable. Are your concerns coming from diet culture? Do you find yourself seeing your child's body changing from a child's to a preteen's? What memories does this phase of development bring back for you? What do you wish someone had said to you, or not said to you, or done more of to support you with, when you were going through that significant time of growth and development?

We've divided up this phase into two subsections: ages five to nine, and nine to twelve.

FIVE TO NINE YEARS

Developmental tasks: Five to nine years

- Developing morals and values.
- Continuing to strengthen existing relationships and branching out to new peer groups and interests.
- Gaining capacity for empathy.
- Building self-confidence.
- Self-soothing, maintaining a sense of internal security.
- Verbally sharing more complex feelings.

Caregiver focus: Five to nine years

- Continue to provide exposure to a wide variety of foods without pressuring.
- Know what is happening with food at other places: school, before- or after-school care, friends' houses, and so on. Convey that you trust them, and show interest.
- See them for who they are and who they are becoming. Validate them.
- Help set them up to have enough food—do they have enough in their lunch?
- Model eating meals and snacks at fairly consistent time intervals—

eating with your kids when you can and not skipping meals is a major behavior to model.

- Provide familiar foods that are tasty as well as new foods. Kids' tastes are still maturing!
- Encourage the routine of everyone coming to the table or eating together when you can, knowing there will be no pressure to eat anything if they don't want it. *The focus is on family connection and positive mealtime experiences.*
- Give your child jobs to do to help with cooking—chopping fruit or vegetables, washing potatoes, shucking corn, making a salad, baking cookies, and so on.
- Do they have snacks packed for after-school or morning break? Will they be with friends for a while and need to bring something to eat?
- Communicate about mealtimes to encourage them showing up to the table comfortably hungry. Let them know what time dinner is, and offer or remind them to have a snack a couple of hours prior.
- Explicitly educate them about body diversity and body respect when they are given encouragement to diet or judge bodies.
- Avoid shaming them for anything they want to eat. Don't punish or reward for what they eat or don't eat.

LUNCH-BOX WOES

Beautifully packed, rainbow-themed bento boxes abound across Pinterest, Instagram, and just about every other parent-focused media outlet you can name. When I (Sumner) see these posts, articles, and images of perfectly curated lunch boxes with just the right amount of various food groups, a sprinkle of sweet and salty, and everything fresh and pretty, complete with clever kid-friendly appeal, I feel a mix of gut-wrenching inner critic (*I'll never be good enough*) and inspiration (*I really should try that*). And then the next moment, I think to myself, *Who are these people? Who honestly has the creativity, the energy, and the time to make lunchbox packing into an art?* I'm over here barely remembering to get to the grocery store for milk before we run out, and these parents are in a race for the gold medal of the lunch-box Olympics. Don't get me wrong . . . *I love them.* I want to eat them all, make them all . . . but let me be clear, I *never* want my kids to see them, because the honest truth is they won't ever be heading to school with a lunch box like that in tow. We (parents) need a reality check. There is *absolutely nothing wrong* with making incredible lunches for your kids. Go for it. And when you do it, take that picture and show it to someone, because only another parent can really appreciate your talent and your dedication for what you've done: you deserve a medal. The point is, we all deserve a medal for keeping our kids fed, and fed with love. It may be that your child eats a nourishing hot lunch every day, and it may be that you pack what you can in two minutes before the bus comes because everyone slept in. However you show the love in your family meals is the right way to show the love. You do not need to be perfect.

The second thought that comes to my mind after I see a picture of the perfectly curated lunch box is: *Do their kids eat it?* Or does it come home full with a few bites taken out here and there? Not every child will eat what is packed for lunch. I (Amee) had a conversation with a fellow parent recently about our kid's lunches. We talked about how funny it can be to see the different foods they actually eat out of their lunch box. My daughter would rarely finish her crackers; her daughter would rarely finish her fruit snacks. No matter how pretty we made it or which fancy or yummy ones we bought, they just wouldn't finish them. The foods would change periodically, which made it harder to keep only the preferred foods in the lunch box. Even if we try, we can't keep up, and the perfect rainbow bento box won't fix that.

Once again, when it comes to packing lunches, we find ourselves at the 3 Keys and thinking about getting them *enough* food for all their needs, promoting satisfaction, and variety. Include your child in the process where you can, and think about how you can tune in to the whole picture of their day rather than just the food.

Lunch-box packing tips

- Focus on providing a mix of food groups. They need lots of energy, including foods that provide carbohydrates, protein, and fat for the day.
- Pack slightly more than you think they may eat (to avoid any chance of them undereating or being too hungry)—give a few choices if you can.
- Include a variety of salty, sweet, crunchy, and soft foods (use what you know about your kid's preferences).
- Some kids eat mostly easier-to-eat-and-digest carbohydrate food sources during the school day, and this is totally fine. They are using a

lot of carbohydrates for the brain work and the physical work of being at school. Don't overanalyze their protein intake. They will likely make up for lower protein lunches and snacks at dinnertime.

- Don't get too concerned about how much they eat: keep your thoughts to yourself as you explore the evidence later that day. Learn from what they tend to eat and keep that in the rotation. Kids whose parents immediately focus on lunch-box contents rather than tuning in about how the day was risk missing out on some important information about what matters most for their child.

- Add new foods often—kids get bored just like adults do. Switch things up.

- If you have serious concerns about your child's eating at school, do contact their teacher, who can observe how lunchtime is going and report back to you.

- Always include at least one or two items you feel are highly acceptable to them, as well as foods that may be more hit or miss.

- Ask for your child's input when you feel a little stumped on what to pack if it seems like they're not eating much lunch. If your child gets really irritated or upset when you ask, that might be an indicator that something about school, or lunch, is bothering them.

NUTRITION EDUCATION

Nutrition education for kids has been hijacked by diet culture. Thanks to two of our colleagues, Anna Lutz and Katherine Zavodni, who have been forging the path of how nutrition education for kids needs to be informed by the science around cognitive development, we know that most nutrition education for kids isn't only inappropriate for their level of cognitive understanding, but it has the potential to—and does—cause real harm. This includes the way we are talking to kids about weight, shape, and BMI as part of lessons on "healthy" eating and exercise.

At the root of it, unsurprisingly, most people, healthcare professionals included, are misinterpreting the weight science—and it's not their (or your) fault. Kids are just as (if not more) vulnerable to the negative consequences of these nutrition lessons than adults are because of the way their brains work. They aren't able to think abstractly about things until about middle school age, and even then it takes about another decade until adolescent brains are fully developed. So, when kids hear something in childhood, they lack the ability to critically analyze that information and determine if it's a safe or smart path for them to take. If they're taught something, generally it's assumed to be absolutely true. One example is teaching kids that sugar is bad for them. We have seen countless families in our practices who have young kids who develop extreme fear and life-threatening eating disorders due to learning about "bad" foods. How much of a mixed message is it to teach kids that sugar is "bad," while we fill their Easter baskets and Halloween bags full of candy, along with celebrating everyone we love on their birthday by making a special cake?

Here are some positive and helpful ways to teach young kids about food and nutrition in their early years:

- How to garden and grow food.
- Where food comes from, such as where does applesauce come from (seed, tree, farm, factory, store, home). Make applesauce together as an interactive lesson.
- How to use frozen fruit to make a smoothie.
- Write stories about a family recipe or a favorite dish.
- Explore how the texture of pasta and beans change from hard (uncooked, inedible) to soft and yummy after cooking.

NINE TO TWELVE YEARS

Developmental tasks: Nine to twelve years

- Increased self-awareness: evaluating one's strengths and weaknesses as compared to others'.
- Concern with popularity, attractiveness, and fitting in with peers.
- Increasing ability to see different points of view.

Caregiver focus: Nine to twelve years (in addition to previously mentioned information for ages five to nine, which all still apply):

- Emphasize open, trusting, and nonjudgmental communication.
- Be the person to talk about puberty and bodies with them.
- Accept that they will start to have independence in when they choose to eat.
- Be prepared for increased eating in general: this is a time of gaining both weight and height.
- Encourage adequate sleep and healthy sleep hygiene.

- Be tuned in to what they are seeing and how they may be influenced by social media.

I (Sumner) can remember really hurtful moments of being judged by peers in my school-age years, and in adolescence. Most kids experience body judgment, to varying degrees—many to a far greater and more harmful extent than I did. This is how weight stigma and discrimination in all forms really shows up for our kids: in peer settings, body judgment and comparison, physical violation, and cyberbullying—something that is extremely high on the radar of kids and parents in school and teen years.

Middle school and high school years can be unsafe for some kids. Bullying and peer pressure have a huge impact on mental health. Feeling awkward in your changing body while also being on the brink of emerging independence means that kids still need parental support even as they want to spread their own wings. We can see why this age is high risk for the development of eating disorders.

This could be the only chapter we really need to write. The part where our kids still need us so deeply, but their life and their separation from us only grows. The part where we have to work harder than we may have ever thought, to stay tuned in, to keep the door open, their dinner warm, our arms open. When our kids are growing older, even before they are ten, they are spending more time away from us, with other people, where we don't know what's being said, or how they are changing inside unless we're talking to them. We have to accept that so many factors will draw your child up and away into their own life, the life where you're a spectator and they are directing the show. And we have to let them.

We (Amee and Sumner) don't have kids at this age yet. However, we have lived it, and we have worked with young people, kids and teens and their families. If we had to emphasize one thing for you to focus on during this phase of your child's life, it would be to have laser focus on Key 1: provide unconditional love and support for your child's body. As they slowly graduate from being a kid in a mostly embodied state (as kids tend to be), they will begin to have increasing awareness of what other people think of them and of their body, and they are constantly receiving messages that make an impression about how their body is expected to look and function to meet societal ideals. Judgment and comparison may begin to seep in.

INTERSECTING IDENTITIES

Many kids may have awareness of their identities from a young age, but some identities might become more obvious to kids around this age. Sexuality is one example of this. Around these school-age and early adolescent years, your child will most likely be coming to recognize and making choices—or at least increasing their awareness about—what their identities are. This stage also covers a vast range of developmental experiences, including their transition from a dependent child to an adolescent approaching or in puberty—broaching independence.

When awareness starts to grow, the most important thing you can do is **support your child as much as you can for who they are.**

WEIGHT GAIN IS NORMAL AND EXPECTED IN LATER CHILDHOOD AND EARLY PUBERTY

Everyone will have a unique experience with when (age) and how (varying degrees and rate of their physical changes) their body and their eating will change related to the onset of early puberty.

Body-fat changes, height gains, and growth patterns are estimated by growth charts (where we actually plot their measures), but remember: *your child's individual growth will likely not follow a distinctly neat and calculated curve*—there is always individual variation, jumps, and plateaus over the years, while generally following a growth curve heading in the direction of increased height and weight throughout puberty, in the big picture. Many but not all kids will gain fat and have increased appetite and intake as their body prepares for a gain in height and maturation that follows. With these natural and expected periods of weight gain and growth, we know their bodies are doing what they're designed to do for developmental reasons: they are increasing fat stores accordingly to fulfill their genetic blueprint of development. Normal hormonal changes rely on adequate calorie intake and adequate fat stores for proper development to take place.

READY YOURSELF TO SUPPORT YOUR CHILD FOR A CHANGING BODY

As your child's body readies itself for physical maturity, they eat more. Their body requires a consistent positive energy balance to allow for healthy development. Positive energy balance means they are eating more calories than they are expending (burning) each day. Studies show that in puberty, metabolic rate increases by nearly 18 percent on average—they are using almost 20 percent more calories daily than they were pre-puberty,[10] and their appetite will reflect it. You can start by preparing yourself mentally to support your child by anticipating that they will gain weight as part of pre-puberty starting at around eight or nine years old (for some not until a few years later). The onset of puberty is largely driven by genetics. Perhaps one of your children will enter puberty slim and tall, and another will be shorter and fatter—there is no better body. Each of these children will still experience an increased need for food for development and continued growth, and each of them will have a different increase in weight and height throughout puberty. As indicated by the AAP suggestions for families, the suggestion that a growing child needs to lose weight is harmful and you don't need to accept it. If there is a nutritional concern, inadequate nutrient intake, medical diagnosis, or disordered eating, those can all be addressed from a weight-neutral approach. This means we don't ignore health and medical concerns simply because weight loss isn't the answer; *we find the ways of actually addressing the health concern*, separate from assuming weight loss is the best thing, because we know that intentionally pursuing weight loss is harmful for children of all ages. It poses a risk in and of itself for worse health outcomes down the line.

Preparing yourself as a caregiver in this stage may include reading about size diversity among kids, informing yourself about body image and adolescence, Health at Every Size, and mental health so that you feel confident rather than insecure about what is normal or what is healthy for kids.

The 3 Keys can help your family with food even now. Make sure your child, who may be experiencing insecurity related to their changing body, knows you want to help them be well fed, and that deprivation is never helpful. Your choices related to dieting, weight management, self-talk, and judging of bodies tells them all they need to know about whether their weight is acceptable to you or not. Speak with care and intention. Tune in to them emotionally when they are upset about a comment made to them about their body or an experience of rejection or judgment. *Know that they are upset because they want to be accepted.* They aren't wrong for having those needs; we all have them. So rather than saying, *You don't need to worry about what other people think of you. Don't let those comments bring you down,* try, *I am here for you every second. I know it hurts when we feel rejected or not good enough. Know that you're always good enough, no matter what you do, or how your body looks. You're good enough because you're you.*

We know it probably doesn't need to be said at this point, but we'll say it anyway to be clear: **Never advocate for or support your child to diet or to lose weight.** Help them see their eating behaviors, even if they are behaviors such as eating to cope, from a different, caring perspective: *I know it feels like you need to diet to seek approval or to change your body, and I always want you to come to me with these thoughts because I understand them. But I can't support you in dieting. I can't let you try to underfeed your body, because it will likely keep leading you to feel worse, not better, and you deserve to feel better. We live in a world that sometimes wants us to feel unlovable. What do you need right now to feel comfortable in your body? What can I/we do to help you? Above everything else, I want you to know I am here for you and I love you in your body today.*

SOCIAL MEDIA

Regardless of age, race, gender, or income, across all demographics, individuals who spend significant time on social media were found to have 2.2 to 2.6 times the risk of developing an eating disorder than peers who spent less time on social media.[11] We have to talk to our kids about this. Have some boundaries around the use of their phone, if they have one. Monitor what they are viewing and who they're talking to. Just because social media platforms are normalized doesn't mean they are safe. Talk about how to remain safe and how to decipher what they are seeing. Suicide is the second leading cause of death among individuals aged ten to twenty-four.[12] There is evidence to show that daily use of social networking sites greater than two hours was associated with fivefold increased odds of suicidal ideation compared to youth who used two hours or less daily.[13] Although the research in this area is emerging and complex, it's critical to be aware of how social media and cyberbullying may be impacting your child's mental health. It's also important to realize that for some kids who may struggle to have meaningful, caring connections with peers around them, social media networking *can also play a protective role*, putting them in touch with groups and communities who they identify with more closely, despite only having a virtual connection. Meaningful connection, in various forms, is protective and supportive for their mental health, underscoring the need for us to talk to our kids, help them find connections that feel authentic and important, and also help protect them from potential harm. This is a really hard thing for parents to navigate—many of us are only the first or second generation of parents who are raising kids that have never known a world without mobile devices and social media, *the world and all its opinions, in the palm of their hand.*

TEACH KIDS ABOUT THEIR BODIES AND DON'T ASSUME THEY'RE LEARNING EVERYTHING THEY NEED TO KNOW IN SCHOOL

Your kids need to know that you, or another trusted adult, are there when they have questions about their bodies. Early puberty can be an opportunity for kids and adolescents to feel even more confident and powerful in their bodies, yet that is nearly impossible when bodies are left mysterious and taboo to talk about. Sonya Renee Taylor gifted the world with her book *Celebrate Your Body (and Its Changes, Too!): The Ultimate Puberty Book for Girls*, which describes how not knowing about our changing bodies is like a feeling of not being able to see in the dark; it causes us to be afraid of our body.[14] Kids should not be in the dark about puberty or the ways that their bodies will undergo changes. Knowledge is power! However, knowledge and health education is often overfocused on food and exercise, which can distract you and your child from other important things we need to be teaching kids on how to take care of themselves. Often, parents may be acutely focused on food but completely ignoring topics like sex, mental health, relationships, self-care, body changes, trust, self-compassion, and fostering interests and passions.

EARLY INTERVENTION ON FOOD RESTRICTION IS IMPORTANT

As your child approaches puberty and adolescence, they're entering the most common life period where eating disorders are likely to surface. Remember: although being underweight can be a scary symptom of an eating disorder, it isn't the greatest risk factor for development of an eating disorder; having higher body weight is.[15,16,17]

If you observe your child's eating changing in a way that reflects anxiety about food or fear of food, or if you have a gut instinct they may be cutting out food groups or skipping meals, not eating at school, or throwing away food and hiding the evidence, *early intervention is a must*. Help is available. Know that a doctor who isn't well versed in eating disorders and Health at Every Size may not be concerned because your child's weight may still be in the "normal" BMI category. This doesn't mean there isn't a problem. Get a second opinion. We've provided a list of resources and directories that can help you find a treatment provider to call for help.

If you aren't necessarily concerned about restriction, but are picking up on your child gaining interest in dieting, know they are trying diets, or are troubled by their body shape or size, we also point families to the *Intuitive Eating Workbook for Teens*, a wonderful self-directed resource that teens can use to help them connect back to Intuitive Eating and understand how diets negatively impact their life.

RELATIVE ENERGY DEFICIENCY IN SPORT (RED-S)

Earlier we talked about the increased calorie needs young people have entering puberty. Along with those increased needs, athletes and active kids have even greater energy needs, and kids of all genders can face severe medical and health consequences by undereating even if they aren't technically "underweight" or diagnosed with an eating disorder. Depression, decreased concentration, interrupted menstrual function, brittle bones, heart concerns, hormonal disturbances, slowed or interrupted growth, and other psychological consequences can all stem from not eating enough to match the energy demands of an athlete for an extended period of time.[18] This condition is known as RED-S and it's something parents of all active and sports-focused kids should be aware of.

One very common negative health consequence from dieting or unintentional undereating, especially among athletes who are assigned female at birth, is amenorrhea, the condition when a period is interrupted. Primary amenorrhea is when an adolescent never starts their period—it's delayed due to hormonal shifts as a result of undereating or overexercising, also known as overtraining. This is a serious and significant hormonal shift that's triggered by the brain when not enough food is consumed over a period of time when the brain recognizes there's not enough food to safely reproduce, or is experiencing an unsafe amount of stress. Hormones return to prepubertal levels as a form of protection. Secondary amenorrhea is when they have had their period, but then stop continuing to have regular cycles or any period at all. Amenorrhea can happen to someone within just a few months of not eating enough to cover their body's calorie needs or from exercising even just a little too much. Your teen also doesn't need to be "underweight" for amenorrhea to set in. Different bodies will shift into amenorrhea at different levels of restriction—it isn't the same for everyone and is mainly determined by genetics. Also, just because someone is still getting a period doesn't mean they are eating enough. Some people with very resilient genetics may continue to get a natural period well into a risky low intake level, low body weight range or low body fat range for their body. Amenorrhea is just one of the many consequences that can happen from well-intentioned dieting and exercise and is a common symptom of disordered eating among adolescents who are assigned female at birth that is often normalized. Parents need and deserve to know that a child with an eating disorder can die of cardiac arrest, at any weight. Doctors and coaches commonly boil an absent period down to "being an athlete," and doctors prescribe birth control to bring back a period, which is actually not a fix for the problem of undereating.[19] Hormonal shifts resulting from food restriction have a detrimental impact on bone formation during the critical period of adolescence through a person's late twenties.

MONITORING GROWTH WITH GROWTH CHARTS

At each visit with a pediatrician your child's weight and length (height) will most likely be measured and plotted on a growth chart. In the United States, the CDC standard recommends the use of growth charts for children and teens from birth through nineteen years.

The curved lines on a growth chart represent percentiles that indicate the rank of a child's measurement, compared to data collected from a reference population of children and teens collected between the 1970s and the 1990s. Interpreting these growth charts can be confusing for anyone who isn't familiar with them—and even for those who are. It can be empowering to have the knowledge to understand growth charts, especially if you're ever faced with a doctor who isn't well informed on Intuitive Eating, or who is fatphobic (typical medical training is weight-centered and fatphobic), and they indicate that you should "control" your child's weight because they are "overweight" or "obese."

The percentile lines you see on a growth chart are references to a sample population. They do not represent the current population measurements of kids today. If a child's measurement, let's say their height, is plotted on the 50th percentile line, it means that fifty out of one hundred children of the same age and sex in the reference population had greater height. If their measurement is plotted on the 95th percentile line, it means that five out of one hundred children of the same age and sex in the reference population had a greater height. Growth charts can plot data using weight, length/height, age, and/or BMI-for-age.

Studies indicate that although it's not commonly thought to be true, young children often *do* cross percentiles and shift up or down to a different growth curve over time—and this doesn't automatically indicate a problem. Growth curves generally can predict growth velocity, but kids are living organisms, not programmed machines. Not every child will stay on one growth curve throughout their development or follow the growth curve exactly. A 2004 study using data collected from the California Child Health and Development Study looked at more than ten thousand children up to sixty months (five years) old. The study concluded that on weight-for-height charts (how much they weigh in reference to other children the same height), "62% of children between birth and 6 months, 20% to 27% of children between 6 and 24 months, and 6% to 15% of children between 24 to 60 months of age crossed 2 major percentiles."[20] The results are significant, as it's common for parents to be counseled by doctors that their child may have a growth or weight concern prematurely, prompting parents to intervene on their child's ability to self-regulate, when in fact there is no problem. Another way weight is commonly misinterpreted as a problem is simply if a child's weight is at a high percentile to begin with. Your child isn't "overweight" if they are born on a high percentile, they are "their weight." **What happens when parents are told their child is either not growing well enough, or they are gaining too much weight?** Parents feel a need to act and control their child's eating as a way to prevent or correct growth problems. We have worked with many mothers who have been "warned" by their doctors that their toddler is too big, growing too fast, and that they recommend withholding snacks or carbohydrates. Parents become concerned about information they don't understand, and they act out of that concern, because they love their child and trust their doctor. They also feel a sense of responsibility and, with that, may feel shame. Parents, however, are often unable to correctly interpret a growth chart, and this becomes problematic by adding to their confusion and their worries. In a 2009 survey conducted with more than one thousand parents, 77 percent interpreted growth charts incorrectly, yet 64 percent thought growth charts to be an important way to identify how their child was growing.[21]

We understand that the intention of doctors to intervene when they see a crossing of percentiles is to help, but there needs to be more careful consideration that growth shifts do not always indicate a problem, and even if there is accelerated weight gain, counseling a parent to attempt weight loss for a child, slowing weight gain, and withholding food are some of the greatest predictors for the development of disordered eating and they are more likely to promote weight gain in the long term.

According to the CDC growth chart standards, a child whose weight is plotted at the 85th to 95th percentile will be labeled as "overweight," even if this is a two-year-old who has remained on or near their same growth curve since birth. *It isn't helpful for a parent to hear that their child's natural weight is diagnosed as "overweight." Over what weight? Do pediatricians help parents to interpret this information, and counsel them to maintain trust in their child's biology and Intuitive Eating abilities? Unfortunately, not always.* Parents are given this information, and feel judged, scared, anxious, and worried that they need to intervene. Think about this: parents (and other adults) have been intervening in children's eating for weight-related reasons earlier and earlier ever since the rise of the "childhood obesity epidemic." Given the data and science we have shared with you throughout this book that shows how weight-loss interventions negatively impact people for the long term, and how these interventions predict weight gain, weight cycling, and disordered eating, we can conclude that the pathologizing of a child's weight can be one of the first points on the eating disorder development trajectory. What's extraordinary about all of this is that the recommendations for weight-reduction feeding practices and withholding food for a child not only go against the American Academy of Pediatrics' recommendations for maintaining healthful weight and avoiding eating disorders, but they are much more likely to be harmful than helpful. These are practices that our children can't and don't consent to in their young age.

GROWTH CHARTS CAN BE IMPORTANT IN EATING DISORDER IDENTIFICATION AND TREATMENT

In early identification of eating disorders, growth charts can be very helpful tools to identify a drop in weight, or slowed growth. Particularly in early puberty, where growth curves predict natural gains in height and weight, a plateau of stature growth or a drop in percentile or BMI is a cause to look closely at what may be influencing the change. There could be an eating disorder or eating disorder secondary to something else. Not every child who has a dip in their growth curve has an eating disorder, but it can be a clue to investigate, and should not be quickly dismissed—no matter what weight or BMI that child is at. A child at "normal" weight, or even "overweight," can still have a life-threatening eating disorder, even if their weight doesn't drop below a "normal" BMI. Don't assume that a child who lives in a larger body is overeating or that they could not have an eating disorder and—this is crucial—*don't congratulate, reward, or commend your child for losing weight or "slimming down" if it happens.*

EARLY PUBERTY AND OTHER CONCERNS

Some kids are going to start puberty before other kids the same age. This can look like growth, hair growth, acne, or body odor. And it can seem pretty overwhelming. But the truth is, kids can start going through changes related to puberty as early as seven or eight. It isn't something that you, as a parent, caused or need to prevent. Kids are so unique and will go through changes at their own pace. (If you're concerned, you can talk to your child's pediatrician.)

SUMMARIZE AND REFLECT

- *Regardless of what age your child is now, you can start to provide them support. Based on your child's developmental stage, what are ways you're already providing responsive feeding and supporting Intuitive Eating?*

- *In what ways can you provide more support to foster Intuitive Eating? What expectations have you set for yourself regarding feeding your child? How have the beliefs that you need to be a "perfect parent" impacted your beliefs about who you actually are?*

WHAT TO DO WHEN THIS FEELS HARDER THAN YOU THOUGHT

In the beginning, as you choose to move you and your family toward a positive relationship with food and body, you might find yourself in uncharted territory. Our culture—diet culture—has not prepared you for this. An all-too-common initial thought when hearing about Intuitive Eating sounds a lot like: *If I don't have rules, how will I know what and how to eat?* Many people have forgotten how to eat without the influence of diet mentality, forgotten that it's something that they can even do. It's safe to say that many parents feel unsure of how to feed their kids or how to help their kids to eat without the influence of diet mentality.

Health doesn't have a look—you may see pictures of white, thin, affluent, cisgender people eating salads, drinking smoothies, and hiking or doing yoga, but that is a stereotype, a trope that has been in our culture for far too long. *Health isn't something you can see. We have been absolutely conditioned to think we can look at someone and, by assessing their weight and their ability, know if they are healthy or not.* You may see a thin person and think they are healthy, when in fact they may be addicted to prescription pills or alcohol, suffering from depression, or have high blood pressure or heart disease. They also could be completely well. **The point is, you cannot see health.** Doing what feels good to you, helping your kids find joy in moving their bodies, enjoying and tasting the food that they have available, and reducing self-blame, body shaming, and weight stigma are all health-promoting things we can do, despite what you eat, how much exercise you do, where you grocery shop, whether you buy organic, or anything else.

THE SPIRAL OF HEALING

Whether you feel you're personally working on your or your child's relationship with food—or both—there is a healing process. It's not as simple as just deciding that things will be different. We know you know that, although it's human to wish it were simple and quick. You may not necessarily set out on the path of Intuitive Eating with kids thinking it will be easy or effortless, yet you may still be surprised by how hard it can feel at times. **It can be helpful to anticipate that you will have tough moments or phases and accept them as normal and even as a helpful part of your process.** The Spiral of Healing[1]—developed by Elyse Resch—describes how challenging experiences aren't a failure on your part. On the contrary, they are important for the big picture of continued upward and onward momentum. The Spiral of Healing shows how when we don't abandon ourselves, we can learn and grow from what happens.

> *The momentum is always upward and onward.*
> *Loops are opportunities for healing.*
> —ELYSE RESCH

The Spiral of Healing is a visual representation of how an experience that feels particularly unpleasant or unproductive can lead to feeling like you're actually taking steps backward. This is the downward-motion feeling of being inside a loop in the Spiral of Healing. If you can allow yourself to sit with these emotions and stay aware of what is happening and how you can respond to it, it starts to feel less all-or-nothing. You might learn something from each experience and become stronger and wiser, instead of completely abandoning your process altogether. *But the key is knowing that tough times will come up,* they are part of the process, and you can troubleshoot and keep going, despite the difficulty. When it feels hard, it doesn't mean you're doing anything wrong. A simple question, *What can I learn from this?*, is often helpful.

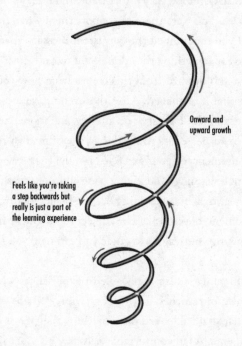

The Spiral of Healing
Originally created by Elyse Resch for The Intuitive Eating Workbook

Onward and
upward growth

Feels like you're taking
a step backwards but
really is just a part of
the learning experience

Imagine you're in front of a large group of people—your extended family, for example—and your child decides they don't want to eat most of what's been prepared for dinner, and they eat two strawberries and a dinner roll, then ask to have dessert. You hear a comment from your sister-in-law, who says to your child, *You can't have dessert, you didn't eat your dinner!* And your child looks at you for reassurance, after you've been telling them for weeks, *You don't have to eat anything you don't want to eat.* You tell them it's fine, they can go ahead and have some of the cookies from the platter. In your head you may think, *Intuitive Eating isn't working. My child won't eat the meals they're offered, and then only wants sweets. My sister-in-law is right, I should not be so lax with my kid. I don't think this is working for us.* You also feel a heavy weight of judgment and criticism from your extended family. It feels like the food police are louder than ever. You feel you have no control, like you're doing this all wrong (*remember, diet mentality gives you the illusion that you have control*). At that moment, you aren't feeling confident in the process. In that moment, your child isn't "eating well" or eating in a way in which diet culture, the food police, and others around you can see how Intuitive Eating is helping your child. You're doubting everything. You feel shame. You doubt that you can trust your child's body. You don't feel you even trust yourself. *It's where you go from here that matters, not that your child had this experience. They did nothing wrong.* In fact, they honored their hunger, didn't eat food they didn't want, and then openly asked for what they did want, cookies. You were there to support them when they looked to you for reassurance and you maintained the consistent message that they aren't pressured or expected to eat something they don't want to eat.

Moving onward and upward from this comes from how you moved through this experience, not that it happened. After this evening, *your child trusts you even more*, which will lead to more honesty, less anxiety, and more trust that their hunger and satiety will be respected by you and that, therefore, *they can respect it too.* It was also a learning moment for your extended family: they saw you in action, not applying pressure, not shaming, and giving your child permission to eat without you being outwardly critical of their eating. It's the bigger picture here that creates the value. In the moment, anything can be subject to judgment from others. Staying present and allowing your values to guide you can help you through hard moments.

The Spiral of Healing is also applicable to experiences where you may feel you've made a mistake, or returned to a past behavior. Perhaps you *did* apply pressure, or your child felt shamed by you for something they ate or you said. You can repair in those moments. As uncomfortable as it may be, you can use your words, apologize to or ask your child about how they felt, and then clarify your intention and acknowledge the impact. Tell them you're going to try to do better next time. That experience of repair will also build trust between you and your child; it will help them sense that you're committed to changing if judgment and shame have been a part of your family's food experiences.

TAKE CARE OF YOURSELF WHEN YOU FEEL OVERWHELMED BY THIS PROCESS

There are so many ways this process can feel overwhelming. It can feel frustrating, even like a personal attack, when your child won't eat food you've taken the time and energy to prepare. You can feel unaccepted when someone makes a judgmental comment about this anti–diet culture approach you're taking. Even something like not being able to find the right words to explain to another person what your values are, or why you're choosing an Intuitive Eating approach for your family, can feel really disheartening and lonely. Understand how these and other circumstances can be an event that quickly leads to your internal narrative of self-criticism, hopelessness, anxiety, and even feeling underappreciated in your role as a caregiver. Realize that in these moments, when you question your process or judge your child's eating or their body—you are vulnerable. You're likely not fully in the present (the present answers the questions: *What is happening in the here-and-now? What is underlying it?* and *Why am I so bothered?*). Instead of being in the present, you may be flashing forward to your worst fear for your kiddo, or you're flashing back to the past, to an experience you had that you want to "fix."

Notice your inner narrative: What is the story you hear? Can you notice that it's an old automatic story? What words can you choose to say to yourself that come from a place of self-compassion for the present moment experience?

Every day we have to engage with diet culture—it doesn't go away just because we've made up our minds to no longer want to be controlled by it. Your children will have to engage with it too. We (Amee and Sumner) have to face it every day, along with everyone else who has chosen to fight back against the oppression. You aren't alone, and yet it can feel very lonely when you challenge norms all around you every day.

Here are some things you can do to proactively build an inner sense of strength and confidence while working on Intuitive Eating:

Find community: Whether it's one person you trust, like a friend or therapist, or an online community where you can turn with questions and struggles, having at least one place to go where you feel you can be transparent and honest is really helpful.

Be mindful of what you take in from social media: You can't control advertisements and mass media, but you do have some ability to curate your social media feed to be a more inclusive and body-diverse source of information. Stop following diet accounts, "fit-spo," and anything that doesn't help you feel calm or connected to your truth. One of the most common things we hear that has helped people to be more accepting and respectful toward their bodies is seeking out and following more diverse bodies and accounts that celebrate diversity and size acceptance. **Regularly seeing bodies of all races, shapes, sizes, abilities, and ages can have a substantial impact on how you feel about your own body.** Over time, you can shift your inner dialogue from one of judgment and not-enoughness to one of appreciating diversity and understanding that health is truly not about weight, and that you're more than your health status and your appearance. When your attitude and views change, it will be reflected in your kids' attitudes.

Give yourself permission to speak up: When you notice a harmful or stigmatizing conversation happening around you or your kids, say what you think. You don't have to go along with harmful narratives, or oppressive stereotypes about bodies and food. You may be able to say something like: *I recently read about Intuitive Eating for kids, have you heard of it? It talks about how rules and overcontrol actually backfires. I'm working on helping my kids to be at peace with food and their body for the long term. Their emotional and mental health can really be impacted by diet mentality.* These conversations are everywhere, so take care of your energy, think about what you feel most called to do or say, and move one step at a time. If someone appears not open to hearing you, you may just decide they're not open and you can't control what other people think. It's okay to reserve your energy and not feel like you're obligated to change anyone's mind.

Give yourself permission to walk away: It won't always feel safe or effective for you to speak up. Trust yourself. Think about what is ultimately best for you and your kids. Sometimes just not saying anything, or walking away, is the best choice.

Read and learn and continue to understand a weight-inclusive approach to health and unlearn diet culture: *See the resources listed at the back of this book.* The more you understand the facts, the more resilient you'll become to diet culture.

Find meaning every day in the things that matter to you that have nothing to do with food and body: This is especially important for parents who may have some history of disordered eating or chronic dieting, and need to really work and fill up your life with things other than a focus on food and body.

If (or when) your child gains weight, it isn't a sign of failure—and the same goes for you. It doesn't mean that allowing them to build trust with their body and stopping controlling their eating was the wrong choice. **We need to normalize changing bodies, fatter bodies.** Body fat is supposed to increase in puberty, and especially for girls and individuals assigned female at birth. We need to get out of our mind, which has been hijacked by diet culture, and have empathy and understanding for our kids. Not only are they not able to control their body or their weight, they should not be expected to. Stay true to your values. Appreciate that their health, their happiness, and their future isn't dependent on the size of their body. They will have the greatest chance at having a healthy relationship with their body and food when you stand up to diet culture, and this goes on to positively impact their physical, psychological, and emotional health.

Come up with a slogan, affirmation, or acronym—something that helps ground you in your beliefs and values about what you want for your children in moments that feel difficult. Take a minute and write out one sentence that feels true to you, in your core, that you can say to yourself when you're feeling the urge to control your child's eating, make a comment about their body, or pressure them to eat. Let this statement guide you and be a truth you can tell yourself when a tough moment arises.

Here are some examples:

I can trust in my child's process.

I am curious about what's happening for them right now.

I trust myself to know what the next best thing is.

When I feel the urge to negatively comment on my child's body or eating, I will resist and instead _____.

I am open to observing how this unfolds if I don't intervene.

I can enjoy and be present with my child, food, and our bodies.

There is little room for their life purpose in the midst of diet culture.

When I overthink their eating, they'll overthink their eating.

WHEN YOU'RE AROUND OTHER PARENTS

Tracy had been working individually with an Intuitive Eating–trained dietitian for a few months and was ready to try a new approach with her seven-year-old son. As she helped him get ready for his friend's birthday party, she was reflecting on an experience they had had last year at the same friend's birthday. The party had been at lunchtime, and when they arrived, there was a buffet of lunch items spread out and parents were making plates for the kids. As someone in a larger body, Tracy often became self-conscious about other parents' judgments of what her son ate, because a part of her told a story that said that how he ate reflected her parenting, how good a mother she was, whether or not she was prioritizing his health, and whether or not she was going to allow him to grow up *to be like her*. Tracy had really been working on that story in her individual work with her dietitian. They had been discussing how Tracy's body isn't a reflection of mistakes, and that her body isn't a problem.

Her body is her body—and she values it. They have been through a lot together. Tracy spent years—most of her life, really—hating her body, hiding her body, and avoiding living her life. Tracy also learned that the more she tried to diet and exercise her way to a smaller body, the worse her relationship with food and movement became. She knows she gained weight over the years, more after each dieting attempt. This had become so confusing to her: How was it that everyone around her was always dieting, and everything she read claimed that if she just followed the diet rules, she would lose weight? Well, what Tracy had finally discovered in her nutrition therapy work was that feeding her body and making peace with food was what was allowing her to feel the best, most settled, and most comfortable in her body she could ever remember feeling. She still noticed when she was being judged, and noticed old thoughts and beliefs popping up—especially in certain circumstances, like at parties—but overall, she had learned the power of an intuitive relationship with food and body. She had never been more at peace with eating. She was ready to begin changing the ways she was parenting her son around food, in order to give him the same gift. The birthday party presented an opportunity to try something different.

Back at the buffet, she recalled how last year, she had said repeatedly that he could only have one piece of pizza, and needed to eat all the vegetables (dry, no dip) and fruit she put on his plate before he could have cake. She remembers he was hungry, it was later than usual for lunch, and he hadn't eaten since breakfast. She can see how limiting his pizza, and forcing him to eat something that didn't taste good to him, was restrictive and controlling. He was hungry for more, and he wanted the satisfying pizza, not the dried-out vegetables. Yet she thought she was doing the *right thing*. She believed she was showing proof, to all the other parents, that she wasn't feeding her child "the wrong way," that she was dedicated to keeping him healthy, preventing him from having *her* body. That she was *in control*. But now, after making sense of her own dieting past, she could see how what she was doing was playing out *what diet culture wanted her to do*. She was not making any space for him to direct his own eating based on his hunger. She was restricting him, and creating a very charged food experience that would stick with him—that would likely create an urge to get as much pizza as he could when she wasn't around. The party this year would be different. Tracy was excited to give her Intuitive Eating skills and perspective a try. She also knew it wouldn't be easy. When they arrived, Tracy felt the old familiar rush of body judgment and looks from other parents. Instead of believing the lies her defensive, diet mind was telling her—that there was something wrong with her appearance—she chose another way of self-talk: *I respect myself, and I'm going to show my son his mom respects herself. I will show up here today and not make this about food.* These thoughts gave Tracy a lot of mental power. She still felt a level of nervousness, a level of discomfort, but she also felt a new strength she didn't usually have in situations like this. As soon as she heard these new thoughts, she was able to relax and remind herself to let her son eat what he needed and wanted, and let him have a good time without adding extra stress or emphasis on his eating. She released the need to "prove" anything to any of the parents. The priority was on her son having a good time, not on what he was eating.

As it came time to eat, small shifts made a big difference. Instead of putting a limit on how many pieces he could have, she asked, *Would you like one or two?* She put some of everything on his plate: two pieces of pizza, some pretzels, fruit, and carrots, and then let him take it from there. She watched him eat two pieces of pizza and a juice box, and none of the other food. He asked for a third piece, she gave it to him, and he ate most of it, before losing interest and running off to join his friends. Her fear that he would never stop if she let him eat as much as he wanted didn't come true. He did stop. He was satisfied. It was no big deal. All the pressure, rules, and limits she had placed on him in situations like this weren't needed. She started to see that deciding what and how much was not her job at all—it was his. His body had all the wisdom to help direct him. If he didn't eat the fruit on his plate, it didn't mean he would never eat fruit again; it just meant that in that moment, he didn't want it. That's all. The most meaningful difference this year was that Eli had a better experience at the party—a memory not overtaken by shame around food. Tracy left the birthday party feeling confident she could make more changes over time. She felt a deep sense of hope and strength that although it's hard, she could let go of old diet thinking, and that this would make a positive difference in her son's life and his confidence around food as he matures.

FACING BARRIERS TO INTUITIVE EATING FOR YOUR FAMILY

Stress comes from many sources and in varying intensities. Divorce, job stress, health concerns, addiction struggles, and grief are all examples of some of the very real-life experiences we know parents and families are living with. Some of these issues may take up so much time that feeding and focusing on your child's relationship with food will not feel like a priority. That doesn't mean that colluding with diet culture, or weight shaming, need to be accepted. The reality often is, this process will look like one or two changes at a time, not a huge overhaul of everything we've talked about. Giving yourself grace, knowing and admitting when something is too much to take on, are important.

WHEN YOUR STRESS IS BUILDING

Stress can be chronic and constant, or it can be moment-to-moment. We all experience tough days, upsetting moments, and depressing, unexpected events. Today, parents are under extreme pressure that is twofold: real and intense pressure from the reality of life, relying on a paycheck, worrying about your child's safety, and having the responsibilities of raising a human, as well as the pressure that is harder to name—the pressure that comes from social media, from perfectionism, from peers, and from the illusion that we can do it all—take care of ourselves, eat right, exercise, go to therapy, and so on—*and get praised for it.* If we perform well enough we might even get enough likes from people we've never met on Instagram. To say the least, there is a lot of real and assumed pressure. This takes away from our ability to attend to our kids and foster that positive feeding relationship. In these scenarios, we are more likely to act on default "autopilot"—and these are likely the behaviors that we experienced growing up, modeled to us by our parents. It often surprises parents how often they say things that they don't actually mean, but that felt like the most natural thing to say: *You can't have your ice cream until you clean your room* (rewarding with food), or *You've had enough, put that away* (controlling and shaming), or *I don't want to hear one more complaint about what's on your plate—eat it or you won't get to go to the sleepover tonight* (punishing with food). We don't think stress and parenting can be separated—they are related. It takes work to notice how you respond to stress, and to identify if there's anything you could be doing differently that could help your kids *and help your relationship with your kids.*

Try to be aware of when your stress is rising or already elevated and then have compassion for yourself, understanding that things will feel harder when you're stressed than they would otherwise—particularly things that involve small people who push back, who are testing the boundaries, or who are at times eating their Choco Chimps at a snail's pace when you need them to hurry up so you can get out the door on time! This isn't easy, folks.

This seems like an important moment to remind every single person here: you're human. You're allowed to be upset. To be mad, sad, angry, frustrated, stressed, or any other emotion that exists. Because you're human. The lie of perfectionism has us believing that if we do "everything right," we will never be upset. We are also conditioned by our culture to only want to experience the "good" emotions. But we feel them all—because we are all human. And that's okay.

Interestingly, stressful experiences are also vulnerable times for anyone who has a history of beating themselves up, talking negatively, or suffering from negative body image for disordered eating behaviors like restriction or binge eating to pop up as coping mechanisms. *When stressed or anxious, you may notice yourself becoming more critical of your child's eating, uncomfortable with their body, or hesitant to give them permission to eat. This is the same way you might automatically respond to yourself when you're under stress.* It's easy to project your inner automatic process onto them.

Here are some suggestions for what to do when your stress is building and you don't want to "undo" all the progress you're making with Intuitive Eating:

1. **Breathe deeply** and tune in to the present moment. Does the story you're hearing in your mind reflect the reality of the present moment, or are you attaching to an old script?
2. **What are you feeling? Name it.** (*I'm feeling really worried I'll be late, and I'm worried that my lack of pressure on or control of my child's eating isn't working.*)
3. **What do you need right now?** What would feel helpful right now? Even if you can't give it to yourself. (*I need my child to stop throwing a fit about breakfast.*)
4. **Remind yourself there is no "perfect"** in this moment—what is the priority? (*The priority is that we try to leave on time, we arrive safely to our destination, and that I don't say or do things I don't mean.*)
5. **Tune in to your kid's needs.** If you're stressed because your kid is stressed, can you focus on supporting them, knowing you can take

care of you ASAP? (*If I slow down, I can help my child not spiral into a meltdown that will mean it takes us longer to get going.*)

6. **Do what you can** and don't overthink the meal or snack. Know that no one meal, or even one week of eating, will impact your child's health (*unless we're talking about a food allergy*). Accept that if they don't finish their breakfast they will be okay. Stop fighting with them about the food.

7. **Relax.** This is a process, not a destination. How can you remind yourself of that? (*Whatever happens right now is just about right now, it's not indicative of their entire future. I am not a bad parent. My child is exhibiting normal behavior and is likely responding to my stress.*)

8. **Reflect** after your stress has deescalated. What was it that was really bothering you? Was your child eating a lot of candy, triggering you to have diet thoughts, and you were believing that your child's eating reflects your value as a parent?

FOOD INSECURITY OR FINANCIAL STRAIN

In many homes, there isn't always enough food to go around or enough room in the budget to have a lot of variety. Food insecurity and hunger interrupt Intuitive Eating just as much as dieting does. The three biggest barriers to food security are income, proximity to a store with fresh food, and having a vehicle. Other major barriers include age, physical disabilities, and cost of living. **If we're working this hard to dismantle diet culture—to help people thrive—we need to be working equally hard to improve food access and fight hunger.**

If your family faces food insecurity, consider some or all of the following reminders and suggestions:

- It's not only okay to eat fast food, it can be important if it helps you or your child get enough to eat. Enough food is the first goal, before "healthy food."
- If you can, incorporate foods that are lower in cost and higher in nutrition, such as eggs, peas, beans, lentils, oats, and cereals.
- Eggs are relatively less expensive compared to meat and fish and provide protein, fat, and vitamins and minerals.

- Opt for frozen or canned fruits and vegetables instead of fresh produce that can go bad quickly.
- If you're consistently seeing that your child doesn't finish their food, try serving food family style instead of serving portions for them and be sure to let them know they can have more if they want it, rather than plating food that will get thrown away.
- If you experience pressure or guilt about the quality of food you're providing—such as being told you should only buy organic milk that costs three times as much as the non-organic brand, give yourself permission to save the money. More money in the food budget to get enough food is more important than buying organic food.

Note on organic: The decision to buy organic food is a personal one, but it's important to know that it's a myth that organic food is more nutritious than conventionally grown food, even though organic foods can be significantly more expensive. Organic food does have about 30 to 50 percent lower pesticide residue than conventional foods, but in general, both organic and conventional are reported to have pesticide levels that are within allowable safety limits. If you cannot afford organic it's far better to consume conventionally grown fruits and vegetables for the nutritional benefit than to avoid them.

These aren't simple solutions, but there are some services that may be able to create a slight ease in your financial burden, if they are available to you and if you feel comfortable accessing them:

- See if you're eligible for SNAP and WIC benefits.
- Consider utilizing a local food bank (many don't have income requirements).
- If you have any area farmers' markets, contact them to see if they donate unsold food.
- Is there a summer feeding program through the public-school system in your area? Many children rely on free school breakfast and lunches.
- Are there any Mobile Market routes in your area?

YOU'RE NOT READY TO STOP DIETING

If you notice you don't want to, don't feel capable of, or have personal reasons why you want to continue to diet or try to lose weight, we see you. You may feel that you accept and want to do everything you possibly can to help your child be an Intuitive Eater and have a positive, embodied experience; believing that the same is right or even possible for you, however, may not be so easy. *We suggest you start by not blaming yourself. You aren't the problem, and you never have been the problem. We are all existing inside bigger systems that influence us and our environment.* All of your struggles and your limits are being reinforced by systems of oppression that operate to keep you feeling powerless or unworthy. You do not bear the weight of the responsibility to make this world safe for your child; that is a collective responsibility.

No one gets to tell you how you should feel in or about your body, period.

The thing about this process is that it's not all-or-nothing. That even if today you don't feel like you're ready to walk away from dieting, we encourage you to be open to the possibility that one day you may feel ready. Empower yourself, seek supportive relationships, make peace with your past, explore different ways of taking care of your body and soul, ask for help if you can. Body image distress and disordered eating are extremely complicated patterns. Give yourself the space and time you need to decide what your next step will be.

WHEN YOU WANT TO EMBRACE AN INTUITIVE EATING APPROACH, BUT EVERY HEALTHCARE PROVIDER AND DOCTOR YOU SEE ALWAYS BRINGS UP WEIGHT LOSS

Many doctors and providers aren't well versed in the literature and science of dieting and weight control, for two reasons: (1) they are educated within a weight-centric medical model, meaning they are taught from an evidence base that is biased against higher-weight bodies and is inherently racist, and (2) they are humans who also live inside diet culture and many have been exposed to it since they were born. They can't see what they don't know.

Medical research fails higher-weight people and people of color, among other marginalized groups, again and again. It's systematically discriminatory[2] in terms of what topics receive funding for health research. Obesity research receives a hugely disproportionate amount of research dollars, making it exceedingly difficult to publish studies that look at less popular paradigms, such as Health at Every

Size and issues surrounding nutrition-related conditions and the social determinants of health.

When this is your experience, we want you to consider some options for how to move forward.

1. You may be direct and clear with your doctor: tell them what your experience with dieting and focusing on weight has been like for you and then ask for what you want:

   I hear you're concerned about my weight. Concern for my weight has never helped me—in fact, it's made things worse. One of the ways I am taking care of myself now is to eat, move, and take care of my body by doing what feels best, and feels energizing. Please stop recommending weight loss, since the statistical chances of me being able to lose weight and keep it off are close to zero. I am not willing to engage in disordered eating in order to lose weight, which isn't even guaranteed to improve my health. I'm open to hearing your thoughts and suggestions for how to take care of my body in ways other than the pursuit of weight loss.

2. You might not feel capable of being that direct—and that is okay. We encourage you to be yourself. Spend a little time prior to the appointment thinking of what would be most helpful and would come from a place of self-care when you are face-to-face with a provider. Consider something like:

   I've realized that trying to lose weight is really backfiring, and has been harmful for me. I've decided to focus on behaviors that I feel are helpful for my health and self-care, without a focus on weight loss. I hope that you can work with me around this goal.

We recognize that when you as a parent are feeling pressured to diet or lose weight, it can make for an extremely difficult state of mind to completely embrace Intuitive Eating for your child. Be gentle with yourself.

WHEN ANOTHER PERSON IS NEGATIVELY INFLUENCING YOUR CHILD

The impact other adults have on our kids can't be ignored, and it also can't be completely prevented. There likely are some adults whose actions *do* influence what your child thinks about food and body. When you're aware something is being done or said that you feel is problematic, first take a breath and know that you will never be able to control everything that is done around your child. Next, realize that every bit you do and have done to help them have resilience is valuable. Then determine what you want to do about it. Is this a situation where you can prevent further harm from being done by talking to this person? Are they reachable? If yes, then it's probably worth the effort to begin opening a dialogue with them about your specific concerns, and suggestions for what would be a better alternative. Many people are very defensive about their nutrition and food beliefs, so we encourage you to come to these conversations prepared to not take their response personally, and to know that it can often take multiple attempts for them to really hear you. Intuitive Eating is so counter to the prevailing culture that we need to step into conversations with people fully understanding they may not "get" the harm right away.

You may think "It's just one comment"—and that one comment from one person isn't enough to be concerned about. People who are around your child regularly are going to have more of an influence and impact than a total stranger—and you won't ever be able to completely save your child from hearing something that may hurt them or confuse them or make them fear their body or eating. These people may make comments about weight, calories, or fat that they think are harmless—but trust us, we've worked with enough young people to have heard countless stories about how there was one defining moment, when a friend or relative warned them about gaining "too much weight," or teased them for noticeable weight gain or body changes around early puberty, for example. This can be enough to alter a person's relationship with their body and food for life.

We know from our work with parents, and from having school-aged kids ourselves, that food policing at school, during lunch or after-school care, as well as in health curriculums, happens. In the eating disorder treatment field, stories about the negative effects of food policing and fearmongering in health class are a daily occurrence. We don't believe food policing of lunch boxes, or of any food, is safe, helpful, or acceptable in a school setting. If you agree, you can be proactive and talk to your child's teacher, or their school principal or counselor, about your concerns. We've included a lunch box card template created by Katja Rowell on page 330 as a way for you to communicate clearly with your child's teacher around your wishes for them to not food police your child.

Be proactive and talk to people before problems come up, including doctors, co-parents, other caregivers, teachers, coaches, and babysitters. Talking to teachers or other caregivers *before* something comes up, although it does take some time and energy, gives you two big benefits: (1) It establishes a good rapport with the person with whom your child spends time with. This creates a sense for your child that you're involved and invested in what is going on in their life. (2) It will make it easier for you to reach them for a follow-up to talk about anything concerning or curious as it comes up over time. With teachers, principals, or other school contacts, it's great to have a relationship with them so that you can be a resource to them, and help them learn what they may not know, but perhaps are actually really open to. At parent–teacher conferences, ask how nutrition lessons are taught. Ask for the curriculum. Introduce yourself to the wellness or PE teachers and school counselor. As parents and caregivers, the "work in the trenches" to break down diet culture happens inside our communities, in real life. This is how we can make a direct positive difference in our children's environment, and although we can't fix everything, or change everyone's minds, we can chip away at the cultural bias and problematic norms. Along the way, you're bound to encounter others with shared views, also building a supportive community or circle of people, so that you don't have to feel alone in your efforts. We are often surprised by how many people are receptive to learning about weight stigma and eating disorder awareness, which reflects just how many people have been impacted over the course of their lives and now want to help address the issues for future generations.

> Lunch Box Card: from *Love Me, Feed Me: The Adoptive Parent's Guide to Ending the Worry About Weight, Picky Eating, Power Struggles, and More*, by Katja Rowell, M.D.
>
> Copy, fill in, and laminate the lunch box card on page 330 . Place it in your child's lunch box and tell them that if an adult asks them to eat certain foods, they should hand over the card. This is hard to ask a child to do, but it may work for some.

FEAR OF BRINGING FOODS INTO THE HOUSE

If you notice you have a literal fear of bringing certain foods into your house, we want to encourage you to pause here and really notice that. If you feel strongly about the power of those foods, or have an intense fear of you or your child eating those foods, you may need some individual support with an Intuitive Eating counselor

Dear Friend of _____,
Please allow _____ to decide how
much to eat, and in what order, from what
I have packed. Even if that means all
_____ eats for lunch is "dessert," or if
_____ starts with dessert. I trust that
_____can rely on hunger and
fullness signals to know how much to eat.
Please call my cell _____ if you
have any questions. The nice thing is,
this should be less work for you. If _____
needs help opening containers, I thank
you for that help, otherwise,
_____ should be good to go.
Thank you for all you do for our children.

or dietitian. We won't tell you what you need to do, but we do feel there's a lot of value in you looking at that fear, and unpacking it. Consider breaking this down into more digestible steps. Can you begin to take your child out for a meal or snack of their choice outside the house, as a way to explore permission to eat? Let them choose what they want, and eat how they want, without you intervening. Focus on enjoying the experience with them. It will be very noticeable and very different for them initially if you begin to bring more foods into the house than you previously allowed. Expect your child to have a reaction, and expect that they may be very drawn to those foods. If you're having your own parallel process of making peace with food, you may want to use the *Intuitive Eating Workbook* (there is a version for teens and a version for adults, but the teen version works for adults too—we all have our inner child!) to help you feel some needed support as you and your family adjust. We want you to know that not everyone reacts the same to having more permission and freedom. Feelings we address with our clients range from experiencing thrills to excitement and surprise that their kids didn't think it was a big deal, to feeling anxious, nervous, or binge eating.

THIS TAKES TIME: GIVE SPACE FOR CHANGE TO EMERGE, AND BE PATIENT

What you're setting out to do, to divest from diet culture, to lay brick after brick down for your child for a safer, better path into their future, is hard work. Many of you reading this will be in the midst of realizing that your child's inner Intuitive Eater has been covered up by a way of eating and relating to bodies that is steeped in judgment, emotional avoidance, perfectionism, control, rigidity, or pressure. **You aren't alone.** If you can see that your child's relationship with food and body is off course, one of the greatest gifts you can give them is to help them find their way back. This takes time. Inside that gradual shift are messy moments. You may have conflicting thoughts: *I want to give my child permission to eat, and it feels really hard to do so. I want to stop weighing myself, but I feel scared about not relying on the scale.*

Allow yourself to release the rigidity a little bit at a time, to find more comfort in flexibility. Feel the discomfort of the process. There is no end to relating to food and body; it's an ongoing, lifelong process. Take it one day at a time.

ACTING USING THE INTUITIVE FOOD AND BODY RELATIONSHIP MODEL

Bringing this back to the Intuitive Food and Body Relationship Model from chapter 3, recall how necessary it is to know that our relationship with food and body isn't all-or-nothing. It's very fluid, changing day to day, based on our environment and our experiences. You may find yourself getting stuck in thoughts like *I'll never have a good relationship with food* or *This is impossible, I hate my body* on a day when you're feeling more of the negative elements. Notice how those thoughts alone keep you moving down a certain path, believing a certain story. Or with respect to your child, perhaps you hear a thought like *I can't handle the fear and anxiety of allowing them to eat intuitively.* These thoughts help you tap into what your suffering is, what you need.

Once you notice the thoughts, remember that it's how you respond to those thoughts that can be so important for what happens next. When you hear a thought like *I hate my body,* explore what it feels like to respond with *I notice the thought I'm having—that I hate my body. I wonder what is happening right now that led to that thought. What is it that I really mean when I say I hate my body? Is that fully true? How is it helpful for me to believe that? What do I ap-*

preciate about my body, to help me realize I don't actually hate it, but that I am suffering right now?

Using the Intuitive Food and Body Relationship Model, consider how if you're feeling a lot of one negative element, such as mistrust (you feel like you can't trust your body), you might be able to lean in to the positive action of a different element, such as comfort. That might sound and look like this: *What can I do to seek comfort in my body, given that I feel like I can't trust it? How can I take care of myself right now?* This can be helpful, because when we can start to experience any more of even one positive element of the model, the negative experience we're having gradually (or suddenly) begins to lessen.

WHY KIDS NEED RESILIENCE

Building resilience involves knowing that there will be strong diet mentality influencers encountered in life—it could be their best friends' parents, a babysitter, social media, a teacher, or a peer. What you say and do at home will be challenged by what your child's friends' parents say and do, or what their teacher or coach says and does. This is reality.

Broadly speaking, independence, or a version of independence, is what most kids, and most parents, are striving for as kids age. At some point, they'll need to have trust in themselves. Within what may feel like the blink of an eye your child will be eating away from you 90 percent of the time. You won't be there to direct choices, to make comments, or to influence how, what, when, how much, or why they eat. This is why we equip them to have practiced listening to their bodies and respecting their bodies: *because it's the most protective thing we can do.*

ANTICIPATING COLLEGE

College is a big life transition and is known to be one of the most vulnerable life phases for the development of disordered eating simply because it's a scary time, full of uncertainty, and likely unfamiliar territory. It's a phase in life when bodies are scrutinized and pressure in terms of academics and achievement reaches an all-time high.

The highest prevalence rates of dieting and disordered eating behaviors of any population are among college students. In particular, there are real reasons to be concerned about the combination of dieting behaviors and alcohol use.

A 2020 study examined alcohol-related disordered eating among nearly five hundred undergraduate students. It's well known that for many, arriving at college is synonymous with arriving to a new level of independence and freedom—for those who diet already, it can push dieting behaviors to the extreme at the same time binge drinking is introduced. Research tells us that nearly 30 to 40 percent of college students binge drink—consume five or more alcoholic drinks at one time—and separately we know that at least one-third are using unhealthy weight-control behaviors. College is a time when these two risky behaviors collide, often causing young adults to become more concerned about weight due to increased calorie intake from alcohol. The more alcohol they plan to drink, the less they plan to eat. Along with the risks of this combination of behaviors, known as food and alcohol disturbance (FAD), comes increased risks for other negative alcohol-related consequences, such as physical injury to self, doing something they regret, and having forced sexual intercourse.[3]

HAVE A STRENGTHS-BASED LENS

Sometimes, behaviors we see in our kids are framed as "negative" or harmful, yet they can be behaviors that are adopted out of strength and resilience. In truth, these behaviors have been lifesaving, particularly for anyone who may have developed them as coping responses from trauma—both single-event trauma, as well as more chronic trauma experiences such as having a body that is oppressed and stigmatized by society, living with a parent struggling with addiction, or experiencing emotional neglect at a young age. Eating disorder behaviors are often much more about trauma than they are about food. Remember that both adaptive eating behaviors and maladaptive eating behaviors can be strengths-based. People do things to protect themselves, avoid emotional or physical pain, or to soothe and escape what feels intolerable. Additionally, eating more after any period of deprivation or restriction is a *predictable eating response*. It's our body's natural defense against the perceived or real threat of not getting enough food. You may see an older child who is shaming or blaming themselves about how they eat or look, and you may be able to draw from a strengths-based perspective to help them see the humanity of what they're doing—that of course they long to be accepted and belong. We all do. **But you still don't need to collude with their diet mentality.** This can help to begin to break down the shame and help them see what is happening through a different lens. If you have a hard time allowing your child to do something, such as eating in a way you're uncomfortable with, without trying to intervene, it can help to think, *How has this* served them? Is it reasonable or fair to expect them not to do this, given their past experiences? What can I do to help my child feel they can get their needs met without having to turn to food in a way that makes them feel unwell or restrict their eating, to avoid what they're feeling?

TALK DIRECTLY AND CLEARLY TO YOUR CHILD AND LET THEM KNOW YOU ACCEPT, APPRECIATE, AND LOVE THEIR BODY

Don't assume they feel this from you—*tell it to them directly and often*. What we have learned from hearing about the experiences of so many people is that if a young person is lucky enough to be deeply validated and seen for who they are as a whole person, early in life, it matters a lot. If we have even just one caring adult who helps us to see that we are important, good enough, and beautiful in our body because of who we are, not according to society's standards. If we feel capable, and loved by someone who doesn't impose the harsh body judgment that the culture around us does, we have more of an opportunity to stay on our own team. We may not turn on ourselves as early or as harshly, mind against body. We need guidance and care from someone to help us learn how to question when we are sold the lies and fantasies of diet culture.

Help your child know they are valuable, special, and worthy no matter what, and when they encounter someone who says otherwise they will see it as a conflicting message rather than reinforcing what they may have already been told.

Talk to them about how bodies are presented in the media, and how rarely we see the real diversity of bodies. Talk about how you love people for who they are, not how they look. One of the best ways you can help your child know that people aren't better or worse humans based on their appearance is by letting them observe your relationships with other people who have diversity in appearance.

SUMMARIZE AND REFLECT

- *What are your opportunities to be more direct in letting your child know you accept, appreciate, and love their body?*
- *How are you feeling about bringing "off-limits" foods back into your house? What first steps do you want to take toward allowing more foods into your family's routine?*

- *Who are other adults or influencers in your child's life that are important to talk to about Intuitive Eating, or your general requests about how they talk about food and body?*
- *Is there anyone at your child's school who might be a good ally?*
- *If you know that your child is experiencing disordered eating, what do you believe this behavior could be about? How does it help them?*

CONCLUSION

You're allowed to decide how and what to feed your child in any way you want—but ultimately, if your child doesn't feel that you *love them, respect them, and unconditionally support them in their here-and-now body*, and as their body changes, they may not learn to provide their own self with the same love, respect, and unconditional support. You have the ability to set your child on a course toward positive embodiment.

All children deserve to live knowing they are worthy, lovable, and capable of living a full, meaningful, and enjoyable life no matter what, especially with any body size or health status among other identities they may hold. Parents deserve to know they can support this for their child without question.

When you start to see what is going on in our culture, you will get angry. You will want to defend everyone, most of all your children, from diet culture. The good in our world gets blocked out too early in our lives, when a young person loses sight of their worth. That's a costly price to pay for the promises we are sold every day by diet culture.

It's not our place to tell you who to be angry at—but we understand this emotional response. Parents can't dictate what their child's experience will be in their body, just as they can't control the size, shape, health, or ability of their child's body. **The belief that we do have that level of control, and that we can assert control over or "manage" our kids' bodies without doing harm, is an illusion.**

Oppression hangs out and thrives inside illusions, systems that keep you from accurately perceiving reality. Diet culture is one of those oppressive systems: it has created a massive illusion with healthism as its greatest tool. Diet culture doesn't exist without its centuries of white supremacist roots and its goal of silencing, shrinking, and withholding power. The illusion is that we are broken, need constant improvement, and that our body needs to be fixed. This illusion erases our true needs of healing from trauma, feeling grief, or receiving the help for our suffering that we inherently deserve. No, we often don't get to the deep interconnectedness, healing, or progress that we really want to be living for, because it's so hard to hear those needs inside the noise of misogyny, trolling, and the medicalization of body size. The illusion keeps us from perceiving the things we actually need and deserve to make this life matter to us. We can learn a lot from the clarity that children enter the world with before they learn to judge themselves and others.

Even though our society is consumed with diet culture, inside all of us is something more soulful, more powerful, more true: our real self. Let's help our kids run confidently and bravely forward; the future relies on them.

Here's the thing we want to leave you with: **You are—and always will be—the decision maker of what foods and what values you want to bring into your home.** No one can take that away from you. It's your responsibility to raise your kids the way you believe is best for them. We want you to be able to do that, to make informed decisions about the feeding relationship between you and your child—the language you use, the food you serve, and the choices you encourage and model. We want you to be able to make whatever decisions feel right and true for you, in the context of having information about what can help and what may harm.

Parenting is never easy. We hope that by understanding some of the long-term potential consequences of deprivation, overcontrol, and diet mentality you can feel confident and empowered to help your child grow into themselves in a way that fosters body respect, autonomy, choice, confidence, and self-compassion. We hope you now can include all the information about how to approach feeding and bodies as you come to your own conclusions and values that will be what your child takes with them when they're no longer under your wing. When you look back on these years of having some say and some influence over how they view and relate to their one precious body, you will know that you valued their whole self, their natural body, and that you didn't let diet culture come between you and your beloved baby.

We've been told the years go quickly. We hope you will allow joy, love, and respect to sit as the centerpiece of your family table. You have one incredible and special opportunity to support your child and shape some of the experiences that ultimately become how they will see themselves—or how they may return to seeing themselves—in a world that will call into question their worth time and time again. Your child looks to you, they seek the wisdom you have, and they seek your unconditional love and support.

We can do this.

ACKNOWLEDGMENTS

We want to say thank you to all of the people who contributed to this knowledge before us. To Elyse Resch, for assisting us over many hours and reviewing concepts of this model from day one, and for your steady love and support as we wrote the book. Also thank you to Evelyn Tribole, who with Elyse paved the way for this work and has had such a remarkable influence on the world of nutrition and dietetics. To Katja Rowell and Jo Cormack, who generously offered expertise and input, enhancing our knowledge of responsive feeding, for your support of this book to become another tool to add to the toolbox. To the EDRD Pro and Body Trust Communities, Tracy Tylka, Ellyn Satter, Lindo Bacon, Christy Harrison, Naureen Hunani, Sonya Renee Taylor, Ragen Chastain, and so many others, including all of our incredible colleagues fighting diet culture. None of our words are unique. So many people are out there already doing this work and fighting to make this world a safer place for our children and their bodies. We are just continuing the fight. Special thanks to Anna and Gina for your wholehearted contributions. Thank you also to our editor Sallie Lotz for supporting us, brilliantly editing, and keeping this whole project moving in the right direction. We are so grateful for your talent and contributions.

I also want to thank my family for putting up with my long sleepless nights of writing mid-pandemic. My friends, who encouraged me and read my notes and sent me encouraging texts and messages along the way, Bailey, Shira, Jack, and many others. My therapist, for listening to my stress and anxiety about this project. And my dad, Paul, and brother, Nik, for encouraging me and even contributing some anecdotes. My mom, Jeannie, for being the kind soul that she was—and setting me down the path to this. My daughter, Kahlan, who taught me all the patience I have now, all the love I needed, and for being the coolest and most confident kid I've ever met. Her compassion surpasses her years. And my partner, my husband—Nick. He put up with a lot of inattention and late nights. Thank you for being the rock I needed. And finally, Sumner—my coauthor and friend—for being the exact person I needed to write this book with. Your knowledge and resourcefulness are unmatched. I'm grateful to have done this work with you.

—Amee

I'm immensely grateful to my incredible daughter, Scarlett, for gifting me with your unwavering trust and love on your birthday. And for showing me that our future world really is worth fighting for. And to Sawyer-boy, thank you for always showing us what the joy of eating is, and for all of the light you give to my life daily. To my husband, Bryan: this book would not exist without your encouragement, and the time and space you patiently and generously helped me find when it seemed nowhere to be found in the midst of 2020. Thank you to my parents, Sarah and Bill, for teaching me to view all people with compassion. My sisters, Jessica and Hannah, who have always been there for me showing me how to be a better human. Patti, my mother-in-law, for your limitless encouragement and always offering a positive outlook. The Murphys—for generously sharing your piece of heaven on earth with me to write in peace and quiet. To so many of my dear friends for your words of encouragement and support. Thank you to Greta Jarvis for all the support and assistance. And a huge thank-you to my friend Amee, for bravely agreeing to join me on this ride. I admire you enormously. What an honor it has been to work with you in bringing this book to life.

—Sumner

RESOURCES

BOOKS FOR CAREGIVERS AND CLINICIANS

A Clinician's Guide to Gender-Affirming Care: Working with Transgender and Gender Nonconforming Clients, by Sand C. Chang, PhD, Anneliese A. Singh, PhD, LPC, and lore m. dickey, PhD.

Becoming an Ally to the Gender-Expansive Child: A Guide for Parents and Carers, by Anna Bianchi.

Belly of the Beast: The Politics of Anti-Fatness as Anti-Blackness, by Da'Shaun L. Harrison.

Body Kindness: Transform Your Health from the Inside Out—and Never Say Diet Again, by Rebecca Scritchfield, RDN.

Body Respect: What Conventional Health Books Get Wrong, Leave Out, and Just Plain Fail to Understand about Weight, by Lindo Bacon, PhD, and Lucy Aphramor, PhD, RD.

Born to Eat: Whole, Healthy Foods from Baby's First Bite, by Leslie Schilling, MA, RDN, and Wendy Jo Peterson, MS, RDN.

Eat to Love: A Mindful Guide to Transforming Your Relationship with Food, Body, and Life, by Jenna Hollenstein.

Fat, Pretty, and Soon to Be Old: A Makeover for Self and Society, by Kimberly Dark.

Fearing the Black Body: The Racial Origins of Fat Phobia, by Sabrina Strings, PhD.

Helping Children Develop a Positive Relationship with Food: A Practical Guide for Early Years Professionals, by Jo Cormack.

Helping Your Child with Extreme Picky Eating: A Step-by-Step Guide for Overcoming Selective Eating, Food Aversion, and Feeding Disorders, by Katja Rowell, MD, and Jenny McGlothlin, MS, SLP.

Intuitive Eating for Every Day: 365 Daily Practices & Inspirations to Rediscover the Pleasures of Eating, by Evelyn Tribole, MS, RDN, CEDRD-S.

Intuitive Eating: A Revolutionary Anti-Diet Approach (4th edition), by Evelyn Tribole, MS, RDN, CEDRD-S, and Elyse Resch, MS, RDN, CEDRD-S, FAND.

Love Me, Feed Me: The Adoptive Parent's Guide to Ending the Worry About Weight, Picky Eating, Power Struggles, and More, by Katja Rowell, MD.

No Bad Kids: Toddler Discipline Without Shame, by Janet Lansbury.

Radical Belonging: How to Survive and Thrive in an Unjust World, by Lindo Bacon, PhD.

Raising My Rainbow: Adventures in Raising a Fabulous, Gender Creative Son, by Lori Duron.

Real Kids Come in All Sizes: Ten Essential Lessons to Build Your Child's Body Esteem, by Kathy Kater.

Self-Compassion: The Proven Power of Being Kind to Yourself, by Kristin Neff, PhD.

The Body Is Not an Apology: The Power of Radical Self-Love (2nd edition), by Sonya Renee Taylor.

The Gender Creative Child: Pathways for Nurturing and Supporting Children Who Live Outside Gender Boxes, by Diane Ehrensaft, PhD.

The Intuitive Eating Workbook: Ten Principles for Nourishing a Healthy Relationship with Food, by Evelyn Tribole, MS, RDN, CEDRD-S, and Elyse Resch, MS, RDN, CEDRD-S, FAND.

The Power of Showing Up: How Parental Presence Shapes Who Our Kids Become and How Their Brains Get Wired, by Daniel J. Siegel, MD, and Tina Payne Bryson, PhD.

The Transgender Child: A Handbook for Families and Professionals, by Stephanie A. Brill and Rachel Pepper.

Unapologetic Eating: Make Peace with Food and Transform Your Life, by Alissa Rumsey, MS, RD.

Vitamin A to Z, by Fiona Sutherland, APD.

What We Don't Talk About When We Talk About Fat, by Aubrey Gordon.

BOOKS TO READ WITH KIDS

Amanda's Big Dream, by Judith Matz.

Big Hair, Don't Care, by Crystal Swain-Bates.

It's Okay to Be Different, by Todd Parr.

Love Your Body, by Jessica Sanders.

Shapesville, by Andy Mills and Becky Osborn.

The Skin You Live In, by Michael Tyler.

What I Like About Me!, by Allia Zobel Nolan and Miki Sakamoto.

Your Body Is Awesome: Body Respect for Children, by Sigrun Danielsdottir.

BOOKS FOR TEENS

Celebrate Your Body (and Its Changes, Too!): The Ultimate Puberty Book for Girls, by Sonya Renee Taylor.

No Weigh!: A Teen's Guide to Positive Body Image, Food, and Emotional Wisdom, by Shelley Aggarwal, Signe Darpinian, and Wendy Sterling.

The Intuitive Eating Workbook for Teens: A Non-Diet, Body Positive Approach to Building a Healthy Relationship with Food, by Elyse Resch, MS, RDN.

BOOKS ABOUT EATING DISORDERS

A Hunger So Wide and So Deep: A Multiracial View of Women's Eating Problems, by Becky W. Thompson.

Binge Eating Disorder: The Journey to Recovery and Beyond, by Chevese Turner and Amy Pershing.

Finding Your Sweet Spot: How to Avoid RED-S (Relative Energy Deficit in Sport) by Optimizing Your Energy Balance, by Rebecca McConville, MS, RD, LD, CSSD, CEDRD.

How to Nourish Your Child Through an Eating Disorder: A Simple, Plate-by-Plate Approach to Rebuilding a Healthy Relationship with Food, by Casey Crosbie, RD, CSSD, and Wendy Sterling, MS, RD, CSSD.

Nourish: How to Heal Your Relationship with Food, Body, and Self, by Heidi Schauster, MS, RDN, CEDRD-S.

Sick Enough: A Guide to the Medical Complications of Eating Disorders, by Jennifer Gaudiani, MD, CEDS, FAED.

The Parent's Guide to Eating Disorders: Supporting Self-Esteem, Healthy Eating, and Positive Body Image at Home, by Marcia Herrin, EdD, MPH, RD, and Nancy Matsumoto.

When Your Teen Has an Eating Disorder: Practical Strategies to Help Your Teen Recover from Anorexia, Bulimia, and Binge Eating, by Lauren Muhlheim, PsyD.

PODCASTS

Body Kindness, with Rebecca Scritchfield.

Comfort Food, with Amy Palanjian and Virginia Sole-Smith.

Food Psych, with Christy Harrison.

Love, Food, with Julie Duffy Dillon.

Mom Genes, with Rachel Coleman and Tina Laboy.

Respectful Parenting: Unruffled, with Janet Lansbury.

Sunny Side Up Nutrition, with Elizabeth Davenport, Anna Lutz, and Anna Mackay.

The Full Bloom Podcast, with Leslie Bloch and Zoë Bisbing.

BLOGS AND ONLINE RESOURCES

American Academy of Pediatrics Infant Food and Feeding: https://www.aap.org/en-us/advocacy-and-policy/aap-health-initiatives/HALF-Implementation-Guide/Age-Specific-Content/Pages/Infant-Food-and-Feeding.aspx.

Crystal Karges Nutrition Blog: https://www.crystalkarges.com/blog.

"Does the Idea of Addressing Your 'Thin Privilege' Make You Uncomfortable? Read this," The Everybody Is Beautiful Project: https://theeverybodyisbeautifulproject.com/blog/2019/12/4/your-intro-to-thin-privilege.

EDRD Pro Recommended Books: https://edrdpro.com/resources/recommended-books/.

Fed Is Best Foundation: https://www.fedisbest.org/.

FEDUP: "Fighting Eating Disorders in Underrepresented Populations: A Trans+ & Intersex Collective": https://fedupcollective.org.

Healthy Bodies, Healthy Minds: A Comprehensive Curriculum to Address Body Image, Eating, Fitness, and Weight Concerns in Today's Challenging Environment: http://bodyimagehealth.org/.

"Help! My kid has been sent home with a serve of diet culture. Your guide to keeping your sh*t together AND taking effective action," The Mindful Dietitian: https://www.themindfuldietitian.com.au/blog/help-my-kid-has-been-sent-home-with-a-serve-of-diet-culture-your-guide-to-keeping-your-sht-together-and-taking-effective-action?rq=school.

"Intuitive Eating Studies," The Original Intuitive Eating Pros: https://www.intuitiveeating.org/resources/studies/.

Intuitive Eating Moms: https://www.intuitiveeatingmoms.com/.

Joyful Eating for Your Family with Nicole Cruz Facebook Group: https://www.facebook.com/groups/joyfuleatingforyourfamily/.

La Leche League International: https://www.llli.org/.

"Let's Make Our Classrooms and Schools Free of Diet Talk," Sunny Side Up Nutrition: https://sunnysideupnutrition.com/wp-content/uploads/2018/09/Let%E2%80%99s-Make-Our-Classrooms-and-SchoolsFree-of-Diet-Talk-Weight-Neutral-Body-Positive-1.pdf.

More Than a Menu Newsletter, by Leslie Schilling: https://www.leslieschilling.com/newsletter.

"National Weight Control Registry: Skydiving Without a Chute," by Ragen Chastain, Dances With Fat: https://www.danceswithfat.org/2012/12/27/national-weight-control-registry-skydiving-without-a-chute/.

"Please Don't Teach My Kids to Diet: 5 Resources to Give Teachers and Schools," by Anna Lutz, Sunny Side Up Nutrition: https://www.sunnysideupnutrition.com/diet-free-resources-for-schools/.

"Sexual Orientation and Gender Identity Definitions," Human Rights Campaign: https://www.hrc.org/resources/sexual-orientation-and-gender-identity-terminology-and-definitions.

Yummy Toddler Food Blog, by Amy Palanjian: https://www.yummytoddlerfood.com/blog/.

WEBSITES FOR LOCATING SERVICES TO HELP WITH FOOD ACCESS

"Find Your Local Food Bank," Feeding America: https://www.feedingamerica.org/find-your-local-foodbank.

Women, Infants, and Children: Food, Education, and Support (WIC): www.signupwic
.com.

FIND A PROFESSIONAL

Certified Intuitive Eating Counselor Directory: https://www.intuitiveeating.org/certified
-counselors/.

Eating Disorder Registered Dietitians and Professionals (EDRD Pro) Provider Directory: https://edrdpro.com/professional-directory/.

FEDUP Support: https://fedupcollective.org/resources.

International Federation of Eating Disorder Dietitians (IFEDD) Treatment Finder:
https://www.eddietitians.com/treatment-finder/.

NOTES

CHAPTER 1: THE PROBLEM YOU'RE NOT ABLE TO SEE

1 Harrison, C. (2020). *Anti-Diet: Reclaim Your Time, Money, Well-Being, and Happiness Through Intuitive Eating.* New York: Little, Brown Spark.

2 Barry, V. W., Baruth, M., Beets, M. W., Durstine, J. L., Liu, J., & Blair, S. N. (2014). Fitness vs. fatness on all-cause mortality: A meta-analysis. *Progress in Cardiovascular Diseases, 56*(4), 382–390. doi:10.1016/j.pcad.2013.09.002.

3 Dhurandhar, E. J., Kaiser, K. A., Dawson, J. A., Alcorn, A. S., Keating, K. D., & Allison, D. B. (2014). Predicting adult weight change in the real world: A systematic review and meta-analysis accounting for compensatory changes in energy intake or expenditure. *International Journal of Obesity, 39*(8), 1181–1187. doi:10.1038/ijo.2014.184.

4 Statistics & Research on Eating Disorders. (2020, May 8). Retrieved January 16, 2021, from www.nationaleatingdisorders.org/statistics-research-eating-disorders.

5 Lowes, J., & Tiggemann, M. (2003). Body dissatisfaction, dieting awareness, and the impact of parental influence in young children. *British Journal of Health Psychology, 8*(2), 135–147. doi:10.1348/135910703321649123.

6 Deleel, M. L., Hughes, T. L., Miller, J. A., Hipwell, A., & Theodore, L. A. (2009). Prevalence of eating disturbance and body image dissatisfaction in young girls: An

examination of the variance across racial and socioeconomic groups. *Psychology in the Schools, 46*(8), 767–775. doi:10.1002/pits.20415.

7 Hudson, J. I., Hiripi, E., Pope, H. G., & Kessler, R. C. (2007). The prevalence and correlates of eating disorders in the national comorbidity survey replication. *Biological Psychiatry, 61*(3), 348–358. doi:10.1016/j.biopsych.2006.03.040.

8 Reba-Harrelson, L., Holle, A. V., Hamer, R. M., Swann, R., Reyes, M. L., & Bulik, C. M. (2009). Patterns and prevalence of disordered eating and weight control behaviors in women ages 25–45. *Eating and Weight Disorders—Studies on Anorexia, Bulimia, and Obesity, 14*(4), 190–198. doi:10.1007/bf03325116.

9 Abramovitz, B. A., & Birch, L. L. (2000). Five-year-old girls' ideas about dieting are predicted by their mothers' dieting. *Journal of the American Dietetic Association, 100*(10), 1157–1163. doi:10.1016/s0002–8223(00)00339–4.

10 Eating Disorders. (n.d.). Retrieved January 16, 2021, from www.nimh.nih.gov/health/topics/eating-disorders/index.shtml.

11 Chesney, E., Goodwin, G. M., & Fazel, S. (2014). Risks of all-cause and suicide mortality in mental disorders: A meta-review. *World Psychiatry, 13*(2), 153–160. doi:10.1002/wps.20128.

12 Pont, S. J., Puhl, R., Cook, S. R., & Slusser, W. (2017). Stigma experienced by children and adolescents with obesity. *Pediatrics, 140*(6). doi:10.1542/peds.2017–3034.

13 Salas, X. R., Forhan, M., Caulfield, T., Sharma, A. M., & Raine, K. (2017). A critical analysis of obesity prevention policies and strategies. *Canadian Journal of Public Health, 108*(5–6). doi:10.17269/cjph.108.6044.

14 Major, B., Hunger, J. M., Bunyan, D. P., & Miller, C. T. (2014). The ironic effects of weight stigma. *Journal of Experimental Social Psychology, 51*, 74–80. doi:10.1016/j.jesp.2013.11.009.

15 Tomiyama, A. J., Carr, D., Granberg, E. M., Major, B., Robinson, E., Sutin, A. R., & Brewis, A. (2018). How and why weight stigma drives the obesity "epidemic" and harms health. *BMC Medicine, 16*(1). doi:10.1186/s12916-018-1116–5.

16 Vadiveloo, M., & Mattei, J. (2016). Perceived weight discrimination and 10-year risk of allostatic load among US adults. *Annals of Behavioral Medicine, 51*(1), 94–104. doi:10.1007/s12160-016-9831–7.

17 McEwen, B. (2005, September). Stressed or stressed out: What is the difference? Retrieved January 16, 2021, from https://www.ncbi.nlm.nih.gov/pmc/articles/PMC1197275/.

CHAPTER 2: WHY WE NEED TO SAY "NO" TO THE STATUS QUO

1 Whitaker, H. (2019). *Quit Like a Woman: The Radical Choice to Not Drink in a Culture Obsessed with Alcohol.* New York: The Dial Press.

2 Strings, S. (2019). *Fearing the Black Body: The Racial Origins of Fat Phobia.* New York: New York University Press.

3 Wolf, N. (2015). *The Beauty Myth: How Images of Beauty Are Used Against Women* (pp. 191–192). London: Vintage Books.

4 Neumark-Sztainer, D., Wall, M., Larson, N. I., Eisenberg, M. E., & Loth, K. (2011). Dieting and disordered eating behaviors from adolescence to young adulthood: Find-

ings from a 10-year longitudinal study. *Journal of the American Dietetic Association, 111*(7), 1004–1011. doi:10.1016/j.jada.2011.04.012.

5 Ellis, J. M., Galloway, A. T., Zickgraf, H. F., & Whited, M. C. (2018). Picky eating and fruit and vegetable consumption in college students. *Eating Behaviors, 30*, 5–8. doi:10.1016/j.eatbeh.2018.05.001.

6 Yee, A. Z., Lwin, M. O., & Ho, S. S. (2017). The influence of parental practices on child promotive and preventive food consumption behaviors: A systematic review and meta-analysis. *International Journal of Behavioral Nutrition and Physical Activity, 14*(1). doi:10.1186/s12966-017-0501-3.

7 Fisher, J., & Birch, L. (1999). Restricting access to foods and children's eating. *Appetite, 32*(3), 405–419. doi:10.1006/appe.1999.0231.

8 Brown, R. (2004). Children's eating attitudes and behaviour: A study of the modelling and control theories of parental influence. *Health Education Research, 19*(3), 261–271. doi:10.1093/her/cyg040.

9 Brown, R. (2004). Children's eating attitudes and behaviour: A study of the modelling and control theories of parental influence. *Health Education Research, 19*(3), 261–271. doi:10.1093/her/cyg040.

10 Birch, L. L., Fisher, J. O., & Davison, K. K. (2003). Learning to overeat: Maternal use of restrictive feeding practices promotes girls' eating in the absence of hunger. *American Journal of Clinical Nutrition, 78*(2), 215–220. doi:10.1093/ajcn/78.2.215.

11 Farrow, C. V., Haycraft, E., & Blissett, J. M. (2015). Teaching our children when to eat: How parental feeding practices inform the development of emotional eating—a longitudinal experimental design. *American Journal of Clinical Nutrition, 101*(5), 908–913. doi:10.3945/ajcn.114.103713.

12 Thompson, H. R., & Madsen, K. A. (2017). The report card on BMI report cards. *Current Obesity Reports, 6*(2), 163–167. doi:10.1007/s13679-017-0259-6.

13 Kaczmarski, J. M., Debate, R. D., Marhefka, S. L., & Daley, E. M. (2011). State-mandated school-based BMI screening and parent notification. *Health Promotion Practice, 12*(6), 797–801. doi:10.1177/1524839911419289.

14 Ursoniu, S., Putnoky, S., & Vlaicu, B. (2011). Body weight perception among high school students and its influence on weight management behaviors in normal weight students: A cross-sectional study. *Wiener Klinische Wochenschrift, 123*(11–12), 327–333. doi:10.1007/s00508-011-1578-3.

15 Bacon, L., & Severson, A. (2019, July 8). Fat is not the problem—Fat stigma is. Retrieved January 16, 2021, from https://blogs.scientificamerican.com/observations/fat-is-not-the-problem-fat-stigma-is/.

16 Bornioli, A., Lewis-Smith, H., Smith, A., Slater, A., & Bray, I. (2019). Adolescent body dissatisfaction and disordered eating: Predictors of later risky health behaviours. *Social Science & Medicine, 238*, 112458. doi:10.1016/j.socscimed.2019.112458.

17 Jones, A., Winter, V. R., Pekarek, E., & Walters, J. (2018). Binge drinking and cigarette smoking among teens: Does body image play a role? *Children and Youth Services Review, 91*, 232–236. doi:10.1016/j.childyouth.2018.06.005.

18 Fox, M. (2018, February 27). America's kids are obese and it's getting worse. Retrieved February 18, 2021, from www.nbcnews.com/health/health-news/americans-kids-are-obese-it-s-getting-worse-n851246.

19 Crenshaw, K. W. (2019). *On Intersectionality: Essential Writings*. New York: The New Press.

20 Burke, N. L., Schaefer, L. M., Hazzard, V. M., & Rodgers, R. F. (2020). Where identities converge: The importance of intersectionality in eating disorders research. *International Journal of Eating Disorders*, 53(10), 1605–1609. doi:10.1002/eat.23371.

21 Becker, A. E., Franko, D. L., Speck, A., & Herzog, D. B. (2003). Ethnicity and differential access to care for eating disorder symptoms. *International Journal of Eating Disorders*, 33(2), 205–212. doi:10.1002/eat.10129.

22 Report: Economic Costs of Eating Disorders. (2020, August 31). Retrieved January 16, 2021, from www.hsph.harvard.edu/striped/report-economic-costs-of-eating-disorders/.

23 Sala, M., Reyes-Rodríguez, M. L., Bulik, C. M., & Bardone-Cone, A. (2013). Race, ethnicity, and eating disorder recognition by peers. *Eating Disorders*, 21(5), 423–436. doi:10.1080/10640266.2013.827540.

24 Race, Social Class, and Bulimia Nervosa. (n.d.). Retrieved January 16, 2021, from http://ftp.iza.org/dp5823.pdf.

25 Swanson, S. A., Crow, S. J., Le Grange, D., Swendsen, J., & Merikangas, K. R. (n.d.). Prevalence and correlates of eating disorders in adolescents. Results from the national comorbidity survey replication adolescent supplement. Retrieved January 16, 2021, from https://pubmed.ncbi.nlm.nih.gov/21383252/.

26 Feldman, M. B., & Meyer, I. H. (2007). Eating disorders in diverse lesbian, gay, and bisexual populations. *International Journal of Eating Disorders*, 40(3), 218–226. doi:10.1002/eat.20360.

27 Hadland, S. E., Austin, S. B., Goodenow, C. S., & Calzo, J. P. (2014). Weight misperception and unhealthy weight control behaviors among sexual minorities in the general adolescent population. *Journal of Adolescent Health*, 54(3), 296–303. doi:10.1016/j.jadohealth.2013.08.021.

28 Diemer, E. W., Grant, J. D., Munn-Chernoff, M. A., Patterson, D. A., & Duncan, A. E. (2015). Gender identity, sexual orientation, and eating-related pathology in a national sample of college students. *Journal of Adolescent Health*, 57(2), 144–149. doi:10.1016/j.jadohealth.2015.03.003.

29 Duffy, M. E., Henkel, K. E., & Earnshaw, V. A. (2016). Transgender clients' experiences of eating disorder treatment. *Journal of LGBT Issues in Counseling*, 10(3), 136–149. doi:10.1080/15538605.2016.1177806.

30 Milano, W., Ambrosio, P., Carizzone, F., Biasio, V. D., Foggia, G., & Capasso, A. (2020). Gender dysphoria, eating disorders, and body image: An overview. *Endocrine, Metabolic & Immune Disorders—Drug Targets*, 20(4), 518–524. doi:10.2174/1871530319666191015193120.

31 Hub: Young Women with Physical Disabilities: 10.1097/00004703–200004000–00002. (n.d.). Retrieved January 16, 2021, from https://sci-hub.scihubtw.tw/10.1097/00004703–200004000–00002.

32 Mayes, S. D., & Zickgraf, H. (2019). Atypical eating behaviors in children and adolescents with autism, ADHD, other disorders, and typical development. *Research in Autism Spectrum Disorders*, 64, 76–83. doi:10.1016/j.rasd.2019.04.002.

33 Morgan, C. (n.d.). Center for Disability Rights. The Unacknowledged Crisis of Violence Against Disabled People—Center for Disability Rights. www.cdrnys.org/blog /advocacy/the-unacknowledged-crisis-of-violence-against-disabled-people/.

34 Addressing Eating Disorders, Body Dissatisfaction, and Obesity Among Sexual and Gender Minority Youth. (n.d.). Retrieved January 16, 2021, from www.lgbtqia healtheducation.org/wp-content/uploads/2018/04/EatingDisordersBodyImageBrief .pdf.

35 Diemer, E. W., Grant, J. D., Munn-Chernoff, M. A., Patterson, D. A., & Duncan, A. E. (2015). Gender identity, sexual orientation, and eating-related pathology in a national sample of college students. *Journal of Adolescent Health, 57*(2), 144–149. doi:10.1016/j. jadohealth.2015.03.003.

36 Ward, Z. J., Rodriguez, P., Wright, D. R., Austin, S. B., & Long, M. W. (2019). Estimation of eating disorders prevalence by age and associations with mortality in a simulated nationally representative US cohort. *JAMA Network Open, 2*(10). doi:10.1001/jamanetworkopen.2019.12925.

37 Puhl, R., & Suh, Y. (2015). Health consequences of weight stigma: Implications for obesity prevention and treatment. *Current Obesity Reports, 4*(2), 182–190. doi:10.1007/ s13679-015-0153-z.

38 Rothblum, E. D. (2018). Slim chance for permanent weight loss. *Archives of Scientific Psychology, 6*(1), 63–69. doi:10.1037/arc0000043.

39 Jacquet, P., Schutz, Y., Montani, J., & Dulloo, A. (2020). How dieting might make some fatter: Modeling weight cycling toward obesity from a perspective of body composition autoregulation. *International Journal of Obesity, 44*(6), 1243–1253. doi:10.1038/s41366-020-0547-1.

40 Rozin, P. (1996). Towards a psychology of food and eating: From motivation to module to model to marker, morality, meaning, and metaphor. Retrieved January 16, 2021, from https://journals.sagepub.com/doi/10.1111/1467-8721.ep10772690.

41 Fothergill, E., Guo, J., Howard, L., Kerns, J., Knuth, N., Brychta, R., . . . & Hall, K. (2016, May 2). Persistent metabolic adaptation 6 years after "The Biggest Loser" competition. Retrieved January 16, 2021, from https://onlinelibrary.wiley.com/doi/full /10.1002/oby.21538.

42 Golden, N. H., Schneider, M., & Wood, C. (2016). Preventing obesity and eating disorders in adolescents. *Pediatrics, 138*(3). doi:10.1542/peds.2016-1649.

43 Portzky, G., Van Heeringen, K., & Vervaet, M. (2014). Attempted suicide in patients with eating disorders. *Crisis, 35*(6), 378–387. doi:10.1027/0227–5910/a000275.

CHAPTER 3: THE PATH FORWARD

1 Hazzard, V. M., Telke, S. E., Simone, M., Anderson, L. M., Larson, N. I., & Neumark-Sztainer, D. (n.d.). Intuitive eating longitudinally predicts better psychological health and lower use of disordered eating behaviors: Findings from EAT 2010–2018. Retrieved January 16, 2021, from https://pubmed.ncbi.nlm.nih.gov/32006391/.

2 Lipson, S., & Sonneville, K. (2017). Eating disorder symptoms among undergraduate and graduate students at 12 U.S. colleges and universities. *Eating Behaviors, 24,* 81–88. doi:10.1016/j.eatbeh.2016.12.003.

3 Chastain, R. (2015, March 26). National Weight Control Registry—Skydiving Without

a Chute. Retrieved January 16, 2021, from https://danceswithfat.org/2012/12/27/national-weight-control-registry-skydiving-without-a-chute/.

4 Clinical practice guidelines for the management of overweight and obesity. (1970, January 1). Retrieved January 16, 2021, from www.nhmrc.gov.au/about-us/publications/clinical-practice-guidelines-management-overweight-and-obesity.

5 Tribole, E., & Resch, E. (2020). *Intuitive Eating: A Revolutionary Program That Works*. New York: St. Martin's Essentials.

6 Piran, N., & Tylka, T. L. (2019). *Handbook of Positive Body Image and Embodiment: Constructs, Protective Factors, and Interventions*. New York: Oxford University Press.

7 Taylor, S. R. (2020). *The Body Isn't an Apology: The Power of Radical Self-Love*. Oakland, CA: Berrett-Koehler.

8 Piran, N., & Tylka, T. L. (2019). *Handbook of Positive Body Image and Embodiment: Constructs, Protective Factors, and Interventions*. New York: Oxford University Press.

CHAPTER 4: GETTING TO KNOW YOUR OWN INNER CHILD

1 Compassion. (2018, March 6). Retrieved January 16, 2021, from https://self-compassion.org/.

2 McLeod, S. (n.d.). Erik Erikson's stages of psychosocial development. Retrieved January 16, 2021, from www.simplypsychology.org/Erik-Erikson.html.

3 Gaudiani, J. L. (2019). *Sick Enough: A Guide to the Medical Complications of Eating Disorders*. New York: Routledge.

4 Siegel, D. J. (2021). *The Power of Showing Up: How Parental Presence Shapes Who Our Kids Become and How Their Brains Get Wired*. New York: Ballantine.

CHAPTER 5: EMBRACING YOUR ROLE
AS AN IMPERFECT PARENT

1 Katzman, D., & Steinegger, C. (2010). Faculty Opinions recommendation of family weight talk and dieting: How much do they matter for body dissatisfaction and disordered eating behaviors in adolescent girls? *Faculty Opinions—Post-Publication Peer Review of the Biomedical Literature*. doi:10.3410/f.5368961.5320062.

2 Abramovitz, B. A., & Birch, L. L. (2000). Five-year-old girls' ideas about dieting are predicted by their mothers' dieting. *Journal of the American Dietetic Association*, 100(10), 1157–1163. doi:10.1016/s0002–8223(00)00339–4.

3 Calzo, J. P., Sonneville, K. R., Haines, J., Blood, E. A., Field, A. E., & Austin, S. B. (2012). The development of associations among body mass index, body dissatisfaction, and weight and shape concern in adolescent boys and girls. *Journal of Adolescent Health*, 51(5), 517–523. doi:10.1016/j.jadohealth.2012.02.021.

4 Nagoski, E., & Nagoski, A. (2020). *Burnout: The Secret to Unlocking the Stress Cycle*. New York: Ballantine.

5 Autonomy. (n.d.). Retrieved January 16, 2021, from www.merriam-webster.com/dictionary/autonomy.

6 CSDH (2008). *Closing the Gap in a Generation: Health Equity Through Action on the*

Social Determinants of Health: Final Report of the Commission on Social Determinants of Health. Geneva: World Health Organization.

7 McGonigal, K. (2021). *The Joy of Movement: How Exercise Helps Us Find Happiness, Hope, Connection, and Courage*. New York: Avery.

8 Draxten, M., Fulkerson, J. A., Friend, S., Flattum, C. F., & Schow, R. (2014). Parental role modeling of fruits and vegetables at meals and snacks is associated with children's adequate consumption. *Appetite, 78*, 1–7. doi:10.1016/j.appet.2014.02.017.

CHAPTER 6: THE DOUBLE-EDGED SWORD
OF PARENTAL CONTROL

1 What is "responsive" feeding therapy? (2017, November 7). Retrieved February 18, 2021, from www.extremepickyeating.com/what-is-responsive-feeding-therapy/.

2 Brehm, J. W. (1966). *A Theory of Psychological Reactance*. New York: Academic Press.

3 Reynolds-Tylus, T. (2019). Psychological reactance and persuasive health communication: A review of the literature. *Frontiers in Communication, 4*. doi:10.3389/fcomm .2019.00056.

4 New study shows tobacco control programs cut adult smoking rates. (2008). *PsycEXTRA Dataset*. doi:10.1037/e408892008–001.

5 Reynolds-Tylus, T. (2019). Psychological reactance and persuasive health communication: A review of the literature. *Frontiers in Communication, 4*. doi:10.3389/ fcomm.2019.00056.

6 Eat and feed with joy. (n.d.). Retrieved February 18, 2021, from www.ellynsatterinstitute .org/

7 Cormack, J., Rowell, K., & Postăvaru, G. (2020). Self-determination theory as a theoretical framework for a responsive approach to child feeding. *Journal of Nutrition Education and Behavior, 52*(6), 646–651. doi:10.1016/j.jneb.2020.02.005.

8 Finnane, J. M., Jansen, E., Mallan, K. M., & Daniels, L. A. (2017). Mealtime structure and responsive feeding practices are associated with less food fussiness and more food enjoyment in children. *Journal of Nutrition Education and Behavior, 49*(1). doi:10.1016/j. jneb.2016.08.007.

9 Hurley, K. M., Cross, M. B., & Hughes, S. O. (2011). A systematic review of responsive feeding and child obesity in high-income countries. *Journal of Nutrition, 141*(3), 495–501. doi:10.3945/jn.110.130047.

10 Grolnick, W. S. (2009). *The Psychology of Parental Control: How Well-Meant Parenting Backfires*. New York: Psychology Press.

11 Deci, E. L., Cascio, W. F., & Krusell, J. (1975). Cognitive evaluation theory and some comments on the Calder and Staw critique. *Journal of Personality and Social Psychology, 31*(1), 81–85. doi:10.1037/h0076168.

12 Fisher, J. O., & Birch, L. L. (1999). Restricting access to palatable foods affects children's behavioral response, food selection, and intake. *American Journal of Clinical Nutrition, 69*(6), 1264–1272. doi:10.1093/ajcn/69.6.1264.

13 Johnson, S., McPhee, L., & Birch, L. (1991). Conditioned preferences: Young children prefer flavors associated with high dietary fat. *Physiology & Behavior, 50*(6), 1245–1251. doi:10.1016/0031–9384(91)90590-k.

14 Crum, A. J., Corbin, W. R., Brownell, K. D., & Salovey, P. (2011). Mind over

milkshakes: Mindsets, not just nutrients, determine ghrelin response: Correction to Crum et al. (2011). *Health Psychology, 30*(4), 429–429. doi:10.1037/a0024760.

PART III: EMBRACING A NEW PATH: THE 3 KEYS

1 Zhang, C., Leeming, E., Smith, P., Chung, P., Hagger, M. S., & Hayes, S. C. (2018). Acceptance and commitment therapy for health behavior change: A contextually-driven approach. *Frontiers in Psychology, 8.* doi:10.3389/fpsyg.2017.02350.

CHAPTER 7: KEY 1: PROVIDE UNCONDITIONAL LOVE AND SUPPORT FOR YOUR CHILD'S BODY

1 Lowes, J., & Tiggemann, M. (2003). Body dissatisfaction, dieting awareness, and the impact of parental influence in young children. *British Journal of Health Psychology, 8*(2), 135–147. doi:10.1348/135910703321649123.

2 Wolf, N. (2015). *The Beauty Myth: How Images of Beauty Are Used Against Women* (pp. 191–192). London: Vintage Books.

3 Siegel, D. J., & Bryson, T. P. (2021). *The Power of Showing Up: How Parental Presence Shapes Who Our Kids Become and How Their Brains Get Wired.* New York: Ballantine.

CHAPTER 8: KEY 2: IMPLEMENT A FLEXIBLE AND RELIABLE FEEDING ROUTINE

1 Resch, E., & Tribole, E. (2020). Intuitive Eating: A revolutionary program that works [Introduction]. (2020). *Intuitive Eating: A Revolutionary Program That Works* (p. 253). New York: St. Martin's Essentials.

2 Coyne, L. W., Gould, E. R., Grimaldi, M., Wilson, K. G., Baffuto, G., & Biglan, A. (2020). First things first: Parent psychological flexibility and self-compassion during COVID-19. COVID-19 Emergency Publications. doi:10.31219/osf.io/pyge2.

CHAPTER 9: KEY 3: DEVELOP AND USE YOUR INTUITIVE EATING VOICE

1 Der, K. B. (2015). *The Body Keeps the Score: Mind, Brain, and Body in the Transformation of Trauma.* London: Penguin Books.

2 Kroon Van Diest, A. M., & Tylka, T. L. (2010). The caregiver eating messages scale: Development and psychometric investigation. *Body Image, 7*(4), 317–326. doi:10.1016/j.bodyim.2010.06.002.

3 Epstein, L. H., Carr, K. A., Lin, H., & Fletcher, K. D. (2011). Food reinforcement, energy intake, and macronutrient choice. *American Journal of Clinical Nutrition, 94*(1), 12–18. doi:10.3945/ajcn.110.010314.

CHAPTER 10: GENTLE NUTRITION

1 CFR—Code of Federal Regulations Title 21. (n.d.).

2 Harris, S. S. (2006). Vitamin D and African Americans. *Journal of Nutrition, 136*(4), 1126–1129. doi:10.1093/jn/136.4.1126.

3 Moraes, J. G., Motta, M. E., Beltrão, M. F., Salviano, T. L., & Silva, G. A. (2016). Fecal microbiota and diet of children with chronic constipation. *International Journal of Pediatrics, 2016,* 1–8. doi:10.1155/2016/6787269.

4 Agans, R., Gordon, A., Kramer, D. L., Perez-Burillo, S., Rufián-Henares, J. A., &

Paliy, O. (2018). Dietary fatty acids sustain the growth of the human gut microbiota. *Applied and Environmental Microbiology, 84*(21). doi:10.1128/aem.01525–18.

5 Makki, K., Deehan, E. C., Walter, J., & Bäckhed, F. (2018). The impact of dietary fiber on gut microbiota in host health and disease. *Cell Host & Microbe, 23*(6), 705–715. doi:10.1016/j.chom.2018.05.012.

6 Sheppard, K. W., & Cheatham, C. L. (2018). Omega-6/omega-3 fatty acid intake of children and older adults in the U.S.: Dietary intake in comparison to current dietary recommendations and the healthy eating index. *Lipids in Health and Disease, 17*(1). doi:10.1186/s12944-018-0693–9.

7 Benton, D., & Young, H. A. (2019). Role of fruit juice in achieving the 5-a-day recommendation for fruit and vegetable intake. *Nutrition Reviews, 77*(11).

8 Keene, D. E., Guo, M., & Murillo, S. (2018). "That wasn't really a place to worry about diabetes": Housing access and diabetes self-management among low-income adults. *Social Science & Medicine, 197,* 71–77. doi:10.1016/j.socscimed.2017.11.051.

9 Shprintzen, A. D. (2015). *The Vegetarian Crusade: The Rise of an American Reform Movement, 1817–1921.* Chapel Hill, NC: The University of North Carolina Press.

10 Sugar. (n.d.). From www.heart.org/en/healthy-living/healthy-eating/eat-smart/sugar.

11 Lansbury, J. (2014). *No Bad Kids: Toddler Discipline Without Shame.* Los Angeles: JLML Press.

12 O'Connor, S. G., Maher, J. P., Belcher, B. R., Leventhal, A. M., Margolin, G., Shonkoff, E. T., & Dunton, G. F. (2017). Associations of maternal stress with children's weight-related behaviours: A systematic literature review. *Obesity Reviews, 18*(5), 514–525. doi:10.1111/obr.12522.

CHAPTER 11: KIDS, MOVEMENT, AND SPORTS

1 Eating disorders & athletes. (2018, April 27). Retrieved February 18, 2021, from www .nationaleatingdisorders.org/eating-disorders-athletes.

2 Jankowski, C. (2012). Associations between disordered eating, menstrual dysfunction, and musculoskeletal injury among high school athletes. *Yearbook of Sports Medicine, 2012,* 394–395. doi:10.1016/j.yspm.2011.08.003.

3 Johnson, C., Powers, P. S., & Dick, R. (1999). Athletes and eating disorders: The National Collegiate Athletic Association study. *International Journal of Eating Disorders, 26*(2), 179–188. doi:10.1002/(sici)1098–108x(199909)26:23.0.co;2-z.

4 Physical activity. (n.d.). Retrieved February 18, 2021, from https://health.gov/our -work/physical-activity.

5 Brawley, L. R., & Latimer, A. E. (2007). Physical activity guides for Canadians: Messaging strategies, realistic expectations for change, and evaluation: Advancing physical activity measurement and guidelines in Canada. *Applied Physiology, Nutrition, and Metabolism, 32*(S2E). doi:10.1139/h07–105.

6 Annesi, J. J. (2005). Correlations of depression and total mood disturbance with physical activity and self-concept in preadolescents enrolled in an after-school exercise program. *Psychological Reports, 96*(4), 891. doi:10.2466/pr0.96.4.891–898.

7 Goldfield, G. S. (2009). Predictors of response to an intervention modifying physical activity and sedentary behavior in overweight/obese children: Attitudes vs. behavior. *Journal of Physical Activity and Health, 6*(4), 463–466. doi:10.1123/jpah. 6.4.463.

8 Norris, R., Carroll, D., & Cochrane, R. (1992). The effects of physical activity and

exercise training on psychological stress and well-being in an adolescent popula-tion. *Journal of Psychosomatic Research, 36*(1), 55–65. doi:10.1016/0022–3999(92)90114-h.

9 Fedewa, M. V., Gist, N. H., Evans, E. M., & Dishman, R. K. (2013). Exercise and insulin resistance in youth: A meta-analysis. *Pediatrics, 133*(1). doi:10.1542/peds.2013–2718.

CHAPTER 12: COMMON MEDICAL AND HEALTH CONCERNS

1 U.S. Department of Health and Human Services. (1999). Mental health: A report of the Surgeon General. Retrieved January 30, 2017, from www.surgeongeneral.gov/library/mentalhealth/home.html. Rockville, MD: HHS.

2 Piran, N., & Tylka, T. L. (2019). *Handbook of Positive Body Image and Embodiment: Constructs, Protective Factors, and Interventions.* New York: Oxford University Press.

3 Gaudiani, J. L. (2019). *Sick Enough: A Guide to the Medical Complications of Eating Disorders.* New York: Routledge.

4 Puhl, R. (2013). Weight-based victimization: Bullying experiences of weight loss treatment-seeking youth. Retrieved February 18, 2021, from https://pubmed.ncbi.nlm.nih.gov/23266918/.

5 Wentz, E., Lacey, J. H., Waller, G., Råstam, M., Turk, J., & Gillberg, C. (2005). Child-hood onset neuropsychiatric disorders in adult eating disorder patients. *European Child & Adolescent Psychiatry, 14*(8), 431–437. doi:10.1007/s00787-005-0494-3.

6 Zucker, N. L., Losh, M., Bulik, C. M., LaBar, K. S., Piven, J., & Pelphrey, K. A. (2007). Anorexia nervosa and autism spectrum disorders: Guided investigation of social cog-nitive endophenotypes. *Psychological Bulletin, 133*(6), 976–1006. doi:10.1037/0033-2909.133.6.976.

7 Kavuri, V., Raghuram, N., Malamud, A., & Selvan, S. R. (2015). Irritable bowel syn-drome: Yoga as remedial therapy. *Evidence-Based Complementary and Alternative Med-icine, 2015,* 1–10. doi:10.1155/2015/398156.

CHAPTER 13: DEVELOPMENTAL STAGES OF RAISING AN INTUITIVE EATER

1 Erikson, E. H. (2014). *Childhood and Society.* London: Vintage Digital.

2 About/FAQs: Fed Is Best. (n.d.). Retrieved February 18, 2021, from https://fedisbest.org/about/.

3 Black, M. M., & Aboud, F. E. (2011). Responsive feeding is embedded in a theoretical framework of responsive parenting. *Journal of Nutrition, 141*(3), 490–494. doi:10.3945/jn.110.129973.

4 Birch, L. L. (1991). The variability of young children's energy intake. *New England Jour-nal of Medicine, 324*(25), 1816–1817. doi:10.1056/nejm199106203242518.

5 Walton, K., Kuczynski, L., Haycraft, E., Breen, A., & Haines, J. (2017). Time to re-think picky eating?: A relational approach to understanding picky eating. *International Journal of Behavioral Nutrition and Physical Activity, 14*(1). doi:10.1186/s12966-017-0520-0.

6 Rowell, K. (2012). *Love Me, Feed Me: The Adoptive Parent's Guide to Ending the Worry About Weight, Picky Eating, Power Struggles, and More.* St. Paul, MN: Family Feeding Dynamics.

7 Wolstenholme, H., Kelly, C., Hennessy, M., & Heary, C. (2020). Childhood fussy/

picky eating behaviours: A systematic review and synthesis of qualitative studies. *International Journal of Behavioral Nutrition and Physical Activity, 17*(1). doi:10.1186/s12966-019-0899-x.

8 Mallan, K. M., Jansen, E., Harris, H., Llewellyn, C., Fildes, A., & Daniels, L. A. (2018). Feeding a fussy eater: Examining longitudinal bidirectional relationships between child fussy eating and maternal feeding practices. *Journal of Pediatric Psychology, 43*(10), 1138–1146. doi:10.1093/jpepsy/jsy053.

9 Palanjian, A. (2020, September 23). How to help toddlers with texture aversions and improve picky eating. Retrieved February 18, 2021, from www.yummytoddlerfood.com/advice/picky-eating/feeding-toddlers-with-texture-issues/.

10 Cheng, H. L., Amatoury, M., & Steinbeck, K. (2016). Energy expenditure and intake during puberty in healthy nonobese adolescents: A systematic review. *American Journal of Clinical Nutrition, 104*(4), 1061–1074. doi:10.3945/ajcn.115.129205.

11 Sidani, J. E., Shensa, A., Hoffman, B., Hanmer, J., & Primack, B. A. (2016). The association between social media use and eating concerns among US young adults. *Journal of the Academy of Nutrition and Dietetics, 116*(9), 1465–1472. doi:10.1016/j.jand.2016.03.021.

12 Biernesser, C., Sewall, C. J., Brent, D., Bear, T., Mair, C., & Trauth, J. (2020). Social media use and deliberate self-harm among youth: A systematized narrative review. *Children and Youth Services Review, 116*, 105054. doi:10.1016/j.childyouth.2020.105054.

13 Sampasa-Kanyinga, H., & Lewis, R. F. (2015). Frequent use of social networking sites is associated with poor psychological functioning among children and adolescents. *Cyberpsychology, Behavior, and Social Networking, 18*(7), 380–385. doi:10.1089/cyber.2015.0055.

14 Taylor, S. R., Laureano, B. I., & Brennan, C. (2018). *Celebrate Your Body (and Its Changes, Too!)*. Emeryville, CA: Rockridge Press.

15 Lipson, S., & Sonneville, K. (2017). Eating disorder symptoms among undergraduate and graduate students at 12 U.S. colleges and universities. *Eating Behaviors, 24*, 81–88. doi:10.1016/j.eatbeh.2016.12.003.

16 Ackard, D. M., Fulkerson, J. A., & Neumark-Sztainer, D. (2011). Stability of eating disorder diagnostic classifications in adolescents: Five-year longitudinal findings from a population-based study. *Eating Disorders, 19*(4), 308–322. doi:10.1080/10640266.2011.584804.

17 Prevalence, severity, and unmet need for treatment of mental disorders in the World Health Organization world mental health surveys. (2004). *JAMA, 291*(21), 2581–90. doi:10.1001/jama.291.21.2581.

18 Mountjoy, M., Sundgot-Borgen, J., Burke, L., Carter, S., Constantini, N., Lebrun, C., . . . & Ljungqvist, A. (2014). The IOC consensus statement: Beyond the female athlete triad—relative energy deficiency in sport (RED-S). *British Journal of Sports Medicine, 48*(7), 491–497. doi:10.1136/bjsports-2014-093502.

19 Gaudiani, J. L. (2019). *Sick Enough: A Guide to the Medical Complications of Eating Disorders*. New York: Routledge.

20 Grummer-Strawn, L. M., & Mei, Z. (2004). Does breastfeeding protect against pediatric overweight? Analysis of longitudinal data from the Centers for Disease Control and Prevention Pediatric Nutrition Surveillance System. *Pediatrics, 113*(2). doi:10.1542/peds.113.2.e81.

21 Ben-Joseph, E. P., Dowshen, S. A., & Izenberg, N. (2009). Do parents understand

growth charts? A national, internet-based survey. *Pediatrics, 124*(4), 1100–1109. doi:10.1542/peds.2008–0797.

CHAPTER 14: WHAT TO DO WHEN THIS FEELS HARDER
THAN YOU THOUGHT

1 Tribole, E., & Resch, E. (2019). *The Intuitive Eating Workbook: Principles for Nourishing a Healthy Relationship with Food*. Brattleboro, VT: Echo Point Books & Media.

2 Ginther, D. K. (2011). Study finds racial disparity in NIH funding. *PyscEXTRA Dataset*. https://doi.org/10.1031/e519412012–006.

3 Horvath, S. A., Shorey, R. C., & Racine, S. E. (2020). Emotion dysregulation as a correlate of food and alcohol disturbance in undergraduate students. *Eating Behaviors, (38)*, 101409. doi:10.1016/j.eatbeh.2020.101409.

INDEX

shame (*Continued*)
  weight/size-based, x, 16, 19, 59–61, 95, 97, 100, 102–3, 108, 112–3, 115, 122, 156–9, 167–8, 191, 253, 257, 259, 322, 333
Sick Enough (Gaudiani), 107–8
Siegel, Daniel, 4, 109, 162, 164
snacks, 172–9, 181, 184–8, 193–4, 203–4, 231–3, 290–1, 296
SNAP benefits, 325
sneaking food, x, 7–8, 107, 132, 139, 166, 174, 191
social issue(s)
  accessibility of fresh/healthy foods as, 3, 69, 122, 171, 224–5, 235–7, 241, 261
  bias as, 3–4, 28–31, 37–8, 52–9, 80, 97, 119–20, 157, 235–7, 241–2, 256, 283, 285–6, 326, 338
  economic inequity as, 236–8, 241–2
  food insecurity as, 2, 3–4, 56, 95, 106–9, 122, 171, 324–5
social media, 303, 306, 317, 322, 332
Sonneville, K., 74–5
Spiral of Healing, 314–6, *315*
sports, 244–7, 250, 308–9
stigma, weight, 21, 25, 29–31, 34, 46–8, 55–6, 59, 62, 68, 75, 84, 236, 242, 257, 258–60, 303, 314, 317, 329
stress, 30, 84, *84*, 85–6, 146, 166, 174, 184, 217, 224, 269, 293
  parental, 242, 322–4
Strings, Sabrina, 37
sugar, 8, 28, 35, 47, 53, 88, 146, 166, 200, 235–7, 240–2
  acceptance of, 101–3, 205–8
  ADHD and, 238–9
suicide, 4, 27, 68, 255, 306

talking, 127, 334. *See also* Intuitive Eating phrases
  positive self-, 113–5, 305, 321
  about shame, 157, 161
  about weight, 63–4, 90–1, 112–4, 115, 125, 143, 167–8, 288, 305
Taylor, Sonya Renee, 81, 307
thin privilege, 62, 65, 115, 211
thoughts, 5, 6, 141–2, 152, 160–1, 279–80
3 Keys to Intuitive Eating, xii, 3, 17, 22–5, 27, 67, 75–6, 79, 87, 89, 100,

104, 129, 149–212, *153*, 254, 275, 291, 293–5, 300, 305. *See also* Key 1: unconditional love and support; Key 2: flexible and reliable feeding routine; Key 3: Intuitive Eating voice development/utilization
Toddlers and Early Childhood development stage (two to five)
  autonomy's emergence in, 203, 286, 288–9
  body awareness origins in, 285–7
  flexible and reliable feeding introduced in, 287–91, 294
  food preference changes in, 291–7
trauma, 58, 89, 96, 109, 118, 191–2, 195, 257, 263–4, 333, 338
Triad of Connection, 162–5
Tribole, Evelyn, ix, 4, 73, 75, 88
trust, 83–4, *84*, 86, 103–4, 126–8, 142, 173, 202, 205, 263–4, 269, 312, 315–6, 318–9, 332
  in developmental stages, 275–84, 287–8, 293, 298, 302, 307, 310
Trust vs. Mistrust stage, 103–4
Tylka, Tracy, 4

unconditional love/support. *See* Key 1: unconditional love and support

values, parenting, 180–3, 194, 205, 206, 283, 290, 297, 316, 319
van der Kolk, Bessel, 191
vegetarianism/veganism, 269
vitamin C, 225–6, 229, 233, 294
vitamin D, 225, 226–7
vitamin E, 294

weight, 248, 304, 307–8. *See also* body image
  bias, 28, 29–31, 283
  bullying, 259–60, 303, 306
  childhood obesity concerns and, 22, 26, 28, 38, 52–3, 59, 171, 236, 242, 259–62, 309–11
  cycling of, 21, 48, 52, 63–4, 141, 171, 237, 311
  genetics/outside factors influencing, 20–2, 47, 48

Make peace with food!

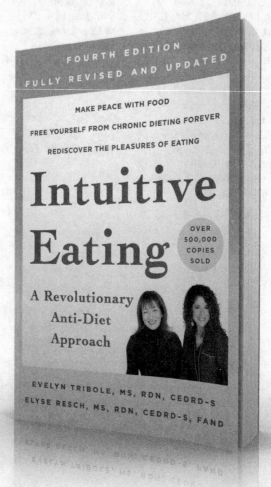

FOURTH EDITION
FULLY REVISED AND UPDATED

MAKE PEACE WITH FOOD

FREE YOURSELF FROM CHRONIC DIETING FOREVER

REDISCOVER THE PLEASURES OF EATING

Intuitive Eating

OVER 500,000 COPIES SOLD

A Revolutionary Anti-Diet Approach

EVELYN TRIBOLE, MS, RDN, CEDRD-S
ELYSE RESCH, MS, RDN, CEDRD-S, FAND

The classic bestseller about rejecting diet mentality.

Now revised and fully updated for the intuitive eaters of today.

ST. MARTIN'S
ESSENTIALS